Y0-BQJ-628

IF YOU ARE:

young or old
pregnant or raising a child
an athlete or a desk person
worried about cholesterol
calorie or carbohydrate conscious
suffering from any food-related disease
a vegetarian or natural foods devotee
overweight or underweight
just right

and want to know all you can about the food you eat and what it does for you and to you

this book, by acclaimed nutritionists and authors of *The Supermarket Handbook,* was written especially for you.

THE DIETER'S COMPANION
A Guide to Nutritional Self-Sufficiency

"A REAL WINNER, one that you'll want around for constant reference for a long, long time!"—LET'S LIVE

"A sensible guide which takes the high-pressured hoopla out of dieting."—KIRKUS REVIEWS

The Very Best On Nutrition and Diet from SIGNET

☐ **THE SUPERMARKET HANDBOOK: Access to Whole Foods by Nikki and David Goldbeck.** Revised and expanded. The most valuable food guide ever written for the consumer. Information about nutritious foods, saving money on your food budget, label reading, recipes, and brand-name recommendations for each region of the country. (#J7233—$1.95)

☐ **CONFESSIONS OF A SNEAKY ORGANIC COOK . . . OR HOW TO MAKE YOUR FAMILY HEALTHY WHEN THEY'RE NOT LOOKING by Jane Kinderlehrer.** An excellent guide to healthy eating and cooking for anyone interested in reviving the nutritive value of foods that have been processed, devitalized, and loaded with additives. Filled with valuable tricks and healthy gourmet recipes. (#W7204—$1.50)

☐ **THE SOUP-TO-DESSERT HIGH-FIBER COOKBOOK by Betty Wason.** The important new high-fiber, low-calorie diet that adds flavor and good health to every meal you eat! Low calorie menus, hundreds of recipes, food composition charts, and a fiber diet dictionary. The essential kitchen companion for every cook who cares about good health and good eating. (#J7208—$1.95)

☐ **THE LOS ANGELES TIMES NATURAL FOODS COOKBOOK by Jeanne Voltz, Food Editor, Woman's Day Magazine.** Discover the joys of cooking and eating naturally with this book of over 600 savory, simple-to-follow recipes. Whether you are concerned with taste or nutrition, these delicious and healthy recipes—high in fiber content—will delight everyone from the gourmet chef to the dedicated dieter. (#E6815—$2.25)

THE NEW AMERICAN LIBRARY, INC.,
P.O. Box 999, Bergenfield, New Jersey 07621

Please send me the SIGNET BOOKS I have checked above. I am enclosing $_____(check or money order—no currency or C.O.D.'s). Please include the list price plus 35¢ a copy to cover handling and mailing costs. (Prices and numbers are subject to change without notice.)

Name_____

Address_____

City_____State_____Zip Code_____
Allow at least 4 weeks for delivery

THE DIETER'S COMPANION

A Guide to Nutritional Self-Sufficiency

Nikki and David Goldbeck

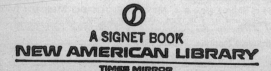

A SIGNET BOOK

NEW AMERICAN LIBRARY

TIMES MIRROR

NAL BOOKS ARE ALSO AVAILABLE AT DISCOUNTS IN BULK
QUANTITY FOR INDUSTRIAL OR SALES-PROMOTIONAL USE.
FOR DETAILS, WRITE TO PREMIUM MARKETING DIVISION,
NEW AMERICAN LIBRARY, INC., 1301 AVENUE OF THE
AMERICAS, NEW YORK, NEW YORK 10019.

Copyright © 1975 by Nikki and David Goldbeck

Introduction Copyright © 1977 by Dr. Ross Hume Hall

All rights reserved.
No part of this publication may be reproduced, stored in a retrieval
system, or transmitted, in any form or by any means, electronic,
mechanical, photocopying, recording, or otherwise,
without the prior permission of the publisher. For information
address The New American Library.

Library of Congress Catalog Card Number: 75-11585

A hardcover edition was published by McGraw-Hill Book Company.

Ⓢ SIGNET TRADEMARK REG. U.S. PAT. OFF. AND FOREIGN COUNTRIES
REGISTERED TRADEMARK—MARCA REGISTRADA
HECHO EN CHICAGO, U.S.A.

SIGNET, SIGNET CLASSICS, MENTOR, PLUME AND MERIDIAN BOOKS
are published by The New American Library, Inc.,
1301 Avenue of the Americas, New York, New York 10019

First Signet Printing, March, 1977

1 2 3 4 5 6 7 8 9

PRINTED IN THE UNITED STATES OF AMERICA

Contents

*Introduction to the Signet Edition, by
Dr. Ross Hume Hall*   vii

Introduction: The Way You Eat   xi

I. THE DIET DIGEST

Weight Control   3

Low-Calorie Dieting 6   •   Weight Watchers 12
•   Low-Carbohydrate Dieting 19   •   Crash
Diets 31   •   Liquid Diets 34   •   How to
Gain Weight 38

Natural, Whole, and Organic Food Diets   43

The Basic Natural Foods Diet 44   •
Vegetarianism 51   •   Yoga Foods 57   •
Macrobiotics: A Philosophical Diet 61
•   The Bircher-Benner Method 65

Eating American-Style   70

A Balanced Diet and the RDA 70   •   Nutrition
in Pregnancy 76   •   Diet for the Nursing
Mother 82   •   Feeding Young Children 86

Food for Health   93

Control of Heart Ailments 94   •   Diabetes 101
•   Hypoglycemia 106   •   Gout 110   •
Allergies 111   •   How Food Affects Mental
Health 113

II. THE DIET SURVEY

Learning to Evaluate Your Diet   121

How Your Diet Measures Up 122

Design Your Own Diet   143

    You Too Can Be a Dietician 143

III. THE TABLES OF FOOD CONTENT

The Nutritive Value of Foods   161

    Meat, Poultry, and Fish 164 • Eggs 198 •
Milk and Dairy Products 200 • Fruit and
Fruit Products 207 • Vegetable and Vegetable
Products 220 • Flours, Cereal Grains, and
Grain Products 236 • Legumes and Nuts 256
  • Fats and Oils 265 • Sugars and Sweets 270
  • Alcoholic and Carbonated Beverages 274 •
Soups 276 • Baby Foods 281 •
Miscellaneous 286

APPENDIX

Recommended Daily Dietary Allowances 291
  • Minimum Daily Requirements 292 • Why
Eat? The Elements of Food 293 • A Summary
of Nutrients 309
INDEX 315
DIET SURVEY FORMS 323

Introduction to the Signet Edition

by
Dr. Ross Hume Hall

Have you ever tried to sort your way through the vast number of diet recommendations touted in books and magazines? There seem to be so many authorities, so many recommendations, so much confusion. Each recommendation pushes a particular point of view claiming particular advantages for its devout followers. Nikki and David Goldbeck take you behind the stage scenery of these diet manuals and show you how many of the more popular diets are constructed. And, having done this, they give you some principles on which you can construct your own personal diet, tailored to your body and to your psyche. Eating is more than just a cultural experience; its primary purpose is to satisfy the body's biological needs. Some people swear by corn flakes for breakfast, others by oatmeal, and yet others by fried ants. Although in each case the consumer has had a satisfying breakfast, all these items vary considerably in their quality of nourishment. Everyone, for some reason or other, follows a definite eating pattern, choosing a range of items prepared in a definite fashion from among a vast spectrum of potentially edible substances. Note that I didn't say nourishing substances, for the fact that a food in the supermarket is edible does not make it nourishing. This is what concerns the Goldbecks, because regardless of why you choose to eat a food, the ultimate goal as far as your body is concerned is nourishment. *The Dieter's Companion* gives you a set of principles of food selection that while allowing great variation in choice of food will enable you to nourish your body wisely.

Why should there be such a profusion of dietary recommendations, many stated with assumed scientific and medical authority? Scientific knowledge of human nutrition is actually poorly developed, and only in the broadest terms can science outline what human nutrition is all about. Far more is known about how to nourish your cat than you. But then that is understandable, because scientists can run experiments on cats and if the experimental diet doesn't work the failures can be burned. To really understand how a particular dietary regimen is working out in humans it would have to be carried out over a lifetime, in fact over two or three life-spans. Instead of waiting for their grandchildren to finish off the experiment, nutritionists try to do short-term experiments on human volunteers, and they try to extrapolate results from their animal models. Not very satisfactory, so consequently the scientific base for human nutrition remains weak and open to a variety of interpretations. The available scientific information can be used effectively, though, if it is treated as only the partial picture it is. Many people, including some scientific authorities, treat the known knowledge of human nutrition as if it were the complete picture, and, as a consequence, their recommendations, if followed, distort the balanced nourishment your body craves.

Superimposed on the uncertainty of nutritional science is the way in which food is grown, processed, and distributed in North America. The food-processing industry has undergone radical change since the end of World War II. Prior to that time it used the same techniques used at home—canning, heating, grinding, mixing. All that changed when the industry embraced chemical technology. The new technology enables the industry to engineer foods at the molecular level and to fabricate products much as if they were fabricating an outboard motor for a runabout. The final product form of the new foods remains unchanged but their basic biology is radically altered, and that is what counts when assessing their nourishing value. Nutrition science lacks, however, the techniques to assess the nutritional quality of the new foods. *The Dieter's Companion* addresses these changes in food processing by providing guidelines that help you to avoid the excesses of the industry.

Human nutrition is an individual experience. Everyone has a distinct personality, a unique face, and just as unique a body biology, which means your nutritional requirements will be just as extraordinary. Scientific nutrition has been unable to address this reality; it cannot advise what your personal nutritional needs should be. Nikki and David Goldbeck's book recognizes the individuality of eating and nourishing your body. Its commentary helps you to develop a common-sense basis for applying to your individual needs the available scientific information, together with general principles that have worked for centuries.

It seems as if almost every American wishes to lose weight. Perhaps, to put it more precisely, most people want to continue eating in the old pattern and at the same time possess that svelte body they believe they should have, but that nature has tricked them out of. Most people do one of two things. Many seek a crash diet that will suck off mounds over a short period of time, then they revert to their old eating habits and the mounds reappear. Others attempt to maintain their accustomed eating pattern, while just seeking the one gimmick that will knock off those pounds. Should weight reduction be your goal, or should your goal be health and vitality through a vigorous life? This book will tell you that if you seek the latter, weight control will come almost automatically. But if weight control obsesses you, you risk disturbing a sane and balanced diet.

The Dieter's Companion dissects some of the better-known weight-loss diets, pointing out their characteristics, their claimed advantages, and their nutritional pitfalls. With this knowledge you can choose from such diets the elements that appeal to you, although that doesn't necessarily mean selecting the alcohol from the drinking man's diet while ignoring the rest of it. This book also describes dietary regimens that don't concern weight loss but that advocate a whole way of life, letting you in on the spiritual meaning underlying these diets. Some of these diets originated in the East, and this book will help you to adapt their requirements to the practicalities of obtaining certain foods in North America. Because these diets require adopting a particular way of life to be effective, you risk nutritional harm if you follow them only partially. Nikki and David Goldbeck wisely counsel you on this point, for many Westerners have got into nutritional difficulties with some of these diets, not because they are necessarily deficient but because people don't follow them adequately.

Vitamin-pill popping seems as much a part of the American way of life as attempted weight loss. Vitamins and minerals are indeed essential, and knowledge about these nutrients is perhaps the most important achievement of nutrition science. Science, however, doesn't know everything about vitamins and minerals. There may be many unknown vitamins waiting to be discovered, and, moreover, science has yet to work out the effective combinations of vitamins and minerals you require. These essential nutrients act in your body as a team, and like a chain, the team is no better than its weakest link. Pill manufacturers and corn flakes' fortifiers can only put in what is known, and at that they tend to put in only those vitamins and minerals that are easy to make, compound, and package. Because of the uncertainties of the balance of vitamins and minerals your body actually needs, Nikki and David Goldbeck point out that you should seek them in real food, not in pills and in foods fortified with selected minerals and vitamins.

Quite a bit is known about the mineral and vitamin content of most American foods—at least for those deemed essential by the United States Department of Agriculture (USDA). This book lists the content in common foods of five vitamins and four minerals, based on the USDA tables. The principle behind using this chart is that if you select from a variety of natural foods, you will not only get the listed vitamins but all the rest, known and unknown. In contrast, if you select fabricated foods in which the listed nutrients have been artificially added, the label may make the product sound magnificently nutritious but the contents will deprive you of the unlisted and just as essential nutrients. I often wonder how some essential nutrients are supposed to be more essential than others. Nutrition science just has not advanced to the point where it can specify how to make a food totally nutritious. One could argue that you eat a variety of foods, but if the variety is all fabricated then that is no variety at all. Through the chemical wizardry of fabrication the original vitamin and mineral content of all these foods slips away.

If there is a bias in this book, it is toward common sense. The human race has chosen its diets and survived quite handsomely for a few million years without the benefit of nutrition science. The common sense of our ancestors still works very well. *The Dieter's Companion* draws on this common sense, and together with the basic information of nutrition science as an indicator of the nutritional quality of food, it aids you in selecting your own personal diet. The goal is health and vitality, and only you can select the dietary program that works best for you. The principles herein will give you the basis for a wise selection.

McMaster University
Department of Biochemistry
Hamilton, Ontario, Canada

FOOD CONTENT. In addition, we have added sample work sheets at the end of the book and easy-to-follow guidelines.

THE TABLES OF FOOD CONTENT have been prepared from research done by the United States Department of Agriculture, published in *Agriculture Handbook No. 8, Composition of Foods* and *Home and Garden Bulletin No. 72, Nutritive Value of Foods*. To make the original tables more useful to you, we have expanded them to include everyday measures and portions. The tables offer the complete nutritional breakdown of the most common foods available in terms of calories, protein, fat, carbohydrate, calcium, iron, sodium, potassium, vitamin A, thiamine, riboflavin, niacin, and vitamin C. By converting these elements of food into standard units you are provided with a simple, practical way of measuring and comparing both individual foods and entire food plans. Most food ingredients and many prepared foods are listed. The introduction of nutritional labeling for many packaged foods hopefully will supplement this information.

The choice of diets in THE DIET DIGEST is based on a broad spectrum of popular eating plans. While these diet reviews do not supply all the particulars of a diet, as previously mentioned, they do provide a complete summary. Of special note is the application of THE TABLES OF FOOD CONTENT as an aid in fulfilling each food plan.

Before you embark on any diet you should read a good deal of the literature available about it. To help you in this pursuit a list of representative readings for each section is included at the end of each section.

If, perchance, the diet you may be considering has not been included in the digest, this does not preclude the applicability of the tables. The materials and approach provided here should permit you to obtain the maximum potential from *any* diet by using the tables to analyze its nutritional value to determine whether it fulfills your personal objectives. You may also use the tables to help select foods which are in accord with the rules of that diet.

To give you even greater flexibility there is a special chapter, *Design Your Own Diet*, which actually shows you how to create a diet for yourself. If you have particular food preferences, or special needs—if you are for example, an athlete, or someone recuperating from an illness, or are just not satisfied with any prepared diet—this section is for you. If followed properly, it can help you "tailor-make" a diet to suit any qualifications and taste preferences.

For those who would like to pursue the subject of nutrition in greater depth, we have added an appendix, *Why Eat? The Elements of Food*. While this understanding of nutrition is not essential if you are simply following the dictates of a ready-made diet, you can be much more flexible in your choice of foods and at the same time protect yourself against inadequate nutrition if you know how the foods you eat affect you. If you wish to maximize your present diet or adapt one of the food plans discussed here to your own tastes, begin with the appendix *Why Eat? The Elements of Food*. But if you are more concerned with putting a diet into immediate action, save this chapter until your interest is more aroused and plunge first into THE DIET DIGEST and THE TABLES OF FOOD CONTENT which compose the heart of *The Dieter's Companion*.

NIKKI GOLDBECK
DAVID GOLDBECK
Woodstock, N.Y.

PART I

THE DIET DIGEST

Weight Control

───◆───

Weight regulation ranks among the least understood of the body processes, and as anyone who have ever attempted to lose weight knows, keeping it off is often as hard as getting it off. Hence the wide assortment of diets claiming to be the only sure way to weight control.

One of the things we do know is that the food we eat is burned as fuel to maintain body temperature and the basic life processes, and to supply the energy for physical activity. If all our food is used as fuel, weight remains constant. But to the dismay of many this is not what necessarily happens. Rather, we convert food to fuel according to our bodily demand for energy and store all the excess as fat, regardless of whether the food in its original state is primarily protein, carbohydrate, or fat.

As complicated as the weight-loss process is, the desire and need to lose weight is uppermost in the minds of millions of Americans daily. Usually they are motivated by the desire for a fashionable, trim figure, but more important, people are becoming increasingly aware of the health hazards involved in being overweight. Such adversities as diabetes, heart and circulatory ailments, complications of pregnancy, and early death are all associated with obesity, and even if too much fat is not the cause of illness, it constitutes an added risk.

To really succeed in losing weight it is helpful to understand the "whys" of eating. Eating to satisfy actual hunger rarely leads to extreme overweight. But more often we eat to be sociable, to relieve frustrations and boredom, for the sensual pleasure of it, or simply because the food is there and most of us have been prodded from childhood to clean our plates. As a matter of fact, although few of us realize it, eating is as much an emotional response as it is a physical process.

3

Whatever influences your dietary habits, there is no escaping the reality that your body must have energy to function. However, the amount of energy, measured in terms of calories, that each of us needs varies greatly with age, size, body composition, hormonal factors, and activity. Although body type is determined by the genes, all too often heredity is used as an excuse for being overweight. Most likely what is inherited is not obesity, but poor food habits leading to an overweight condition.

While there are no absolute criteria for judging obesity, most people become aware of the need to reduce when they are honest with themselves about the way they feel and look. With children the problem is somewhat more complex since it often takes time for a child's height to catch up to his width. Nevertheless, overeating and gross overweight are apparent at any age to anyone willing to recognize them. Some idea of just how fat you may be can be gleaned from consulting the Table of Desirable Weights (page 5). Although there is some leeway in assessing "frame size," this table provides a good guideline and helps set realistic goals. Remember—the first step toward control of overweight is prevention, and this makes it a matter of some concern to everybody.

Misunderstanding of foods is one common contributor to unnecessary weight gain. Many people have a mental image of certain foods based on an ignorance of true caloric values. Bread, for instance, is thought of as a high-calorie food, while in reality one slice of rye bread provides only 56 calories, barely more than one small orange. Meat, on the other hand, often enjoys an elevated position in the diet of those seeking weight reduction. Most calorie tables consider a serving of meat to be 2 or 3 ounces of lean meat. This is misleading since most people consume easily twice this amount in a sitting. A generous restaurant serving of beef can furnish 1,100 calories—just about half the total daily energy requirement of most adults. But, our food habits have been with us since our first days of life and it takes both awareness and determination if we expect them to change. If consciousness does not change, weight loss will never be successful, for the measure of success is not in the losing, but in the maintenance of that loss.

Before you embark on any reducing diet you must realize that restricting food intake is bound to create stress—both

TABLE OF DESIRABLE WEIGHTS*

Height (without shoes)	Weight (without clothing)		
	low	average (pounds)	high
Men			
5 feet 3 inches	118	129	141
5 feet 4 inches	122	133	145
5 feet 5 inches	126	137	149
5 feet 6 inches	130	142	155
5 feet 7 inches	134	147	161
5 feet 8 inches	139	151	166
5 feet 9 inches	143	155	170
5 feet 10 inches	147	159	174
5 feet 11 inches	150	163	178
6 feet	155	167	183
6 feet 1 inch	158	171	188
6 feet 2 inches	162	175	192
6 feet 3 inches	165	178	195
Women			
5 feet	100	109	118
5 feet 1 inch	104	112	121
5 feet 2 inches	107	115	125
5 feet 3 inches	110	118	128
5 feet 4 inches	113	122	132
5 feet 5 inches	116	125	135
5 feet 6 inches	120	129	139
5 feet 7 inches	123	132	142
5 feet 8 inches	126	136	146
5 feet 9 inches	130	140	151
5 feet 10 inches	133	144	156
5 feet 11 inches	137	148	161
6 feet	141	152	166

* Based upon data on heights and weights of individuals twenty to thirty years old, as obtained by the United States Department of Agriculture. The USDA table assumes that the weight that is desirable in your midtwenties is the best weight for later years too.

physical and emotional. While many diets help you lose initially, often they do not prepare you to continue to lose or stick with the loss. Since all people are different, you must discover the plan that is best for you. Often quick results are enough to inspire you to go on, although crash diets cannot be depended on to reeducate your dietary habits. Some people need strict rules to follow, while others do best with a more flexible plan; for some dieters skipping meals is the answer, while for others spreading the food into five or six small meals throughout the day is more feasible. Many people find outside support gives them the necessary momentum they need.

No matter which dieting plan you decide to try, it is only effective if you are well acquainted with the procedures and the consequences involved. Basically, any diet pattern is fine as long as it is nutritionally adequate. But no diet is magic. There is no easy way to weight loss and the only way you can make it easier for yourself is by wanting to lose weight more than you want to eat.

Here are some of the more popular food plans which have been effective in bringing about desired losses. Once you have made your choice, THE TABLES OF FOOD CONTENT will aid you in selecting foods that are in accordance with the rules of that diet.

1. LOW-CALORIE DIETING

Energy Input and Outflow

The most conventional scheme of weight reduction is the low-calorie diet. This is a gradual path toward weight loss through the restriction of food intake to a point where the body energy you generate daily exceeds the energy the food you eat is able to provide. With this form of dieting the actual choice of foods can be left to the dieter, although selection of low-calorie, high-nutritive foods is recommended and planned menus are available.

Low-calorie traditionalists insist that weight control cannot be a battle against food, for then you are likely to become irritable, discouraged, and soon revert to former eating habits. It is their conviction that if you cut down on calories by reorganizing consumption of familiar foods, you can lose weight gradually, sensibly, and at the same time develop new and better food habits.

As explained in the appendix *Why Eat? The Elements of Food*, a calorie is a measurement of the energy value of foods. Any diet low enough in caloric value will force body fat to be converted to energy. If during this time all other nutrients are kept at levels adequate to maintain good nutrition, weight reduction can be achieved with a minimum of stress on the body.

It is estimated that a moderately active person expends 12 to 15 calories daily for each pound of body weight. Therefore, under normal circumstances, someone who weighs 150 pounds can burn up to 2,250 calories per day. Of course this is only a general estimate and as activity decreases and age increases the amount of energy one requires goes down considerably. Also, due to individual differences in metabolism some people can burn up whatever they eat no matter what or how much, while others just "think" about eating and gain weight.

Assuming an average energy expenditure, in order to lose weight you must sufficiently lower calories to cause body fat to be burned (or oxidized) for fuel. Since 1 pound of body fat represents about 3,500 calories of stored energy, for each 3,500 calories of energy used by your body beyond that provided by the food you eat, you can expect to shed 1 pound. Therefore, if you are overeating or currently overweight and calorie counting, you must cut well below the calorie expenditure that corresponds to your present weight. For an acceptable level of calorie intake, determine your desired weight (see Table of Desirable Weights, page 5), multiply this by 12 (calories per pound per day) and you will know the approximate number of calories you can use from your food supply to maintain this weight. Any deficit below this figure will mean the oxidation (burning) of body fat to make up for calories lacking in your diet—and, a resultant weight loss. Since 3,500 calories add up to 1 pound of fat, a daily deficit of 800 calories can mean 5,600 calories worth of fat will be gone by the end of a week, or about 1½ pounds. At this rate, in twenty weeks you can expect to shed 30 pounds. Naturally, the greater the calorie restriction the faster you lose, although too drastic a cut will sabotage health.

---

approximate number of calories
you can convert to energy daily
$$= \text{desired weight} \times 12$$

approximate number of calories
you can convert to energy daily
$$+ 3500 = 1 \text{ pound weight gain}$$

approximate number of calories
you can convert to energy daily
$$- 3500 = 1 \text{ pound weight loss}$$

As you become slimmer you will find your need for energy decreases, so that the rate of loss may diminish slightly. Moderate exercise, however, can increase the amount of energy your body uses, particularly if this activity becomes a daily ritual.

To best accomplish weight loss on a low-calorie diet, protein, vitamins, and minerals should be kept at high levels to insure vitality and preserve your health.

Make Calories Work to Your Advantage

Many low-calorie diets propose a menu to follow which is well endowed with all nutrients yet limited in calories.

A balanced low-calorie diet is aimed at meeting the dictates of good nutrition. It emphasizes: lean meats, fish, poultry; low-fat milk and cheeses; whole-grain breads and cereals; fruits and vegetables, and a moderate amount of nut or vegetable oil. Fat, mostly unsaturated, accounts for about 30 percent of the total calories, and carbohydrates comprise 20 percent of the daily calories. Of course, pasta, rich cream soups and sauces, cream cheese and butter, cakes, cookies, candies, and other similar items can add up to a low-calorie day if eaten to the exclusion of other foods, but they will not add up to good nutrition and therefore do not contribute to the effectiveness of balanced dieting.

As it turns out, most diets which profess "calories don't count" and outline specific patterns of food consumption would prove to be dependent on calorie cutback if analyzed. Only *you* don't have to count because the repetition of certain foods naturally limits the amount you can eat. But if you actually do the calorie computations yourself, you can select the foods you like, eliminate only those highest in calories, and then limit the overall quantity of what you eat to achieve the same ends. Moreover, as you do so, you will begin to understand the relationship between food and physique, which will be a great assistance in maintaining the loss.

On a low-calorie diet plan you can arrange your meals in any way you like. One popular variation of traditional low-calorie dieting is "snack dieting" in which the daily calorie allotment is divided not only into breakfast, lunch, and dinner, but stretched out over a midmorning, midafternoon, and bedtime snack as well. In this manner food is continually being digested, energy levels are kept up and there is less chance to experience hunger pangs.

When following a low-calorie diet weigh yourself only once a week at the same hour, on the same scale, in the same manner of dress. Daily weighing reflects daily swings due to water retention and water loss and does not give you an accurate measure of your progress; it will only be discouraging to an anxious dieter.

Once you have reached your desired weight, by following the guideline of 12 to 15 calories per pound per day you should be able to hold this weight constant. If you find you are gaining a bit, cut down gradually again until your weight is stabilized. Since individual differences cause calorie expenditure to vary from person to person, this figure may need some adjustment. Remember too, as you grow older your calorie needs decrease; to avoid putting on unwanted weight, with each adult birthday cut 10 calories off your daily total.

Is This the Diet for You?

A diet based on calories alone, rather than any set menu, allows a wide variety of food choices. If such a diet is approached with an eye toward good nutrition it can bring with the weight loss new food awareness, better food habits, and thus a good chance of maintaining your new weight.

A balanced low-calorie diet exerts the least amount of stress on your system and if all essential nutrients are kept at a high level you should enjoy excellent, perhaps even improved, health. Many physical ailments like diabetes, hypoglycemia, and high blood cholesterol are often brought under control during balanced dieting.

Since a low-calorie diet is based on familiar foods, it is easy to stick with and gives you more leeway in social situations. When dining with others daily, as in a family situation, the person on a low-calorie diet can enjoy the same foods as others by simply eating small portions or bypassing the higher-calorie items like the sauces, salad dressings, butter, syrups and sweet spreads, fried foods, and rich desserts on the menu.

What Are the Possible Pitfalls?

Many people who find food too great a temptation need strict guidelines as to what they can and cannot eat in order to lose weight. For these people, counting calories is often not effective; they give way to the tendency to consume all their calories in one sitting or in ice cream sundaes, fudge cake, vichyssoise, fried chicken in gravy, or in one of the other foods that brought their original downfall. This *may* be cutting calories, but it does not offer the body any of the other benefits that accompany a balanced low-calorie regimen.

Another deterrent to successful low-calorie dieting is hunger. When food intake is limited, hunger (sometimes real and sometimes imagined) convinces the food lover that restricting food may be a big mistake. Diets which allow unlimited eating are therefore apt to be more appealing.

Without accurate tables of food values people can fool themselves into believing a food is more "dietetic" than it may actually be, and often act on misfounded images of some foods being high or low in calories. In reality, a small amount of any food cannot be the cause of obesity, while overconsumption of almost anything will generate too many calories.

Unless you plan meals to include adequate amounts of other nutrients, too drastic a cut in calories can lead to decreased resistance to infection and a general lack of spirits.

Initial weight loss on a low-calorie diet is slow, so that it is easy to become discouraged. In the long run, however, weight loss will be equal to that of any other diet.

Using The Tables of Food Content

Anyone anxious to lose weight while continuing to maintain their freedom of food choice, will find that THE TABLES OF FOOD CONTENT offer complete information about the foods they might select, thus helping them to stay within calorie restrictions while discovering foods with high protein, vitamin, and mineral content.

Before you begin your diet you can compute your present calorie consumption with which you have been gaining or maintaining your overweight to help you determine just how drastic your calorie reduction must be. If you are heavier than you care to be, but are not continuing to gain weight, any deficit below your present calorie level should lead to weight loss. If you are putting on weight you must cut back far enough to stop the gain and then some to create a "fat loss."

By planning the size of your servings from the values on the tables, you can enjoy all your favorite foods. Just keep meals within the proper calorie limits and make sure you are getting the recommended balance of protein, fat, and carbohydrates plus vitamins and minerals.

Once you have reached your goal, you can stabilize your weight by using the tables to plan meals with the correct level of calories for your new weight and lifestyle.

Representative Readings

Good Housekeeping. *Cooking for Calorie Watchers*. The American Heart Association.

Iowa State Department of Health. *Simplified Diet Manual*. 3d ed. Ames, Iowa: Iowa State University Press, 1969.

Jolliffe, Norman. *Reduce and Stay Reduced on the Prudent Diet*. Rev. ed. New York: Simon & Schuster, 1965.

Lamb, Lawrence. *Metabolics*. New York: Harper & Row, 1974.

2. WEIGHT WATCHERS

Mind Over Matter

The Weight Watchers diet is actually a well-supervised version of the balanced low-calorie diet. As its name implies, Weight Watchers is dedicated to helping obese people "watch their weight"; that is, reduce. The Weight Watchers plan is aimed at educating overweight people to eat a regular diet of low-calorie foods so that weight loss is gradual and permanent. Once the desired loss is effected, Weight Watchers maintain their trim figures by remaining conscious of how they ate in order to lose and by planning future menus with the same tactics in mind. The aim of Weight Watchers as a group is to give members emotional support and to replace the desire for food with the desire to be thin and attractive.

Weight Watchers, founded by "formerly fat housewife"

Jean Nidetch, is based on the principle that being fat comes from "overeating the wrong foods." People who are fat, the organization feels, are compulsive eaters and, since compulsive eating is an emotional problem, Weight Watchers brings fat people together in regular meetings to openly discuss the reasons for and solutions to their problems. This is particularly beneficial to those who feel they are alone with these problems, for with the understanding of people in similar situations, they can begin to help each other and themselves.

Behind the diet itself is the theory that you must restrict calories to lose weight, but only in such a sensible manner that the other essential food elements remain adequate. The Weight Watchers diet recognizes that you can lose weight on any weird eating plan but, "sometimes you don't feel well, often you don't look well." The Weight Watchers diet is designed not only so people will lose weight, but so they will maintain both the loss and good health. The formerly fat people on Weight Watchers have discovered that to keep off lost weight *a new food consciousness must be developed*. Because food is a source of satisfaction for overeaters, vanity as an alternate form of self-fulfillment is emphasized and the dieters are taught to desire a sylphlike figure above all else.

How Weight Watchers Eat

The Weight Watchers diet itself is fashioned after a diet developed by Dr. Norman Jolliffe for the Obesity Clinic at the New York City Department of Health. On this diet the participant must have three meals daily, strictly outlined but with a good variety of food choices within the set menu plan. There are, additionally, unlimited snacks from the foods listed in the "free" category. There are no substitutions permitted and all foods suggested on the diet must be consumed. The point is to avoid being hungry. Because the foods you are allowed to eat are carefully enumerated there is no need to count calories, although in fact this diet is based on a low-calorie, high-nutrient intake. Since body weight normally fluctuates from day to day, dieters are counseled to weigh themselves only once a week at group meetings.

The daily Weight Watchers menu for women is outlined as follows*:

Morning

Juice or fruit
Choice of: Cheese, 1 ounce hard *or* 2 ounces farmer *or*
        ¼ cup cottage or pot cheese
               OR
        Fish, 2 ounces
               OR
        Cereal, 1 ounce with skim milk
Bread, 1 slice
Beverage, if desired

Noon

Choice of: Fish, meat, or poultry, 4 ounces
               OR
        Meat alternatives, 7 ounces except soybeans,
        6 ounces
               OR
        Cheese, 2 ounces hard *or* 4 ounces farmer *or*
        ⅔ cup cottage or pot cheese
               OR
        Eggs, 2
At least one "#3 vegetable" (including, for example, most
        leafy greens, mushrooms, peppers, sprouts,
        radishes, etc.)
4 ounces "#4 vegetable," if desired (including, for example,
        more of the colored vegetables like beets,
        carrots, pumpkin, tomato, yellow squash, etc.)
Bread, 1 slice
Beverage, if desired

* This material is extracted from the most recent *Weight Watchers Program Handbook for Ladies* and is incomplete. Its purpose is illustrative only, i.e., to give an idea of the nature of this diet. The "#4 foods as explained to members.
vegetable," for example, refers to a Weight Watchers classification of

Evening

Choice of: Fish, meat, or poultry, 6 ounces
OR
Meat alternatives, 10 ounces except soybeans, 9 ounces
4 ounces "#4 vegetable" (if not eaten at noon)
Reasonable amounts of "#3 vegetables"
Beverage, if desired

(Note: For men the daily allowance is increased to four slices of bread, five fruits or the equivalent, and 8 ounces of meat at dinner. Children are permitted three slices of bread and five fruits daily.)

Each day the menu must include 1 tablespoon vegetable oil, margarine or mayonnaise, or 2 tablespoons diet margarine; two 8-ounce glasses skim milk (four for children) or 8 ounces evaporated skim milk or 12 ounces buttermilk; three fruits (five for men and children); two "#3 vegetables" and 4 ounces "#4 vegetables."

The weekly menu must feature liver at least once; a maximum of three servings from the meat group including beef, frankfurters, and lamb; four eggs, and fish at least five times.

If you wish, you can add bouillon or broth, tomato juice, club soda, coffee, tea, or water to the daily menu.

You may not eat or drink any of these foods:

alcoholic beverages
bacon or fat back
butter
cake, cookies, crackers, pies
candy, chocolate
chili sauce
coconut or coconut oil
corn
cream (sweet or sour)
cream cheese
fried foods
dried beans or peas
dried fruit or fruit canned in syrup
ice cream, ice milk, ices, sherbet
ketchup
jam, jelly, preserves
luncheon meats
muffins, biscuits, rolls, specialty breads
nondairy creamers or toppings
olives or olive oil

pancakes, waffles
peanut butter
peanuts and other nuts
pizza
popcorn, potato chips, pretzels
pork and pork products
puddings, custards, fruit-flavored gelatin
raw fish

raw meat
salad dressings
sardines
smoked fish (except finnan haddie and salmon)
smoked meat
soda, ades, punch
soup
sugar
syrups

The fruits, vegetables, and meats that you may eat and the amounts prescribed for each are all included in the program booklet which is given to all members. Numerous sources of recipes, such as the *Weight Watchers Cookbook* and *Weight Watchers Magazine*, are available for creative meal planning.

Is This the Diet for You?

One of the most significant advantages of the Weight Watchers diet is the group support and encouragement it provides. This psychological element is certainly important to some prospective dieters.

The diet itself is based on a plan you could comfortably live with for the rest of your life. It does not consider merely calories, but the amount of nutrients you get from these calories. This is one of the primary reasons no substitutions are permitted.

On this diet you need not experience hunger. If you feel the familiar dieter's pangs you can reach for a stalk of celery, a can of mushrooms, a dish of bean sprouts, spinach, pickles, or other "free" foods, and you can keep eating these until your hunger (real or emotional) is satisfied.

This diet allows, actually requires, you to eat three ample meals a day. Portions of meat are large to compensate for the starchy vegetables that are missing. You are free to snack on the "unlimited" foods all day long if you desire.

Weight loss is slow on this diet, giving the body a chance

to adjust to its new weight. At the same time, new eating habits are instilled.

Although the foods you are permitted are quite restricted, the abundance of original recipes prepared in conjunction with the Weight Watchers diet provides for interesting and varied meals nonetheless.

It is also fairly easy to maintain this diet away from home.

What Are the Possible Pitfalls?

If you intend to join the Weight Watchers organization you are required to have a complete physical and a signed doctor's statement that you can satisfactorily sustain such a diet. Nothing, however, prevents people from following this eating plan on their own, or perhaps with a group of friends simulating the organization's techniques. Those who undertake such a venture, however, should be aware that certain physical conditions can preclude them from participating in this diet. An individual with gout, for example, could fare poorly on a food plan so dependent on meat and the high-purine vegetables promoted in the Weight Watchers scheme.

Unless fortified skim or nonfat dry milk is selected and consumed along with food containing fat, vitamin D levels may be lower than advisable.

A line of Weight Watchers products has been developed as an outgrowth of the organization's success, and artificial sweeteners and "diet foods" are promoted in Weight Watchers' menus and recipes. The potential dangers in these chemicalized food items reduces their acceptability for additive-conscious dieters.

Finally, the foods you must avoid are usually the most tempting for the dieter, and thus a good deal of willpower and self-imposed guilt are demanded.

Using The Tables of Food Content

It may seem that in a diet where exactly what you can and cannot eat is carefully specified, THE TABLES OF FOOD CONTENT would have little use. Not so.

Weight Watchers believes that people are overweight because they overeat. Just as the group encourages honesty, the tables convey the basic truths about food. A glance at the charts and you must admit to yourself that many foods offer a lot of calories and little else. The tables increase your knowledge and reduce the temptation to overeat the wrong foods based on ignorance or false notions. They help you to see food as nourishment for the body and a means to better health rather than as a reward. Thus, 3 ounces of potato chips (a "snack-size" bag) can be looked upon as 483 calories, 33.8 grams of fat, and as much as 840 milligrams of sodium, while an average carrot (a "free snack") is a paragon at 17 calories, 140 milligrams of potassium, and 4,500 units of vitamin A.

By calculating for yourself the nutrient value of the foods prescribed by Weight Watchers, you can ensure a high nutrient intake while still losing weight, something that cannot be said for many other reducing plans. And, if by chance you have failed to follow the recommendations—for instance if you proudly passed up your skim milk—you will see for yourself that your calcium (or other) nutrient intake may suffer.

By consulting the tables you will learn that it is not enough to substitute one food for another of equal calories. Unless you replace it with a food that is equal in all nutrients you are not enjoying the same diet.

Once you have graduated to a maintenance diet, the tables will help you check up on foods you are unsure about.

And, of course, if you are gaining (and cheating) the tables will show you why, scientifically.

Representative Readings

Jolliffe, Norman. *Reduce and Stay Reduced on the Prudent Diet.* Rev. ed. New York: Simon & Schuster, 1965.

Nidetch, Jean. *The Story of Weight Watchers.* New York: New American Library, 1972.

Nidetch, Jean. *Weight Watchers Program Cookbook.* Great Neck, N.Y., Hearthside Press, 1973.

Weight Watchers Program Handbook. Weight Watchers International, 1973.

3. LOW-CARBOHYDRATE DIETING

Banting, Stillman, Atkins, et al.

The low-carbohydrate diet is the recurring dietary phenomena of the last hundred years. In the 1860s and 1870s it was the Banting diet; in the 1950s and early '60s it reappeared as the Calories-Don't-Count diet, the Du Pont diet, the Air Force diet, the Mayo Clinic diet, and the Drinking Man's diet, and in the late 1960s and '70s it was with us again as the Stillman Quick-Weight-Loss diet and the Atkins Diet Revolution. In all its forms, the low-carbohydrate diet is aimed specifically at reducing excess poundage and counteracting obesity, the nation's number one health problem. The enormous success that has been claimed with the "diet that saves you from hunger" has given it widespread appeal for desperate dieters.

The Diet with the Secret Ingredient

Those who advocate a low-carbohydrate diet believe that carbohydrate is primarily responsible for forming body fat and that carbohydrate metabolism in the fat person is impaired so that all potential energy (calories) is converted immediately to fat tissue. Only when carbohydrates are sufficiently restricted or removed from the diet, they assert, can body fat be broken down for energy. The proponents explain that a fat-mobilizing hormone is released in the absence of carbohydrate, while the presence of insulin (stimulated by carbohydrate consumption) inhibits this hormone. Thus, they contend, as long as carbohydrate is lacking in the diet you can eat as much protein (and even fat, in some versions) as you like without gaining weight. Most of the champions of the low-carbohydrate diet concede that an additional reduction of calories would accelerate the weight loss, but they feel freedom from hunger is psychologically more important. For most people the high satiety value of the fat and protein stressed at mealtime tends to limit calories instinctively. (This, say critics of the diet, is the real reason for its success. While some of these critics acknowledge the existence of the fat-mobilizing hormone, they insist that unless total calories are restricted as well, the stored fat simply "mobilizes" itself to another site in the body and may move, for example, from the abdomen to the hips, which is no real improvement.)

Since protein, when not combined with fats or carbohydrates, requires more energy to be digested (a process known as *specific dynamic action*) you can burn as much as 275 extra calories daily on a diet that consists exclusively of protein. But because fat and protein are not burned as cleanly as carbohydrate in the body, substances known as *residual fatty acids* and *ketone bodies* accumulate, are brought to the kidneys, and are excreted through the urine. The large quantities of water recommended in the Stillman plan are thought to help flush out this waste. According to Atkins, the presence of these ketone bodies, demonstrated when litmus paper soaked in urine turns purple, is evidence that the body fat is being broken down and a positive sign that the diet is working.

Although most low-carbohydrate diets permit up to 60

grams of carbohydrate in the daily menu, the lower the carbohydrate intake the faster weight loss proceeds. Atkins begins his diet at a base level of zero carbohydrates.

The menu itself varies somewhat with each version of the low-carbohydrate diet, but the basic approach is the same. In the low-carbohydrate diet any amount of protein, and in many cases any amount of fat, can be consumed. The carbohydrate intake is restricted from 0 to 60 grams daily. These diets may indicate the need for some food control, but for the most part you are permitted to eat until you are no longer hungry and then maybe a little more. You are allowed only the foods specified on the complementary guidelines; that is, high-protein items such as meat, fish, and poultry. Bread, crackers, pastry, cereal, grains, potatoes, pasta, fruits and juices, candy and sweets are forbidden. Slight variations are found in each of the menu plans, some including cheese, eggs, and other high-fat proteins; some suggesting pure fats like butter, oil, and cream; some allowing alcoholic beverages; some with a minimum of vegetables, and others forbidding all these items. An outline of some of these restricted menus appears below. Many other variations are in existence.

THE MAYO CLINIC DIET (NOT RECOGNIZED BY OR ASSOCIATED WITH THE MAYO CLINIC).

This daily meal plan is given to those on the Mayo Diet:

Breakfast: ½ grapefruit or unsweetened grapefruit juice
2 eggs, any style, 2 slices of bacon, minimum
(You may eat as many eggs and slices of bacon as you want.)
Coffee or tea, no cream or sugar

Lunch: ½ grapefruit
Meat, any style, any amount
Salad, as much as you can eat with any dressing that contains no sugar
Coffee or tea

Dinner: ½ grapefruit
Meat, any style, any amount, with gravy, providing it is not thickened with flour. Of course, you can substitute fish for meat.

> Any green, yellow, or red vegetables, as much
> as you can eat, and salad as above
> Coffee or tea

Bedtime
Snack: Tomato juice or skimmed milk

1. At each meal you must eat until you are full, until you cannot possibly eat more.

2. Don't eliminate anything; for example, don't skip the bacon at breakfast or omit the salad at dinner. It is this combination of foods that burn up the accumulated fat.

3. The grapefruit is important because it acts as a catalyst that starts the fat-burning process.

4. Cut down coffee. It is thought to affect the insulin balance that hinders the burning-up process. Try to limit yourself to one cup at each meal.

5. No eating between meals. If you can eat the combination of foods suggested until you are stuffed you won't be hungry between meals.

THE AIR FORCE DIET
(DISCLAIMED BY THE AIR FORCE, AND LATER RENAMED THE DRINKING MAN'S DIET).

Although alcohol is not a true carbohydrate, it stimulates insulin production (as do coffee, cola, and other caffeine-containing beverages) and thus inhibits the so-called fat-mobilizing hormone. Therefore, it is excluded from most low-carbohydrate menus. The Drinking Man's diet, however, is one of meat, poultry, limited amounts of egg, cheese, fish, and vegetables, plus hard liquor and dry wine. This diet is very similar to the latest version of the Stillman plan, although it does not deny any foods by name, but rather relies on your counting carbohydrates and imposes an upper limit of 60 grams per day.

THE STILLMAN QUICK-WEIGHT-LOSS DIET
(UPDATED VERSION).

If you follow Stillman's counseling you may eat "satisfying portions" of protein, a limited amount of carbohydrate, and no fat other than that inherent in the protein foods you consume. In terms of actual menu planning, this means:

"Satisfying portions" of:

Skinless chicken or turkey cooked without added fat.
Fresh fish or seafood cooked without fat, or water-packed salmon or tuna.
Lean fresh meat, trimmed of all visible fat, plus variety meats (but only occasional servings of liver) and all-beef frankfurters.
Eggs, cooked without fat, but if you have a cholesterol problem no more than three per week.
Cottage cheese.
Coffee, tea, club soda, and no-cal beverages.

Restricted amounts of:

The following vegetables—asparagus, bamboo shoots, bean sprouts, green, string, and wax beans, beet greens, broccoli, brussel sprouts, cabbage, cauliflower, celery, chard, chicory, Chinese cabbage, chives, collards, cucumber, eggplant, endive, escarole, fennel, kale, kohlrabi, lettuce, mushrooms, mustard greens, parsley, peppers, radishes, sauerkraut, spinach, summer squash, tomatoes, turnip greens, watercress, zucchini.
If the vegetable is eaten as a salad you may use only low-calorie dressing, vinegar, or a wedge of lemon or lime to dress it.
Four ounces each day of skim or buttermilk, or ½ cup plain, skim-milk yogurt.
Up to two slices bread daily.
Up to 3 cups diluted bouillon or consomme.
Up to 1½ ounces pure distilled liquor or very dry wine.
As much as three servings of no-sugar gelatin, a tablespoon of no-sugar jam and up to three unsalted olives.

And sparing amounts of vinegar, mustard, ketchup or cocktail sauce, fresh lemon or lime, and low-calorie dressing.

Salt is best omitted, but may be used sparingly; herbs, pepper, and spices can be added freely.

If you do not bother with any of the "restricted" foods, weight loss will come faster. You must, however, drink *at least* 10 cups of liquid (water plus the permitted beverages) each day, and the more you drink, the quicker success will come.

You may not eat anything other than the items enumerated above, and that means no fruit (other than a slice of lemon or lime), no regular salad dressings, oil, butter, margarine, sauces, pickles, relishes, salty or spiced foods, processed meats, potatoes or other root vegetables, flour, pasta, grains, beans, nuts, cake, cookies, candy, potato chips, pretzels, etc.

Eating takes place three times a day or is divided into six smaller meals. Stillman advises you to weigh yourself each day and continue the diet until your ideal weight is reached. To figure "ideal weight" Stillman provides the following guideline:

Women age twenty-five or over: 5 feet—100 pounds. For every inch above 5 feet add 5 pounds per inch for average weight; from that figure subtract about 10 percent for ideal weight. For eighteen to twenty-five years of age subtract 1 pound for each year under 25.

Men age twenty-five and over: 5 feet—110 pounds. For every inch over 5 feet add 5½ pounds per inch for average weight; from that figure subtract about 10 percent for ideal weight. For eighteen to twenty-five years of age subtract 1 pound for each year.

THE ATKINS DIET.

Atkins includes not only high levels of protein, but high levels of fat in his diet as well. If fat is too low, he says, the diet is not satisfying, variety is lacking, hormone production slackens, and the essential fatty acids which keep the skin healthy are forfeited. Atkins' meals consist of any meat, fish, or fowl (including such unlikely choices as pork, bacon, lobster dripping with melted butter, and duck), two small green salads daily with any rich, creamy dressing you favor, and other supplements of cheese, olives, fried foods, eggs, caviar, beef jerky, and similar high-fat, no-carbohydrate foods. For dessert you can choose artificially sweetened gelatin, whipped cream in your coffee, or the special low-carbohydrate recipes he supplies in the bestseller *Dr. Atkins' Diet Revolution*.

On Atkins' diet you can eat whenever you like, but are advised to start the day with a good hearty meal, perhaps one of steak, bacon, a cheese omelet, and coffee with cream. Each week you may add 5 grams of carbohydrate to the menu until you reach your "critical carbohydrate level" (the point at which the urine test you administer daily no longer registers purple). Then cut back a few grams until the purple color indicates ketone bodies are once more present in the urine. Ultimately you should not exceed 40 grams of carbohydrate daily if you intend to preserve the weight loss. Once you are within 5 to 6 pounds of your ideal weight you add 5 grams of carbohydrate weekly until you are losing no more than 1 pound per week.

THE BOSTON POLICE DIET.

The Boston Police diet is the same as the Atkins diet, perhaps a bit more permissive when it comes to fruits and vegetables. This diet suggests the use of a thyroid supplement to speed metabolism while Atkins strictly forbids any drugs in his plan.

Daily multiple-vitamin tablets are advised on all the low-carbohydrate diets.

What Are the Possible Pitfalls?

The preponderance of nutritional research indicates that carbohydrates are essential to normal body functioning—although this is still subject to controversy. Your body needs 5 grams of carbohydrate for each 100 calories it burns whether these calories come from food or stored fat. Therefore, if you oxidize 2,000 calories to perform your daily activities you should provide your system with 100 grams of carbohydrate. While some dietary protein can be broken down to form the glucose needed for body processes, in doing so nitrogen is released and must be excreted, putting great strain on the kidneys. For some people this strain creates serious, permanent damage. And, since protein used in this manner is not available for tissue maintenance, the brain and nervous system that draw on protein for glucose are, in effect, living off body tissues.

When the body does not have enough food-fuel it compensates by breaking down its store of fat. But in order for fats to be changed to energy smoothly, the compounds of carbohydrate metabolism must be present. If this carbohydrate is not available, certain fatty acids accumulate in the bloodstream, bringing on a condition known as ketosis. While Atkins considers this a positive sign of fat destruction, prolonged ketosis can lead to kidney and liver damage and a build-up of uric acid, which may precipitate gout and associated ailments. The more fat you include in your diet, the more carbohydrate you need for its normal breakdown.

Those who advocate low-carbohydrate dieting have stated that such a food plan can reduce blood cholesterol and triglycerides, both implicated in heart disease, even when fat consumption is extravagant. While some experimentation has shown these blood lipids to be directly related to carbohydrate in the diet, evidence supporting a direct causal relationship between dietary fat and elevated blood triglycerides and cholesterol is equally as weighty. It appears that anyone possessing these symptoms could be running a great risk by following a diet *emphasizing* fat, such as Atkins'.

Although Atkins also recommends his zero-carbohydrate diet for combating low blood sugar, other medical authorities have found that *low* levels of carbohydrate are necessary to trigger glucose metabolism from fats and protein. If glucose is not formed, low blood sugar occurs.

Many essential nutrients are found primarily in carbohydrate foods. Whole grains, nuts, and beans—the richest sources of the B vitamins thiamine and pantothenic acid—are excluded from the low-carbohydrate diet. Fresh fruits and vegetables—essential for vitamin A, vitamin C, potassium, and magnesium—are lacking in this food plan; hence the low-carbohydrate dieter is more susceptible to infection and nervous irritability, and eventually more pronounced symptoms of vitamin and mineral deficiencies. Unless *large* quantities of cheese are consumed, calcium intake may be inadequate and on the low-fat, low-carbohydrate regimens this means as much as 2 pounds of cottage cheese daily.

Although most low-carbohydrate diets advise you to take daily vitamin pills, if you do not know what nutrients are missing in your diet it is difficult to make up for them with supplements. Moreover, if you plan to get your vital nourishment in pill form, why not lose weight on an exclusive diet of Coke and potato chips? The fact is, most overweight people suffer from poor food habits and unless they learn to relate to food primarily as nourishment they will never be cured.

America is indeed a nation of "meat-eaters"; but, to be limited in choice to plain cooked meat, day in and day out, without benefit of salt, gravy, or any of the accompaniments to a meal that make dining interesting, as is the case in the low-carbohydrate, low-fat versions of the diet, is unbearably boring. For anyone who enjoys food, a diet of bland meat (which according to Stillman should be cooked well-done for maximum weight loss) will never be satisfying, no matter how much you eat.

While low-calorie diets include some sugars and starches, the low-carbohydrate method preaches total abstinence because it is argued that just one taste can trigger insulin production and that old sugar craving. In most cases however, the desire for sweets is not eliminated, but is satisfied by artificial sweeteners utilized in many recipes which supplement these diet plans. The most recent revelations now suggest that saccharin, as well as cyclamates, may be related to human cancer.

The lack of roughage from whole grains, fruits, and vegetables may cause constipation and related lower-intestinal illnesses, including cancer.

Claims that this diet is the "only one that works" and that it works "in all cases" are obviously untrue. If this were so, there would be no need for the proliferation of diets on the market. The truth is, many overweight people eat not from hunger, but from anxiety, fear, and the search for love and security. Among the most comforting foods are sweets and snacks. If they could give up these indulgences almost any diet would be productive.

Perhaps even more than on all other diets, you cannot cheat on a low-carbohydrate regime. If you give in the slightest bit to your craving for sweets, or have even an extra slice of bread, you could easily throw the intricate carbohydrate balance off and end up with a weight gain instead of a weight loss. Hidden carbohydrates that you may not be aware of in prepared foods will have the same negative effect.

Finally, the high-protein diet is very expensive, carbohydrates being the most reasonable items and protein the most costly on the food market.

Is This the Diet for You?

Even those who criticize the low-carbohydrate diet will grant that highly refined carbohydrates in the form of sugar, white flour, processed foods, pizza, potato chips, cake, cookies, candy, etc., are not beneficial. While eventually some carbohydrate is returned to the menu in all low-carbohydrate diets, the upper limits are never high enough to allow a reentry of these most offensive foods. If the high-protein diet puts an end to such empty-calorie eating it is indeed a positive influence.

Weight loss on a low-carbohydrate diet, while in the long run no greater than on any other diet, does proceed faster, providing the encouragement many dieters need to go on.

Protein and fats are digested slowly so that the fear of hunger most dieters blame for their past failures is not experienced. Just the knowledge that they can eat as much as they want helps motivate some people who normally resist any food deprivation. For those on the unrestricted-fat regimens the fact that they can sit down to a meal of such "fattening" items as bacon, creamy salad dressing, and butter, with even a drink before dinner and heavy cream in their coffee for dessert, makes the low-carbohydrate diet all the more appealing.

Using The Tables of Food Content

While you don't have to count calories on any of these diets, you do have to count grams of carbohydrate. Unless you are familiar with the carbohydrate content of foods and are attuned to possible hidden setbacks in sauces, gravies, ketchup, milk products, combination dishes, etc., you cannot accurately follow the dictates of this food plan. THE TABLES OF FOOD CONTENT inform you of the carbohydrate content of all common foods so you can enjoy a highly flexible diet within the necessary limitations and still avoid the less obvious carbohydrates in many foods.

While some low-carbohydrate diets advocate high fat intake, others counsel low fat consumption. The tables will help you determine the fat content of foods and distinguish between the essential unsaturated fatty acids and the saturated ones.

All low-carbohydrate diets do allow for some carbohydrate eventually. If you wish to maximize health, those carbohydrates you include should be chosen for their nutritive value. By learning to choose from the table such things as wholegrain breads and cereals, nuts and other vitamin-B-rich carbohydrates over chewing gum, candy, jam, cakes, and other empty-calorie, high-carbohydrate items, you may even bring about improvement in your carbohydrate tolerance.

All low-carbohydrate diets press you to take vitamins. But, unless you know which ones are missing from your diet you may be wasting money on overdoses of some and depriving yourself of others. Evaluate the foods you are eating in terms of vitamin A, vitamin C, the B vitamins, and the minerals calcium and potassium in particular. If any of these fall short of the recommended daily allowance you will then have a basis for proper supplementation, either through those foods permitted in the diet plan or other means.

Once your desired weight is within view, you may wish to continue some modification of this food pattern forever (as Atkins suggests) or you may wish to revert to a more conventional way of eating. In order to prevent a return to your old ways, and your old weight, plan your diet around the elements of food as revealed in the tables. Emphasize foods with relatively few calories and plentiful resources of vitamins and minerals to replenish body stores. Calories do count, although their source may be just as important. The proper balance of nutrients (protein, fat, and carbohydrate) can help you maintain your new, cherished figure. If you find that you have wandered off course, a more restricted food selection in the following days will steer you back in the right direction. This is only possible if you maintain a keen awareness of the potential value of foods.

Representative Readings

Atkins, Robert. *Dr. Atkins' Diet Revolution: The High Calorie Way to Stay Thin.* New York: Bantam Books, 1973.

Baker, Sam S., and Stillman, Irwin M. *The Doctor's Quick Weight-Loss Diet.* New York: Dell, 1968.

Berman, Samuel. *The Boston Police Diet and Weight Control Program.* New York: Frederick Fell, 1972.

Cameron, Robert. *The New Drinking Man's Diet and Cookbook.* New York: Bantam Books, 1974.

Fredricks, Carlton. *Dr. Carlton Fredricks' Low-Carbohydrate Diet.* New York: Award Books, 1970.

Lamb, Lawrence. *Metabolics.* Chapter 39. New York: Harper & Row, 1974.

Mayo Clinic Committee on Dietetics. *Mayo Clinic Diet Manual.* 4th ed. Philadelphia: W. B. Saunders, 1971.

Netzer, Corinne, ed. *The Brand Name Carbohydrate Gram Counter.* New York: Dell, 1973.

Taller, Herman. *Calories Don't Count.* New York: Simon & Schuster, 1961.

Yudkin, John, M.D. *Dr. Yudkin's Low Carbohydrate Diet.* Mayo Clinic Diet Manuals. Philadelphia: W. B. Saunders, 1971.

4. CRASH DIETS

One-Sided Diets

The crash diet (also known as the fad diet or one-sided diet) is designed for quick weight loss. Those who promote the popular crash diets that appear and reappear from time to time (frequently promoted in "women's magazines") feel that immediate weight loss is paramount to other nutritional considerations in dieting.

The crash diet is usually based on a high proportion of food from one category or sometimes even a single food. They all involve eating only the foods specified, often as much as you like, and nothing else.

Beneath the surface of these crash diets lies the knowledge that you can only eat so much of any one food combination, after which either your stomach rebels or your desire to eat dissipates out of boredom. The crash dieter therefore rarely overindulges even in the unrestricted food, which results in an involuntary restriction of calories.

Taking "Inches Off"

Actually, the low-carbohydrate, high-protein diets can be classified as one-sided diets. So can the low-protein, high-carbohydrate food plans. Dr. Stillman's Quick-Inches-Off diet, for example, advocates eating large quantities of fruits and vegetables, unlimited juices and vegetable soups, plus tiny amounts of sugar, butter, pasta, artificially sweetened puddings and beverages, and vegetable oils. No nuts, dried beans, milk, cheese, eggs, meat, fish, fowl, or other protein-rich foods are on the menu. The basic premise of Stillman's diet is that body mass is primarily protein. To take "inches off," a diet lacking sufficient protein to meet daily requirements forces the body to reduce protein tissues in its attempt to fill the gap. (Of course, this doesn't mean you can control the site of the lost inches.)

Other popular versions of the crash diet include: *the egg and grapefruit diet*, which features grapefruit and egg at breakfast, lunch, and again at dinner, sometimes alternated with steak or fish, plus small digressions for celery, spinach, and tomato; *the on-off diet*, on which you limit yourself to 1,000 calories on weekdays and go on a binge for the weekend or similarly carry on a restricted-calorie/free-calorie pattern on a daily rotating basis; *the "sweet-tooth diet,"* basically a low-calorie diet supplemented with lollipops or hard candy to satisfy the craving for sweets; *the banana and skimmed milk diet; the wine and eggs diet; the rice diet*, a menu of fruit, vegetables, rice, and 3 ounces of meat or 4 ounces of fish or poultry daily; *the cottage cheese diet*, made up of 1 cup of cottage cheese, 75 calories worth of fruit and vegetables and 70 calories worth of crackers at each of your three daily meals (or divided into six meals throughout the day); and *the "miracle eggnog diet,"* where a concoction of 4 ounces of orange juice, three eggs, 3 tablespoons of vegetable oil, and 5 cups (1 quart 8 ounces) of skimmed milk is prepared and rationed into seven 6-ounce meals over the course of the day for a total of one month.

At their most extreme, crash diets recommend total fasting.

Is This the Diet for You?

Crash diets usually bring amazingly quick results, however they are not meant to be continued for a prolonged length of time. For many, these diets provide the initial proof that they can indeed lose weight. In rare instances they may even be near adequate in food value.

What Are the Possible Pitfalls?

Since no one food contains all the essential nutrients your body needs to grow, rebuild blood and body tissues, and maintain its overall health, many deficiencies can occur if a one-sided diet is adhered to for long. One week is usually sufficient for health to begin degenerating and those who go on and off such patterns are constantly throwing their systems off balance. Unless such a diet is carefully supervised or of short duration, it is possible to cause serious damage to vital organs by upsetting your body chemistry.

Most crash diets are too monotonous to offer the habitual eater any real satisfaction, so they are rarely continued long enough to be effective.

Sooner or later you must go off the one-sided diet, and while you may be thinner, you have received no long-term solution. It even appears that pounds "crashed off" also "crash on" much quicker than weight slowly shed. So, most crash dieters go through life following one "proven" pound-peeler after another, never becoming at ease with their diet or their weight.

Using The Tables of Food Content

THE TABLES OF FOOD CONTENT are designed to provide you with accurate information on the nutritive value of foods. Before you embark on any crash diet you will find it helpful to analyze it in terms of its food value so you can add vitamin supplements (as specified in many of these diets) which are appropriate to the food plan itself. You may, for instance, find that the egg and grapefruit diet is high in protein, vitamin A, riboflavin, and vitamin C, but lacks calcium, thiamine, and niacin. These then are the nutrients you will seek in a supplement. Conversely, the rice diet, while high in B vitamins, might warrant supplements of iron and calcium.

With careful planning through the tables, you will be able to make some of these diets more nutritionally rewarding (or less harmful). On the cottage cheese diet, for example, you can select fruits and vegetables with an eye toward their vitamin and mineral assets. Rather than receiving concentrated amounts of only one nutrient you can cover a broad spectrum within the restricted food choices.

While you are on a crash program the tables can make

you aware of the deficiencies you are imposing on your system. Once you have brought your weight down, they can help compensate for the nutritional abuse by including foods that provide high levels of essential nutrients, especially foods which remain low in calories so you do not put back the weight you fought to lose. In other words, once only the memory of being fat remains, the tables can be your guideline for staying slim.

Representative Readings

Baker, Sam S., and Stillman, Irwin M. *The Doctor's Quick Inches-Off Diet*. New York: Dell, 1970.

Baker, Sam S., and Stillman, Irwin M. *The Doctor's Quick Weight-Loss Diet*. New York: Dell, 1968.

Bliss, Betsy. *Lose Seven Pounds in Seven Days*. New York: Bantam Books, 1971.

Fiteljorg, Sonja. *Sweet Way to Diet*. New York: Pocket Books, 1971.

Netzer, Corinne. *The Ten-Day Ten-Pounds-Off Diet*. New York: Dell, 1972.

5. LIQUID DIETS

Don't Eat, Drink

Although liquid diets have been recently popularized as a pathway toward body cleansing and renewed health, they are equally useful for weight reduction. Therefore they are placed at this point in the book.

The liquid diet is, in theory, a low-calorie regimen in which sustenance is taken solely in liquid, rather than solid, form. Since water, the basic component of all liquids, has a bloating effect, it is difficult to drink all that much without considerable discomfort. With small servings of the chosen beverage spaced throughout the day, you can remain somewhat satisfied. And, as you can only drink your nourishment, the liquid diet prevents you from straying with some "forbidden food" that is easily sneaked onto the menu and somehow justified in more food-oriented regimes.

In Search of the Perfect Beverage

There is no single liquid diet. For some it is a form of fasting in which only water is taken. When used for spiritual/cleansing purposes, herbal teas may be acceptable too; when strictly a weight-loss tactic, tea, coffee, and bouillon are freely administered.

Some liquid diets center around unrestricted consumption of freshly extracted fruit and vegetable juices. Many people practice this form of dieting on a once-a-week or once-a-month basis to rejuvenate the body systems while simultaneously producing a calorie diminution. Dr. Stillman has proposed a two-week liquid semifast for losing weight.

The once bestselling Rockefeller diet, later expanded into the Metrecal plan, translates the liquid diet into a milkshake of sorts (evaporated milk, corn oil, flavoring, and sugar combined into a 900-calorie drink). Such commercial items as Instant Breakfast and Carnation Slender are in this tradition.

No matter what its orientation, the exclusively liquid diet is followed for a set period of time only, ranging anywhere from one day to one month. Once the food fast is over, it is suggested that solids be reintroduced gradually and the first few meals be bland and moderate in size.

Those who recommend longer fasts to flush out body toxins advise a diet of fruit juice for one week prior to any complete fast. During the fasting period water is taken for thirst or hunger; a gallon a day is suggested. A little lemon juice, honey, or molasses may be added to the water for its laxative effect. A return to fruit juice, one day of juice for each day of fasting, precedes the reentry into the world of solid food. This procedure is known as "scientific" or "rational" fasting.

What Are the Possible Pitfalls?

Although Stillman tells us no serious deficiency will occur throughout the continuance of one month of his liquid diet, some adverse symptoms are more than likely to manifest themselves during this time. This potential depends on body stores previous to the diet, but you can expect protein and calcium inadequacies if the juice diet is pursued for long; low levels of vitamin C, thiamine, and iron on a prolonged milk-based diet; and multiple nutritional deficiencies on a water-coffee-tea regime.

Also, for those who must "eat," a liquid diet may not be emotionally acceptable.

Lastly, while a liquid diet may be effective in taking off pounds, it will not help you to nurture that slim figure in the future.

Is This the Diet for You?

Not all liquid combinations are nutritionally deficient. After all, an infant does most of its growing on a milk formula. A juice diet replete with all essential vitamins and minerals is harmless and in many ways uplifting for short time spans. The lack of protein and certain B vitamins can even be reversed by blending the juice with wheat germ or brewers' yeast. A milk-based drink combined with fruit (a homemade fruitshake) can also provide highly nutritional meals on a limited calorie intake.

Scientific fasting is advised by one school of medicine as a cure for certain ailments, based on the conviction that disease is caused by poisons in the body. Approached in a rational (highly controlled) manner, a cleansing fast has been known to bring relief to sufferers of metabolic disorders which cause overweight and underweight, digestive ailments, respiratory impairments, allergies, recurrent headaches, insomnia, depression, and a host of other illnesses.

For people who cannot resist the temptations of food, the prohibition of all solids often provides the impetus for vital weight loss, but, to repeat, it is only a short-term solution.

Using The Tables of Food Content

Whether or not the liquid diet you select falls into the "sound" or "deficient" category can be determined by THE TABLES OF FOOD CONTENT. Certainly you should be aware of any shortcomings before you begin, and perhaps your awareness of nutritional needs and your previous food history will alert you to any potential hazards such limitations might inflict upon your system. If you suspect your nutritional reserves will not carry you through this period you can then add the appropriate supplements to the beverage.

There is no magic in any liquid diet, including the prepared mixes sold commercially. With a small input on your part you can save money and devise an all-liquid diet of your own which is nutritionally balanced (including protein, carbohydrate, and fat) and yet low in calories. By selecting liquid foods based on the nutritional value they offer, you can formulate concoctions in all your favorite flavors. Use the information in the tables to build the levels of each nutrient to a point acceptable to you. The appendix *Why Eat? The Elements of Food* can help you map out these needs and you can then prepare your drinks accordingly.

Representative Readings

De Groot, Roy. *How I Reduced with the New Rockefeller Diet.* New York: Horizon Press, 1956.

Ehret, Arnold. *Rational Fasting.* Beaumont, Calif.: Ehret Literature Publishing Company, 1971.

Kloss, Jethro. *Back to Eden.* Chapter 5. Santa Barbara, Calif.: Lifeline Books, 1972.

Lamb, Lawrence. *Metabolics.* Chapter 38. New York: Harper & Row, 1974.

6. HOW TO GAIN WEIGHT

Why Some People Weigh Less Than They Should

In a society such as ours where so much priority is placed on being slim, it is inconceivable to many people that others actually face the problem of being underweight. But it is true that there are many who weigh too little to remain in good health and to have the vitality to enjoy life. For those who are underweight, this condition is just as pressing as obesity. With proper diet, however, most cases of underweight can be remedied.

In most instances underweight is the result of your body getting too little food to provide energy equal to daily activity expenditure. Usually the underweight person just doesn't eat enough. However, this is not always so; sometimes the underweight individual does ingest ample calories but due to illness, stress, or some error of metabolism, the food that is eaten cannot be properly assimilated, with the ultimate effect that it is not oxidized to provide the needed energy.

Planning a Diet for Weight Gain

Although diet alone may not cure the emotional or physical impairment that inhibits food absorption, it can often help improve the situation. For those people whose weight deficiency comes from undereating or the aftermath of a depleting illness, diet can certainly be effective in achieving normal weight.

Assuming lack of ample food energy is the cause of underweight, increasing the daily calorie intake is the first step toward its cure.

Just how many calories you need daily differs for each individual. As explained in the section "Low-Calorie Dieting," the average, moderately active person expends 12 to 15 calories per pound of body weight. Some people use more calories due to a high basal metabolic rate (the basic energy utilized in carrying out the essential life processes). Others are sufficiently active to warrant more fuel for their daily activities. People who are constantly in motion burn more calories. (With little body fat in reserve, thin people may even use more body fuel just trying to keep warm.)

In order to find your particular energy requirements you must first compute your present calorie intake by using the diet survey methods described in the chapter *Learning to Evaluate Your Diet*. If your weight is constant, this then will be the base level for maintaining your present (low) weight. If you are losing weight, you can reach your base level by increasing your calorie consumption until your current weight is constant. From this base point, you need approximately 3,-500 additional calories to add one pound of body weight. Depending on how quickly you wish to gain, add an average of 300 calories to the daily menu at first, gradually increasing this as your appetite adjusts. Once you gain several pounds you will find that you'll require a higher base level of calories to maintain the weight and will have to increase your daily intake to continue the gain. Once you have achieved your desired weight you can estimate your new base level so that you can keep your weight constant.

Gaining weight is more than a process of adding high-calorie foods to your diet. In planning the daily menu, consideration should be given not only to the calorie content of foods, but to their nutritional value and how they are prepared. Most people who are underweight are also undernourished and exhibit a relatively low interest in food and nutrition. Actually, poor nutrition may cause the lack of appetite which perpetuates this condition.

The need for protein, vitamins, and minerals in the underweight is therefore usually greater than the National Re-

search Council suggests in the Table of Recommended Daily
Dietary Allowances (see page 291). If you cannot maintain
weight due to poor absorption and metabolism, it is vital that
you be exposed to even larger amounts of each nutrient to
compensate for the unused portions. Given these possibilities,
a diet planned for weight gain should be particularly well endowed with the most nourishing elements in food in addition
to calories. Although empty calories from candy, soda, pretzels, potato chips, pastries, and the like do play a certain role
in increasing total calorie intake, they do nothing to increase
vitamin and mineral reserves in the body and impose the risk
of replacing more body-building foods. No matter what your
weight status, too much sugar and salt are bad for your
teeth, your nervous system, and your digestive system.

The underweight individual, lacking body fat, breaks down
body tissues for energy when ample food is not available
from the diet. Life progresses at the expense of body protein.
To rebuild bones, blood, and all cells, and to create new body
tissues not just pounds of fat, a high protein requirement
must be met during weight gain.

Fat is the most efficient source of food energy, yielding 9
calories per gram. Foods rich in fat can be of considerable
use in adding energy value to the diet; however, these foods
have several drawbacks. Fat is digested more slowly than
other nutrients and may prove so satisfying that the small
eater is not hungry, skips meals, and thereby reduces the
amount of other foods and potential calories consumed.
Moreover, too much fat can be as harmful to the coronary
system of the underweight as it is to that of the obese individual. Therefore the total fat in the diet should still remain
below 35 percent of the daily calories. The largest proportion
of these fats should be of the unsaturated variety, particularly
since fats form such a large part of the menu.

Since carbohydrates are plentiful in the high-calorie diet, B
vitamins become increasingly important; they are the catalysts for carbohydrate metabolism and are needed in increasing proportion to carbohydrate and total calorie intake.

Vitamin A, along with the B vitamins, is said to improve
the appetite, which will encourage you to eat more as
prescribed in a weight-gaining regimen.

As you plan the menu, consider adding sauces, salad dressing, grains, beans, nuts, dried fruits, and whole-grain breads

to round out your meals. Choose whole milk and fruit juices rather than water, coffee, or tea. These will create new food interest while adding nutritionally replete calories. Although meat and cheese are important foods, they should not be overemphasized since their high fat content makes them quickly satisfying and those who have small appetites may consequently eliminate other items on the menu. It is better to have smaller portions of several items than large quantities of one food when trying to gain weight.

What Are the Possible Pitfalls?

By increasing fat and carbohydrate intake without attention to the vitamins and minerals that play a vital role in their utilization, you can throw your system into a state of impaired metabolism. Uncontrolled eating of high-calorie sweets and fats may actually destroy the appetite, and, if done to the exclusion of other foods, is likely to result in malnutrition.

Often people who set out to gain weight overshoot their mark. A diet planned to add pounds should be gradual and should not distort the appetite or you will wind up on the opposite side of the scale.

Is This the Diet for You?

Sensible weight gain results not only in a more attractive physique, but can bring with it improved health and greater physical and mental stamina. When carefully planned, it can also generate renewed interest in good food and set a pattern for future living.

Using The Tables of Food Content

Unless you know your present calorie intake, it is difficult to determine your needs. This is the first step in any weight-control plan and can be discovered by using THE TABLES OF FOOD CONTENT to calculate the energy potential of the meals which have created your current body condition. The chapter *Learning to Evaluate Your Diet* will help you prepare this data. Once you have established your base calorie level (the amount of energy that keeps your weight constant) you can use the calorie listings in the tables to design meals around food combinations which provide at least this much energy, plus extra calories depending on the desired rate of gain.

As you select foods with an emphasis on potential calories, pay attention to their nutrient make-up. In this manner you can stress those rich in protein, unsaturated fatty acids, B vitamins, vitamin A, plus the remaining vitamins and minerals needed to increase body stores and improve health. With the tables you can ferret out the foods which offer calories alone, reserving them for those times all other daily nutritional needs have been fulfilled.

Natural, Whole, and Organic Food Diets

———◆———

The great controversy over processed, prepared foods versus foods in their whole, unrefined state has led to considerable popularity of diets featuring natural foods.

The advocates of natural eating are keenly aware of the body's daily requirements for high levels of essential nutrients. Furthermore, they are of the opinion that foods in their natural form, that is, unprocessed or processed "only enough to render them suitable for eating" retain the highest nutrient content. Much information about food and nutrition is still being uncovered and while further studies are in progress, foods in their whole state are most likely to insure the proper balance of both the known and the as-yet-undiscovered elements that the body needs for top performance. By refining foods, many of these essentials are likely to be destroyed or discarded in the process. Even when nutrients are put back, as in flour and cereal enrichment, they are not replaced in their original form, balance, or amount. Another important aspect of a natural foods diet is the absence of all chemical additives in the form of preservatives, emulsifiers, texturizers, synthetic flavoring, artificial coloring, etc.

Not all natural foods diets are the same. Some stress the importance of high levels of all nutrients. In the belief that poor soil conditions, lengthy storage, improper handling and cooking limit the availability of nutrients in foods, proponents of some natural foods diets may counsel not only a high food intake of many vitamins and minerals, but daily supplementation as well. Other natural foods diets assume that high concentrations of certain nutrients in certain foods (most notably the huge quantities of protein in meat) tax the digestive organs; they therefore promote food plans minus these traditional American foods. Some natural foods diets stress raw foods, while others detail strict cooking procedures.

Despite these variances, all natural foods plans are based on the conviction that the refining of food decreases its inherent nutritional value and therefore processed, prepared foods are eliminated from the menu. There is also general agreement that growing conditions affect the production of nutrients in food, and although these diets are not solely dependent on organically grown foods (that is, foods grown on soil enriched with natural matter—humus—as opposed to chemical fertilizers, and without the use of pesticides) they all prefer organic foods, crediting them with higher nutritional advantage. There is also a strong contention that foods grown without the aid of chemical fertilizers and pesticides are free of toxins associated with many metabolic disturbances.

Other concepts common to all natural foods diets include the beliefs that foods are most nutritious in the fresh rather than canned or frozen state, and then eaten as close to harvesting as possible, and that improper handling is highly destructive of vitamins and minerals. When cooking fruits, vegetables, meat, and grains the lowest possible temperature is suggested along with the least amount of water to prevent loss of heat-sensitive and water-soluble nutrients. Low-temperature oven roasting of meats and quick sauteing or steaming of vegetables are integral parts of natural foods cookery. The juicing of fruits and vegetables is another popular method of preparation in these diets.

1. THE BASIC NATURAL FOODS DIET

Are "Recommended Allowances" Enough?

According to those who have popularized the basic natural foods diet (J. I. Rodale and Adelle Davis, among others), good nutrition is the basis of preventative medicine and its practice can help maintain health and prevent illness. It is the aim of the basic natural foods diet to provide us with *real* sustenance from our food. By selecting foods with discernment, we can enhance the supply of all the elements known to be needed by the body; by choosing foods grown on chemical-free, nutrient-rich soil, as near to their natural state as possible, promoters of natural foods diets feel we will have the greatest chance of getting the still unknown nutrients as well. In this manner, they propose, the body can heal ailments and protect itself against invasion from harmful bacteria, viruses, chemical intoxicants, and pollutants.

The human body is an intricate structure of billions of cells. Food nutrients keep these cells in proper working order; they provide the essential materials for new cells to be built, for maintaining the balance of body fluids, etc. The amount of nourishment supplied to the cells determines our health, and a minor lack of one or more nutrients can greatly damage the cell structure. There are presently over forty nutrients known to be essential to the human cell; many are waiting to be discovered. While single nutritional deficiencies induced in animal experimentation are rarely observed in the human body, multiple deficiencies occur frequently. They are evidenced in a lack of energy, low spirits and less than optimum body functioning; in obesity and heart disease and low blood sugar; in frequent colds, viruses, and temporary and permanent debilitating diseases.

Natural foods theorists believe food processing is largely responsible for the high incidence of malnutrition and the overall poor health status of the American population. The refining of the basic ingredients that compose prepared, packaged foods removes much of the original food value; synthetic food enrichment reinstates high percentages of some food elements, but ignores the simultaneous need for others. Processed foods add excessive quantities of salt and sugar. While not all these foods are harmful in themselves, they may satisfy our appetites and thereby crowd out the use of other more substantial foods. The elaborate marketing and promotion of these largely synthetic, chemicalized foodstuffs eases Americans into believing their food intake is of better quality than it may be. By contrast, natural foods enthusiasts feel our modern reliance on food processing and prepared, packaged foods has made it virtually impossible to obtain adequate amounts of nutrients, particularly within the calorie limits imposed by decreased activity. Even the term "adequate amounts" is felt to be somewhat troublesome; most people who follow the basic natural foods plan believe the Recommended Daily Allowances (RDA) to be extremely unreliable since individuals vary greatly in body needs and daily experience, both prime factors in determining nutrient requirements. Thus, the values expressed in the RDA are considered by them to be minimal.

If wholesome foods were obtainable, they say—meaning fruits and vegetables and grains grown on naturally fertilized soil; untreated milk from animals allowed to graze on green pastures; meat and animal products from uncastrated animals raised on natural grain, free of hormones, antibiotics, and chemical feed—it might be possible for our diet to furnish all the nutrients our bodies need daily in just the right amount. But the use of poor, chemically treated soil for growing produce, the mindless spraying of crops, and the raising of animals with drugs and chemicals, coupled with the lengthy storage of food and improper handling, has reduced the nutritive value even before the processing or cooking begins. As a result, in order to obtain optimum levels of nutrients, the most staunch advocates of natural eating often deem food supplementation a necessary adjunct to eating even the highest quality unrefined foodstuffs available.

Foods Chosen for Their Whole Quality

Since no food element works in isolation, it is important to achieve the *proper balance* of protein, fat, carbohydrate, vitamins, and minerals in as efficient a manner as possible. Three well-balanced meals are recommended daily. Breakfast is considered the most important of these meals since morning food intake determines how you will feel throughout the entire day. The typical American high-starch breakfast gives an initial surge of energy but it is soon followed by fatigue, depression, and a craving for sweets. The aim of the natural-foods-diet breakfast is to balance a high-protein food with some fat and carbohydrate. This provides a gradual re-

lease of sugar into the bloodstream and maintains a high
level of energy over the longest period of time. A minimum
of 22 grams of protein is suggested. Such foods as meat, fish,
fowl, eggs, milk, and cheese, plus less conventional foods
such as soy products and yogurt are promoted as excellent
protein sources that can be further enhanced by the use of
nutritional (brewers' or torula) yeast, dry-milk powder,
wheat germ, soy flour, and ground nuts and seeds in food
preparation.

A natural foods lunch should also contain a good source of
protein, a moderate amount of carbohydrate, and again,
some fat. Although most people get lots of fat in their daily
diet, the kind of fat referred to in the natural foods plan is
unsaturated fat, important as a source of linoleic and linolenic acid, to provide satiety and a slow release of sugar into
the bloodstream, and to transport the fat-soluble vitamins
A, D, E, and K. All hydrogenated fats from processed
peanut butter, processed cheeses, solid cooking fat, and
French fried foods are avoided. Animal fat from beef, pork,
and lamb is limited, replaced by more fish and fowl on the
menu; highly saturated coconut oil and palm oil, found in
imitation cream, filled milk, and infant formulas are rejected.
The highest priority is given to unrefined nut and vegetable
oils.

While in typical American households dinner is the
heaviest meal, dinners on the natural foods plan are light,
following the pattern of lunch.

To obtain the extremely high levels of vitamins and minerals the body needs, carbohydrates come in the form of fresh
fruits and vegetables and in whole, unrefined grains where
they are accompanied by rich supplies of other nutrients
necessary for proper digestion. White flour, white rice, packaged cereals, and white sugar have no place in the natural
kitchen. They are considered poor substitutes for whole-
wheat flour, honey and molasses, brown or converted rice,
and other whole-grain cereals. The aforementioned whole
foods are stressed as vital sources of B vitamins, vitamin E,
calcium, iron, phosphorous, and magnesium. Fresh produce is
rich in vitamin A, vitamin C, potassium, phosphorous, and all
trace minerals. Nuts and beans contribute B vitamins, iron,
magnesium, and trace minerals.

Despite the high level of vitamins and minerals in these

preferred foods, individual stresses, bacterial infections, use of drugs, smoking, plus air- and food-borne chemicals are felt to bring an increased need for nutrients. To provide as much as 20,000 international units (IU's) of vitamin A (recommended by both Rodale and Davis) vitamin supplementation may be counseled. To assure the proper balance of B vitamins, particularly difficult to obtain in a culture where most grains are refined, whole foods can be supplemented with nutritional yeast.

Vitamin-C levels necessary to fight illness may be as high as twenty to forty times the normal recommendation, and since this vitamin is easily destroyed in cooking and by antibiotics and toxicants in the body, a habitual C supplement is considered prudent.

Vitamin D, thought to be supplied by exposure to the sun, knows no concentrated food sources with the exception of vitamin-D-fortified milk; natural food followers believe much time spent indoors, heavy layers of clothing, and air pollution block out the ultraviolet rays of the sun which convert the oils on the skin to vitamin D so there is no longer a reliable source of this nutrient. Consequently, 1,000 units of vitamin D from fish-liver oil in the first year of life, increasing to 1,500 units for the next seven years is often recommended as a dietary supplement. (Adults can tolerate from 4,000 to 5,000 units daily.)

Vitamin E is needed in proportion to the amount of fat you eat, and since it is difficult to obtain unless wheat germ and unrefined oils are included in the diet, vitamin E supplements are recommended. (As much as 1,600 units can be taken daily without fear of toxicity.)

In order for adults to receive at least 1 gram of calcium daily, when a quart of milk is not drunk each day, a calcium supplement might also be added.

And so the trend continues for vitamins and minerals to supplement food elements which should be as plentiful as possible on the daily menu, but which many natural foods dieters may still wish to increase.

What Are the Possible Pitfalls?

Diets are rarely followed in their entirety, and body metabolism being quite intricate, dietary recommendations are frequently subject to confusion. The basic natural foods diet is particularly susceptible to misinterpretation, and consequently the overzealous follower may become a pill-popper without an eye to the essential combination of food nutrients and food supplements in the diet. An oversupply of one nutrient, often leading to depletion of another, is one possible consequence. Money thrown out on supplements that cannot be utilized effectively by the body is another. Furthermore, while vitamin toxicity is rare, it is a definite possibility, particularly in the case of vitamins A, D, and E.

Many people make the mistake of thinking that all foods sold as "health foods" will make them healthier and so consume them in huge quantities. It is important to realize that many natural foods candies, baked goods, even the "natural cereals" still contain a good deal of sweetening and calories and they, too, can be overemphasized in the diet.

Many people fail to note that identical products may be offered in supermarkets and natural foods stores at widely differing prices. They may also accept on faith products labeled "natural foods" as being wholesome, whereas if they read all the small print they might discover such processed ingredients as sugar, hydrogenated vegetable shortening, MSG, corn syrup, etc.

Is This the Diet for You?

The basic teachings of the natural foods diet deserve high praise. With nutrition education sadly lacking, this movement has brought increased food awareness to America. The foods recommended for their whole, natural quality can only add to the nutritional status of the individual. Even the supplementation, if done with moderation, may prove beneficial, and is certainly without harm.

Contrary to adverse publicity, natural foods are more full-flavored than their processed counterparts. They can reduce the craving for sweets and salt, and because they are more satisfying, often lead to desired weight control. By adding more bulk to the diet, natural foods also facilitate elimination.

The consumption of unprocessed foods greatly reduces the amount of chemicals, salt, sugar, and saturated fats you introduce into your system.

Criticized as a costly diet, a natural foods plan is often less expensive than most other food patterns since no money is wasted on high-calorie overprocessed foods with little nutritional value. For each dollar you spend you receive high-nutrient returns. And, say the natural foods advocates, "hundreds of dollars are saved yearly on medical and dental bills." It is true that certain whole foods are more costly than their refined counterparts; on the other hand, prepared dinners, packaged baked goods, and snack foods are among the highest priced items in the food marketplace when you consider their nutritional worth.

Using The Tables of Food Content

In order to know which foods are highest in nutritional value you must have an unclouded picture of their nutrient content. The most complete tables of food composition available are provided here, although some limitations are imposed by variations in food samples and home storage and cooking methods. With THE TABLES OF FOOD CONTENT you can plan your meals around high levels of protein, vitamins, and minerals as recommended in the natural foods plan, and include carbohydrates and unsaturated fats as desired. By calculating the amount of nutrients you thus obtain, you can determine for yourself any need for supplementation.

Using the tables, you can not only select foods but you can actually evaluate your diet to verify for yourself many of the truths in the natural foods philosophy. By assessing your food intake either casually or through THE DIET SURVEY, you will be able to note any deviation from the recommended balance of nutrients and correct it for improved health. Although all the vitamins and minerals advanced under the natural foods concept are not included on the tables (such as magnesium, iodine, the entire B complex, etc.), the introduction to each food group informs you of rich food sources of these additional nutrients.

Representative Readings

Davis, Adelle. *Let's Eat Right to Keep Fit*. New York: Signet, 1970.

Deutsch, Ronald. *The Family Guide to Better Food and Health*. Des Moines, Iowa: Creative Home Library, 1971.

Goldbeck, David, and Goldbeck, Nikki. *The Good Breakfast Book*. New York: Links Books, 1975.

Goldbeck, David, and Goldbeck, Nikki. *The Supermarket Handbook: Access to Whole Foods*. New York: New American Library, 1974.

Hunter, Beatrice T. *Consumer Beware*. New York: Simon & Schuster, Inc., 1971.

Hunter, Beatrice T. *The Natural Foods Primer*. New York: Fireside Books, 1973.

Jacobson, Michael F. *Eater's Digest: The Consumers' Factbook of Food Additives*. New York: Doubleday, 1972.

Jacobson, Michael F. *Nutrition Scoreboard*. Washington, D.C.: Center for Science in the Public Interest, 1973.

Rodale, J. I., et al. *The Complete Book of Food and Nutrition*. Emmaus, Pa: Rodale Books, 1971.

2. VEGETARIANISM

Why No Meat?

Often people choose vegetarian diets because of ethical convictions or religious teachings. (Vegetarianism is practiced

by Buddhists, Seventh-Day Adventists, Hindus, Jains, etc.)
These vegetarians believe that you should not take the life of
another being. Some practitioners, referred to as *vegans*, go
so far as to eschew all animal by-products (found in soaps,
cosmetics, jewelry, household items, and clothing) as well as
any food of animal origin including flesh, milk, and eggs.

Those who choose vegetarianism for health reasons do so
on the theory that animal flesh contains many toxins and stim-
ulants and additionally puts a strain on the body's digestive
organs. Moreover, protein, along with a richer supply of vitamins and minerals, can be obtained from a variety of plant
sources. At the same time the elimination of animal flesh
from the diet means a reduced intake of saturated fats and
cholesterol found primarily in foods of animal origin. Another consideration is the fact that pesticide levels increase as
one organism consumes another. The pesticide residue on
plants and in the environment is transferred to the animal living off these raw materials. The animal thus accumulates the
pesticides and transfers them along the food chain to another
animal or human. Therefore, the lower you eat on the food
chain, or the closer to the original food source (plants or less
predatory animals), the lower the level of pesticides in your
diet. Today's practice of feeding livestock chemically treated
feed and antibiotics adds another dimension to the selection
of a no-meat diet for health.

Many vegetarians have been motivated by ecological factors, for meat is indisputably wasteful of natural resources.
Animal production is dependent on grazing land which might
otherwise be used for agricultural production. Furthermore,
animals raised for food must consume huge quantities of
grain and plant protein that could more efficiently be used in
the direct feeding of people.

Frances Lappé details the economics of protein production
in her book *Diet for a Small Planet.* Among her revelations
is the fact that a cow eats 21 pounds of vegetable protein to
produce 1 pound of protein for man's consumption; other
animals are a bit more efficient: 1 pound of meat protein is
supplied by feeding 8.3 pounds of grain protein to a pig and
5.5 pound of grain protein to a chicken; 4.4 pounds of grain
protein are needed to produce 1 pound of milk protein; and
4.3 pounds of grain protein generate 1 pound of egg protein.
As Lappé further informs us, one acre of cereal can provide

five times the protein of an acre of land devoted to meat production; legumes offer ten times the protein yield per acre, and leafy vegetables yield fifteen times as much protein per acre as land devoted to animal raising.

This waste is compounded by the fact that Americans consume far more protein as a population than any other nation, and, on the average, consume far more protein than the body needs to perform its essential functions. A mere 7 ounces of meat is sufficient to fill your daily protein requirement, assuming you are receiving *no* protein from other foods. All excess protein is burned as fuel (or stored as fat) just like fats and carbohydrates are.

The economics of a no-meat diet is a reflection of these ecological factors. Because meat is wasteful in production, it is expensive to buy. Many people choose vegetarian eating daily, or on a less regular basis, to save on food costs.

The Meatless Menu

Vegetarian diets cover a wide range of eating patterns, which may or may not include fish, poultry, eggs, milk, and cheese. Because fish and poultry are such conventional substitutes for meat, this form of vegetarian diet does not differ greatly from the meat-vegetable-potato pattern of the basic balanced diet.

Most of those who practice vegetarianism (particularly those motivated by the health aspects), do so taking special care to choose as few processed foods as possible. They avoid refined sugars, white flour, excessive salt, and prepared food items. They include whole grains, nuts, fresh produce, and similar whole foods in their meals. Many choose organic foods as well. This category of vegetarians includes strict vegetarians and ovo-lacto vegetarians (those who consume eggs and milk products).

People who become vegetarians by simply deleting the meat portion of the meal are less likely to develop the commendable characteristics and reap the rewards that accompany intelligent vegetarianism, and may continue to eat all the foods that comprise the typical American diet with the exception of animal flesh.

In a well-planned regimen, vegetarians obtain their principal protein from nuts and seeds, legumes, and whole grains, while some will dip into eggs, cheese, and milk. The protein value of eggs and cheese is as high as, and in some cases higher than, that of meat. Nuts, seeds, legumes, and cereals are termed "lower-quality protein foods," referring to the fact that they do not contain enough of all the eight essential amino acids the body needs from food to synthesize protein. Eating large quantities of these foods, however, will provide adequate supplies of protein, and combining them with each other, or with eggs and milk products, greatly elevates their protein potential. This is known as protein complementation. Foods lacking one or more essential amino acids, when eaten together with foods rich in these amino acids, are as high in food value as meat, eggs, and cheese. These foods are best combined during the same meal since amino acids are not stored by the body and all must be present simultaneously to build protein.

Other nutrients generally associated with meat, such as B vitamins and iron, are also obtained from plant sources, as well as from eggs and cheese. Calcium, if not supplied by milk and milk products in strict vegetarian diets, comes from such foods as unhulled sesame seeds, soy products, leafy green vegetables, almonds, sunflower seeds, and other plant foods.

Wheat germ, nutritional (brewers' and torula) yeast and soy flour are used by vegetarians to enhance the nutritional value of their meals in terms of protein and B vitamins. Other popular choices which provide substantial food elements include soybeans and other soy products, whole (brown) rice, whole wheat, cornmeal, oats, bulgar (cracked wheat), millet, bean sprouts, sunflower seeds, sesame seeds, whole-grain breads, raw cashews, yogurt, as well as all varieties of beans, nuts, fruits, and vegetables.

What Are the Possible Pitfalls?

The vegetarian who simply eliminates meat from the menu without changing other food habits may develop a wide range of nutritional deficiencies. For those who become vegetarians following a sound plan, certain areas should be given particular attention to avoid possible inadequacies.

Those whose diets do not include eggs, milk, or milk products should take care to include foods rich in calcium and riboflavin along with the protein-rich items suggested in this section.

The most significant nutrient that may be missing in a diet which includes no animal foods is vitamin B_{12} (not enumerated in THE TABLES OF FOOD CONTENT). This deficiency can be avoided by the use of wheat germ, nutritional yeast, and kelp (unique nonanimal sources of this vitamin).

Suspicious symptoms of inadequate B vitamins and protein include lack of energy, poor health, unusually slow healing, brittle hair or loss of hair, soft nails, rashes or other skin eruptions, and a disagreeable temperament. Consult the tables to remedy these conditions.

As is true of any new diet, switching to a vegetarian regimen requires some initial effort and reeducation in planning and preparing meals. Eventually, though, it can be as natural as any other mode of eating.

Is This the Diet for You?

While protein and B vitamins require particular attention in the vegetarian diet, those who follow a rational vegetarian food plan usually enjoy a higher intake of most other vitamins and minerals, particularly vitamins A, C, E, niacin and thiamine, and phosphorous, potassium, and magnesium.

Less animal fat in the diet means less saturated fat and cholesterol.

Unless a vegetarian goes overboard on "bread and potatoes," a well-planned vegetarian diet also usually means fewer calories. Whole grains, nuts, legumes, and foods made with these items arc quite satisfying and thus are eaten in smaller quantity than the nonvegetarian might realize. This is assuming, of course, that the vegetarian also cuts down on processed foods and limits intake of pastries, candies, and other empty-calorie fare dependent on refined ingredients.

The elimination of meat from the diet means a significant reduction of certain potentially harmful chemicals, hormones, and antibiotics consumed along with meat flesh.

Because vegetarian meals are less costly than meat meals, there is a noticeable monetary saving in this diet as well.

Once the meat-vegetable-potato routine is rejected, a wide variety of new culinary experiences awaits the vegetarian. The many vegetarian and natural foods cookbooks will arouse your interest and help you prepare many of these intriguing new dishes.

Using The Tables of Food Content

The most common question a vegetarian encounters is, "How do you get enough protein?" If you use THE TABLES OF FOOD CONTENT to help you plan your meals you can guarantee a diet sufficient in this nutrient. In addition, other nutrients commonly associated with a meat diet, like iron and riboflavin, can be assured in adequate amounts if you are aware of alternate sources. The strict vegetarian can ensure supplies of calcium by consulting the tables too.

Those interested in further reducing saturated fats and dietary cholesterol willfi nd low-fat dairy products listed in the tables.

Representative Readings

Altman, Nathanial. *Eating for Life: A Book About Vegetarianism.* Wheaton, Ill.: Theosophical Publishing House, Quest Books, 1973.

The Committee on Nutritional Misinformation. *Vegetarian*

Diets. Washington, D.C.: National Academy of Sciences, 1974.

Goldbeck, Nikki. *Cooking What Comes Naturally: A Month's Worth of Natural/Vegetarian Menus,* New York: Cornerstone Library, 1973.

Hurd, Frank J., and Hurd, Rosalie. *Ten Talents.* Collegedale, Tenn.: College Press, 1968.

Lappé, Frances M. *Diet for a Small Planet.* New York: Ballantine Books, 1975 rev. ed.

3. YOGA FOODS

In Pursuit of Prana

Prana, a key word in yoga philosophy, translates loosely as "life force," and the study of yoga is devoted to gaining access to the life force dormant in all of us and to assimilating life force from outside the body. It is part of the belief of the yoga community that the way you look and feel is directly related to what you eat, and therefore an eating pattern based on foods which "regenerate and impart vitality to the body with a minimum of stress, and which will leave the mind clear and elevated" has been composed. Whole foods, and primarily those which are planted, are believed to be a major source of life force, and the yogi aims to incorporate this prana into the body, simultaneously providing an alternative to both chemical additives and denatured foods.

The underlying theory behind the yoga foods plan reflects the entire yogic philosophy—the more life force the body assimilates, the greater the potential for health, vitality, mental clarity, serenity, and self-awareness. Food can either regenerate the body, regulate weight and elevate the mind, or sap the life force, add excess poundage, and bring about premature aging and illness. Eating foods closest to their native state, or prepared only enough to render them digestible, with minimal destruction to their inherent life force has a positive effect on physical and mental well-being. The other foods we eat are merely testimony to the remarkable strength of our bodies and the amount of abuse they can take and continue to survive.

Putting Life Force on the Menu

Natural eating is the basis of the yoga diet, concentrating mainly on foods which are planted, such as vegetables, fruits, herbs, nuts, grains, and legumes, plus certain dairy products. Foods are consumed raw or lightly cooked and most dishes avoid heavy seasoning and sweetening so that the taste of the food itself can be experienced.

The yogi believes the form in which food enters the digestive system is critical. Vegetables should always be fresh, and organically grown produce is deemed superior. Frozen vegetables can be used as an alternative to fresh, but canned vegetables are never acceptable in the yoga diet. At least one meal each day includes raw salad, and one or more servings of cooked vegetables is recommended. Steaming is the best method of vegetable cookery, and all cooking liquid is conserved for soup or other service. Bean and seed sprouts are highly acclaimed.

Since harsh spices can irritate the digestive system and are said to "agitate the mind," only sea salt, vegetable salts, herbs, garlic, onion, lemon, and soy sauce are used to season foods in the yoga tradition.

Meat is excluded from the diet as animal slaughter runs contrary to the yoga belief in the sanctity of life. Additionally, it is thought to be so near decomposition that it places a toxic burden on the body. The yogi counts on legumes, nuts, grains, avocado, yogurt, and cheese to supply protein. Dairy products that are low in fat—nonfat milk or raw milk, cottage cheese, farmer cheese, ricotta and feta cheeses—are all an integral part of the yoga foods regime; yogurt is touted as a boon to both digestion and elimination. Preferred cheeses are unsalted and made with raw or goat's milk; certain other mild, natural cheeses such as Swiss, Monterrey Jack, and cheddar, are permissible in limited quantity. Fertilized eggs are thought to contain all life-supporting elements but play a minor role in the yoga diet; the more orthodox yogi, who follows the Indian example, consumes neither eggs nor milk.

Whole grains, often combined with fruit or yogurt, are a popular morning food. Nuts and seeds contribute the primary plant protein, and are adopted for their high content of vitamins, minerals, carbohydrate, and unsaturated fats. They are considered a "complete" food.

The natural sugar in fruits is used as a concentrated source of energy and dried fruits are stressed instead of candy. Honey, molasses, date sugar, carob, and other unprocessed sweeteners are used with discretion. Fruit and vegetable juices, vegetable broth, and herb teas play an important role in the daily diet.

Is This the Diet for You?

The "life force" component in the yoga philosophy of eating is manifested in the abundance of vitamins and minerals and general low level of calories, particularly those calories which are not coupled with other food value. Since food consumption is minimal and items rich in calories are not part of the plan, the yoga diet incidentally brings about weight loss.

Yoga foods are virtually free of saturated fat, cholesterol, and concentrated sugar, all implicated in heart ailments, diabetes, kidney disease, and many other body disorders.

Food preparation is simple and straightforward and therefore meal planning is not complicated or time-consuming.

Although some of the items on the menu are priced higher than common supermarket fare (organic foods, honey, pure peanut butter, raw nuts, etc.), these costs are more than offset by the savings of a meatless, prepared-food-free diet, so that the yoga food plan is a very economical one.

The potential hazards of chemical food additives, too, are eliminated by the yoga pattern of eating.

What Are the Possible Pitfalls?

Many people who follow a yoga diet without being acquainted with food values unknowingly plan a diet low in certain B vitamins, calcium, iron, and protein. Daily menus must include a well-rounded assortment of the foods which compose the yoga diet. It appears that the yoga plan must be approached with true awareness if it is to be effective.

Using The Tables of Food Content

THE TABLES OF FOOD CONTENT provide the eye-opener most people need to reap the beneficial effects a diet such as this one has to offer. The columns tabulating vitamins and minerals reflect those foods which are high in "life force"; they should be consulted particularly in planning meals based on plant foods which are plentiful in B vitamins, calcium, and protein.

The concentration of one nutrient in a meal does not advance the physical and mental level the yogi seeks. The tables can help you balance your food intake so that a meal is not all protein, all carbohydrate, or all fat, but contains proportions of all food elements.

Since the yoga teaching has its origins in India, many of the foods popular in this diet (tahini or sesame paste, lentils, pine nuts, millet), are foreign to the American table and palate. The tables can provide you with some information about these foods so they can be used knowledgeably.

Representative Readings

Hittleman, Richard. *Yoga Natural Foods Cookbook*. New York: Bantam Books, 1970.
Taylor, Renee. *The Hunza-Yoga Way to Health and Longer Life*. New York: Lancer Books, 1973.

4. MACROBIOTICS:
A PHILOSOPHICAL DIET

Eating with the Environment

The essence of macrobiotics is to "eat within the natural order of the universe." In contrast to our modern techniques of food cultivation and processing which make foreign foods and manufactured foods available at all times, macrobiotic teachings prescribe foods that are native to one's own region and climate. The late George Ohsawa, founder of the movement, propounded the view that we eat in order to keep our body in balance and harmony. Therefore, the foods we choose should be related to our biological needs, well-being, activity, and environment.

The macrobiotic theory is based on the belief that the food animal is an unnecessary intermediary between our bodies and the basic source of food. The animal eats our essential food nutrients for us; by seeking to ingest these elements through animal products, we risk receiving them in an altered, unbalanced form. In addition, the animal flesh contains toxic wastes and bacteria associated with its decomposition. Macrobiotics aim to eat as few animal foods as possible, and then only in the "lowest forms" such as fish, game, and eggs.

Macrobiotics is based on the supposition that a mixed, strictly vegetarian diet of grains, vegetables, beans, and nuts can supply the body with all its nutritional needs. The consumption of foods in their natural form imparts all the inherent nutrients, plus good roughage to keep intestines active, and exercise for the facial muscles through the recommended thorough chewing.

The macrobiotic philosophy also involves intricate methods of food preparation relating to the *Yin* or *Yang* of the food, the time of year, seasonings, and many other variables. The macrobiotic takes all environmental factors into consideration when preparing food.

Yin-Yang Foods

The Yin-Yang method of food selection is based on an ancient Oriental philosophy of dualism which sees opposite forces (Yin and Yang) in all things. In this scheme of balancing, all foods can be placed at varying positions along a "seesaw" with grains, particularly brown rice, which Ohsawa claims are in perfect Yin-Yang balance, at the fulcrum. A general balancing scheme, presented in *Macrobiotics: An Invitation to Health and Happiness*, by George Ohsawa, appears below. To maintain optimal nutrition, foods on one side must be balanced by foods on the opposite side, and selection of inherently balanced foods is preferable to foods at either extreme.

YIN DRUGS SUGAR OIL YEAST HONEY FRUIT WATER NUTS SEA VEGETABLES LAND VEGETABLES BEANS GRAINS SHELLFISH MISO FISH SOY SAUCE CRUDE SALT FOWL MEAT EGGS REFINED SALT YANG

In terms of mineral elements, Yin represents foods rich in potassium, while Yang foods are high in sodium, and it is the proper balance of these that creates the essential acid-base balance in the blood.

To achieve the balance, ten different dietary patterns are proposed, ranging from the lowest level, 3, which consists of 10 percent cereal, 30 percent vegetables, 10 percent soup, 30 percent animal products, 15 percent salad and fruit, and 5 percent dessert, to the highest level, 7, a diet of 100 percent grain. Liquid intake, particularly with meals, is discouraged. To follow the macrobiotic way of life, a novice is expected to start at the lowest level and progress toward level 7 until the desired state of well-being is attained.

What Are the Possible Pitfalls?

One of the most serious problems with the macrobiotic diet is that it requires careful study and understanding and should not be undertaken casually. Failure to comprehend or follow the principles of the diet can lead to serious malnutrition.

Macrobiotics involves a gradual reduction of traditional foods, not a leap into an all-grain diet as many assume. If food consumption is not considered in terms of the participant's own lifestyle, and one advances immediately to the more rigid diet, beyond the "desired state of well-being," such ailments as scurvy, anemia, protein and calcium depletion, and limited kidney function from restricted fluids are likely to result.

The possibility of dehydration is another frequent medical criticism of the macrobiotic diet. But since both grains and vegetables have a high water content, and the salt consumption of a well-controlled macrobiotic diet is quite low, the restricted water intake is not necessarily harmful. A follower of this philosophy who is not 100 percent faithful to its teachings, however, might suffer from dehydration if any deviations are not compensated for.

Among the teachings of macrobiotics is a tradition of self-healing, and complications from unattended illnesses are not uncommon.

Is This the Diet for You?

Those who gain mastery of the macrobiotic diet can greatly expand their eating horizons. They will be introduced to foods uncommon to the typical American diet; foods which are highly nutritious and offer abundant supplies of essential vitamins and minerals. These foods include sesame seeds, tahini (sesame paste), and gomasio (sesame salt), all rich sources of protein, calcium, and iron; nuts and seeds which provide protein, magnesium, calcium, and B vitamins; seaweed, an excellent source of all minerals; soy and soy products like miso (soybean paste), tamari soy sauce and tofu (soy cheese) which possess important minerals and inexpensive protein; esoteric beans and grains of high mineral and protein value. High vegetable intake furnishes all essential vitamins, and although critics of macrobiotics call this diet nutritionally deficient, careful investigation of these foods will prove this untrue.

The macrobiotic enjoys a diet that is low in saturated fat and cholesterol, yet carefully designed to include two tablespoons of unsaturated oil daily.

The macrobiotic diet is also very low in concentrated sugar, with food energy from starch provided in the vegetables and grains consumed.

Because foods are in their natural form, the macrobiotic consumes very few chemicals in his diet.

Although many of the staples are hard to obtain and therefore high priced, this diet is basically low in cost.

Using The Tables of Food Content

Yin and *Yang* do not appear in THE TABLES OF FOOD CONTENT and most other conventional forms of nutrient computation do not apply to the macrobiotic lifestyle. But for those who have trouble with the Yin-Yang idea, yet are still attuned to the balancing concept of this Oriental philosophy, the potassium and sodium values of foods will be quite useful. If you find it difficult to balance the Yin and Yang of a meal, plan your meals around a 5:1 ratio of potassium to sodium for a similar effect.

Unfortunately some of the most beneficial foods common to the macrobiotic diet like tahini, gomasio, and soba (buckwheat noodles) cannot be located in the tables. However, many of the basic ingredients are included, so that a concerned macrobiotic, or one eager to assure others of the nutritional quality of this diet, can use the tables to determine if the diet is sufficient in terms of more traditional nutrition theory.

If illness or other dietary abnormality does occur the tables will help disclose if there are any nutrients lacking in the diet that might be triggering this reaction.

Representative Readings

Abehsera, Michael. *Zen Macrobiotic Cooking*. New York:
Citadel Press, 1971.

Aihara, Cornellia. *The Chico-San Cookbook*. San Francisco:
Japan Publications Trading Co., 1972.

Farmilant, Eunice F. *Macrobiotic Cooking*. New York:
Signet, 1972.

Ohsawa, George. *The Macrobiotic Guidebook for Living*. Los
Angeles: Ohsawa Foundation, 1972.

Ohsawa, George. *Macrobiotics: An Invitation to Health and
Happiness*. San Francisco: Japan Publications Trading Co.,
1971.

Ohsawa, George. *You Are All Sanpaku*. New York: University Books, 1971.

5. THE BIRCHER-BENNER METHOD

The Raw Foods Philosophy

The Bircher-Benner diet was developed in the 1890s by
Dr. M. O. Bircher-Benner in Zurich. The philosophy behind
the Bircher-Benner diet (and related clinic) is to eat to retain
the "vital, curative, and regenerative" quality of food along
with the good taste. We should eat, according to Dr. Bircher-
Benner, "for the health of our body and our spirit." Since
nutrition has a profound effect on our health, a sound diet
must be followed to prevent illness and withstand the diseases
of aging.

It was the belief of Dr. Bircher-Benner, and it is still
maintained by the clinic and his followers today, that overprocessed, rich foods, too highly concentrated in certain nutrients while lacking other essential food elements, lead to
overstimulation of the nervous system. Excess sugar and ex-

ccss protein are a particular burden to the body, 200 grams of sugar alone raising the adrenalin in the blood as much as 30 to 120 percent. Too much protein at once floods the system and overactivates it, resulting in an increased and inefficient use of energy (calories).

Raw foods are the foundation of the Bircher-Benner diet because they retain the highest level of vitamins and minerals. Furthermore, cooking destroys food enzymes which normally begin the breakdown of foods and assume some of the work for the digestive glands; enzymes also promote the growth of beneficial bacteria. According to Bircher-Benner's theory, raw foods do not mobilize white blood cells to the intestine and are therefore left free to defend the body against disease. By beginning each meal with raw foods, the microelectric tension in the cells is increased and cell functions are thereby vitalized.

Green leafy foods are particularly important for the formation of red blood cells, improved nitrogen metabolism, better use of protein, and improved circulation, among other essential functions.

By consuming foods from healthy, preferably organic, soil you can supply your body with all the food elements it needs in the proper balance. Whole grains and uncooked fruits and vegetables satisfy you longer, allowing you to eat smaller amounts of food—a vital step in maintaining and preserving the body.

Less Food, More Nutrition

The Bircher-Benner clinic has established a diet that is based on fresh, unprocessed foods from healthy soil, and consumed largely in the raw state. As a matter of fact, at least half the food eaten on this diet should be raw and each meal *must begin* with a raw food item. Leafy greens, considered among the most tonic foods, are on the menu daily.

Cereals are eaten in the whole-grain form; enriched grains are not considered a proper substitute for them, for they can never recapture the original nutrient balance.

Seasonings are limited to herbs and sea salt, condiments

which emphasize rather than disguise the natural taste of foods. Stronger spices disguise taste and distort the appetite.

Because meat has such a high concentration of one nutrient (protein), and generally contains many toxins, antibiotics, and pesticides, the Bircher-Benner diet contains no meat, fish, or poultry. Meat also tempts the palate and as this diet is based on limited food consumption, meat eating is self-defeating.

The dairy foods preferred are of a fermented variety, that is, yogurt, sour milk, sour cream, buttermilk. Milk itself is an addition to, not a staple of, the Bircher-Benner food plan.

The Bircher-Benner diet is based on an economical intake of food. Protein is limited to 50 grams maximum daily and is best supplied by fermented milk products plus greens, grains, and nuts. Mixed vegetable protein is preferred over animal sources and if the protein is supplied by raw foods, 35 grams daily is said to be sufficient.

Fats high in essential, unsaturated fatty acids that are easily digestible are promoted. Grains, nuts, seeds, vegetable oil, olive oil, and butter are the primary sources. Foods containing unrefined oils are also high in vitamin E.

Vitamins are considered best in their most natural form, that is, within foods. One hundred grams of vitamin C, 2 milligrams of vitamin E, and high levels of vitamins A, B, D, and K are recommended daily.

Calcium is viewed as especially important for growth and as a defense against body degeneration; the amount needed depends on the total diet and the amount of phosphorous in the diet. Approximately 1 gram of calcium daily is advisable, and that in a ratio of 1:1.7, with phosphorous. (The calcium:phosphorous balance in nuts and berries.) Vitamin D is imperative for maximum calcium absorption.

Bircher-Benner calls for .3 grams of magnesium daily; 12 milligrams of iron daily for adults, and up to 15 milligrams of iron for children and pregnant women; plus high levels of all trace minerals. There must be a proper balance of potassium to sodium, with potassium intake high and sodium low. The food pattern consists of one main meal, preferably midday, and two light meals (morning and evening) daily.

Is This the Diet for You?

It should be noted here that Dr. Bircher-Benner founded this diet based on his own medical research when the science of nutrition was in its infancy. Many of his techniques, based on trial and error, later were found to hold up under new-found scientific knowledge. Many more of his ideas, while not yet proven, have certainly not been found to be incorrect or detrimental.

Despite the fact that very little was known about nutrients at the time this diet originated, it is very well endowed with all the essentials, though some may consider protein levels low.

The Bircher-Benner diet is both low in saturated fats and high in essential unsaturated fatty acids.

It is suitable for those seeking to lose weight as well as those who want to maintain their trim figures.

Although many people have the impression that they cannot digest raw foods and whole grains and nuts, *thorough* chewing of food helps minimize this problem and by gradual assimilation of these foods into the diet the Swiss clinic has alleviated many intestinal disorders. For those people whose digestive organs are unaccustomed to such bulk, raw foods can be taken initially in liquidized form. Most systems will soon adjust and regenerate so that very few people inevitably have difficulty coping with foods in their natural state.

As with other natural foods plans, those who eat according to the Bircher-Benner recommendations will be subject to very few harmful chemicals in their food intake.

What Are the Possible Pitfalls?

Anyone on a diet such as this one, limited in animal products, must pay close attention to the protein, calcium, and B vitamins in their meals to avoid deficiencies.

The only other drawback to the Bircher-Benner method of eating is the strong convictions you must hold to be able to sustain the diet outside your own home.

Using The Tables of Food Content

THE TABLES OF FOOD CONTENT have an obvious use in conjunction with the Bircher-Benner diet in that, to accomplish its ends, high levels of vitamins and minerals, with few calories and limited protein are obligatory. By consulting the tables you can determine which foods offer you this kind of sustenance. The incorporation of all the nutrients into your meals at the desired levels and the evaluation of whether you are living up to all of these requirements can be facilitated by the tables.

Representative Readings

Bircher-Benner Clinic. *Bircher-Benner Raw Food and Juices Nutrition Plan.* Los Angeles: Nash Publishing Corporation, 1972.

Bircher-Benner, Ruth. *Eating Your Way to Health.* New York: Penguin Books, 1972.

Eating American-Style

———◆———

The following food plans comply with the basic guidelines set by the United States Department of Agriculture, and the Food and Nutrition Board of the National Research Council, the agency which has been given the responsibility of setting the official recommendations for the nutrient requirements in the United States.

The information provided in this section is based on the research and interpretation of present data in the field of nutrition by these official agencies. It is believed that these dietary standards are suitable for people living in North America with its typical climatic conditions, work patterns, and available food supply. These recommendations are purported to provide practical food guidelines for American families.

Those who had their education in the United States and were taught to eat from the "four food groups" (once known as the "basic seven") will recognize some of the material in this section.

1. A BALANCED DIET
AND THE RDA

Defining Nutritional Needs

All through life our body cells, tissues, and organs undergo constant growth, breakdown, and rebuilding; food provides the materials for all these processes. If food is inadequate, the body cannot perform at optimum level. Only a diet containing high enough levels of the fifty-some-odd known nutrients needed for the system to carry out its work can promote good health. We refer to this nutritionally replete eating pattern as a "balanced diet."

Much research has been done in the field of nutrition over the last fifty years to determine what elements in food are needed by the body and how much of each is required to prevent deficiency diseases and promote good health. The Food and Nutrition Board of the National Research Council has studied the available data and the food-consumption patterns in this country and from this information has computed an officially recognized table of Recommended Daily Allowances (see page 291). This table lists the amounts of each nutrient suggested for people in various age groups and is designed "to *maintain* good nutrition in *healthy* persons in the United States" (emphasis ours). The Recommended Daily Allowance (referred to as the RDA) is supposed to "afford a margin of sufficiency above average physiological requirements to cover variations in individuals." The nutrient levels are said to provide for full growth and serve as buffers against common stress; they do not cover additional needs in times of illness or extreme stress. In planning or evaluating daily food intake, the values expressed in the RDA serve as a general reference point and offer a basis for dietary comparisons.

Additionally, the Food and Drug Administration has established a table of minimum daily requirements (MDR) which specifies the amount of certain major vitamins and minerals which are needed daily to prevent actual signs of deficiency (see page 292).

Both the MDR and the RDA underlie food selection in mapping out a balanced diet.

A Well-Rounded Diet

Five main qualifications must be met in order to achieve a balanced diet. First, the body must have energy (in the form of calories) to meet its daily needs. During times of growth, extreme activity, or underweight, additional energy is called for. Second, the body must have a complete assortment of amino acids in the form of high-quality protein to promote growth and replace the daily protein loss. Third and fourth, many minerals are needed to carry on the life processes, and vitamins are necessary to regulate metabolism and control growth and reproduction of cells. And last, in addition to the bulk or roughage provided by foodstuffs, the body needs water, the main constituent of blood and other body fluids and the regulator of mineral balance. (See the appendix *Why Eat? The Elements of Food* for a discussion of the specific nutrients needed to support good nutrition.)

Since not many people bother to calculate the exact amounts of each nutrient in the foods they consume, four basic food groups have been devised by the USDA and daily menus are planned based on these recommendations, in order to ensure a well-balanced diet. No one who has gone to public school has not heard of the "basic four":

• The Milk Group
• The Meat Group (including eggs)
• The Vegetable-Fruit Group
• The Bread-Cereal Group

Underlying individual choices from these food groups is the fact that the body needs a continual supply of food as a source of energy. Although the amount of fuel each person needs varies according to individual circumstances, the demand never ceases. Since muscular work is done preferably and most economically at the expense of carbohydrates, starch foods are viewed as an important part of a meal. While fat is a concentrated source of energy, fat alone places much strain on the digestive system and results in an 8 percent to 12 percent loss of energy value; however, when fat is combined with carbohydrate the mixture is burned with ease. Protein consumed as the sole source of energy is extremely wasteful; up to 30 percent of the energy value is lost in the body's efforts to use protein as fuel. Protein is used most economically when a small portion is mixed with carbohydrate and fat. Since protein has many more important uses in the body than as a source of energy, fat and carbohydrate should be present so that muscular work is not done at the expense of the (more costly) protein supply.

The recommendations for a balanced diet suggest a *mini-*

mum of 20 percent of the daily calories should come from carbohydrates, 10–15 percent of the daily calories should be provided by protein, and a *maximum* of 35 percent of the daily calories should be supplied by fat, with as much of it as possible coming from an unsaturated source. The remainder of calories come from additional carbohydrates and/or protein. (See page 137 to learn how to compute these percentages.) The exact number of calories (or grams) of each nutrient these figures represent depends on the individual's total energy needs and food consumption. Activity, age, and sex are all-important determinants in finding the right calorie level for your body. These factors also receive consideration in figuring your other nutrient requirements and consequently the table of Recommended Daily Allowances (page 291) is divided by both sex and age group.

In general, a varied selection from each of the food groups is thought to ensure a balanced diet.

Is This the Diet for You?

Those who enjoy a balanced diet can expect to have high energy, be mentally alert, and exhibit all the outward signs of good health, barring any organic difficulties.

A person eating a balanced diet will also have a wide variety of foods to choose from and will be able to select to suit personal tastes. All foodstuffs fall into the category of balanced dieting as long as they are taken in moderation, with an awareness of their nutritional significance.

What Are the Possible Pitfalls?

A major criticism of the balanced diet is that it requires an awareness of the nutritional significance of foods that few people have, particularly with the number of ready-made products on the market today. Since processing often depletes the nutrients in foodstuffs, those who are unaware assume they are receiving more in their meals than they are actually getting. Unless you are familiar with all ingredients (and the amount of each) in a product, calories, sugar, and fat may be (and often are) consumed unknowingly.

Another difficulty encountered in following the "basic four" recommendation results from the different concepts each person has of what constitutes "a serving." Official sources, for instance, consider one serving of meat to be 2 to 3 ounces, boneless lean; most people, however, eat much larger quantities of meat at a sitting.

In addition to the excessive quantities of meat that often result from misinterpretation of the basic four, much of this meat comes in the form of a heavy meal at the end of the day, followed by very little physical activity. This frequently causes restless sleep and strain on the digestive system.

What the term *balanced diet* really implies is adequate amounts of all the essential nutrients as revealed in the RDA. Those who rely on the basic four to fulfill their needs may find their diets are still inadequate unless they include as wide a variety of foods within each group as possible. Otherwise, for example, you may wind up selecting fruits and vegetables which are all excellent sources of vitamin C but which offer no vitamin A. Thus, in order to include the vast array of products on the market, you must have a better idea of the actual nutritional contribution they make.

Although the balanced diet may be high in essential nutrients, it often lacks fiber content. This fiber content, also known as roughage, is essential for bowel activity. The growing incidence of cancer of the colon and rectum is believed to reflect the lack of roughage in the American diet.

Even the Recommended Daily Allowances are subject to misuse and misinterpretation. People who are not in peak health may be shortchanging themselves if they rely on the RDA to satisfy their nutritional needs. And, as the values expressed in the RDA represent an estimated guess, albeit backed by scientific research, these levels, while sufficient for some, may not be for others. In addition, the RDA is not meant to set standards for the ideal diet, for the present knowledge of human needs is not sufficent to make such recommendations. The RDA is merely a *recommended allowance*, not a requirement.

Using The Tables of Food Content

THE TABLES OF FOOD CONTENT present the actual nutritional breakdown of the foods in your diet so you can choose foods and plan menus appropriate to your particular age and sex group. They can help you decide which foods within the "basic four" supplement each other best so that lack of nutrients from one food group can be made up with another.

With the information provided in these tables, foods can be compared to one another so that selection can be made knowledgeably with an eye toward relative calorie and nutrient availability.

Finally, by calculating the nutrients available in the meals you create you can see for yourself if you have indeed supplied the recommended daily allowance.

Representative Readings

Dietary Allowances Committee and Food and Nutrition Board. *Recommended Dietary Allowances*. 8th ed., rev. Washington, D.C.: National Academy of Sciences, 1974.

Fleck, Henrietta. *Introduction to Nutrition*. 2d ed. New York: Macmillan, 1971.

Present Knowledge in Nutrition. 3d ed. New York: The Nutrition Foundation, 1967.

Pye, O. F., and Taylor, Clara M. *Foundations of Nutrition*. New York: Macmillan, 1971.

Stare, Frederick J. *Eating for Good Health*. Rev. ed. New York: Cornerstone Library, 1969.

U.S. Department of Agriculture. *Food for Us All: The Yearbook of Agriculture*. Washington, D.C.: Government Printing Office, 1969.

Your Diet: Health Is in the Balance. New York: The Nutrition Foundation, 1966.

2. NUTRITION IN PREGNANCY

Your Changing Body

Although the concept of "eating for two" has been misconstrued by many a pregnant woman and offered as an excuse to overindulge in previously forbidden foods, it is certainly a fact that the pregnant woman must eat to maintain herself and provide a storehouse of elements which will support the growth of the uterus, placenta, internal membranes, and the fetus. While many complications of birth are inexplicable, it has been proven that a nutritious diet during pregnancy leads to a reduced number of miscarriages, stillbirths, premature births, a lower incidence of mortality, and even a decrease in illness in the first six months of an infant's life. Actually a woman's diet even before conception can influence the course of her pregnancy, for fertility itself can be inhibited by dietary deficiencies. Furthermore, repeated experiments have shown that previously infertile women can be helped to conceive, habitual aborters can be helped to carry to term, and women who have repeatedly produced stillborn babies can be helped to bear live children by proper diet.

Nothing can guarantee a successful birth, but a nutrient-rich diet minimizes the risks involved.

While pregnancy is most certainly a natural process, it does create additional physical and mental stress, so that a diet that was previously adequate may no longer be so. And although pregnancy may increase the body's utilization and storage of certain nutrients, they must first be made available for ingestion.

Many changes take place in a woman's body when she conceives. Hormones, primarily a product of protein and B-vitamin interaction, are called into play; consequently those nutrients needed for hormone production must be provided. The thyroid gland is particularly active so that iodine must be available. Changes occur in blood volume and circulation, and the mother's diet must contain large amounts of iron for hemoglobin production in order to forestall anemia. By the third month, when most expectant mothers begin to show, all the essential amino acids are called upon for enlargement of the mother's breasts and uterus.

One common manifestation of these initial body changes is a mild toxemia, experienced as frequent nausea, and known colloquially as "morning sickness." It is believed now that high levels of thiamine may prevent this discomfort.

Your Baby Is What You Eat

During pregnancy, a mother's diet must provide all the growth-producing substances for the newly conceived child. Development of the placenta, the source of food for the fetus, takes place during the first half of pregnancy. Nutrients stored during this time are drawn from the placenta in stages as the fetus forms.

Calcium is the basis of an infant's teeth and bones. At birth the first twenty teeth are already inside the baby's jaw and this development depends not only on calcium, but also on phosphorus, and the presence of vitamin D which makes conditions favorable for utilization of these minerals.

By the fourth month, rapid fetal growth is in progress and additional protein is needed for formation of the baby's tissues. If this protein is not available directly from the mother's diet it will be drawn from the mother's tissues, resulting in possible anemia in both mother and child. Protein is also responsible for the growth of brain cells in the fetus. A lack of protein has been demonstrated to inhibit the number of brain cells the child can develop.

It is not only the expectant mother who requires an increase in iron, but the child as well. Prenatal feeding must provide a reserve for the first three to five months of life, when the diet is low in this vital mineral.

Vitamin A is particularly important for the formation of epithelial cells and bone-building protein tissue. Vitamin-C deficiency may limit the growth potential of the child in the uterus, and levels must again be high enough to impart the large quantities of vitamin C needed by the infant at birth. Both these vitamins provide resistance to infection and thus

RECOMMENDED DAILY DIETARY ALLOWANCES DURING PREGNANCY* (Seventh edition, 1968.)

	AGE	WEIGHT	HEIGHT	CALORIES	PROTEIN	CALCIUM	PHOSPHORUS	IODINE	MAGNESIUM	IRON	VITAMIN A	VITAMIN D	VITAMIN E	VITAMIN C	NIACIN	RIBOFLAVIN	THIAMINE	VITAMIN B12	VITAMIN B6	FOLACIN	ZINC
	years	pounds	inches		grams	mg	mg	mcg	mg	mg	IU	IU	IU	mg	mg	mg	mg	mcg	mg	mg	mg
Pregnancy	19–22			2,400	76	1,200	1,200	125	450	18	6,000	400	15	60	16	1.7	1.4	4	2.5	.8	20
	22–50			2,300	76	1,200	1,200	125	450	18	6,000	400	15	60	15	1.5	1.3	4	2.5	.8	20

*Published by National Academy of Sciences, National Research Council, Food and Nutrition Board.

reduce the possibility of maternal illness which can bring about malformations of the fetus. The B vitamins are associated with protein for the formation of the infant's tissues and must be increased proportionately. Moreover, levels of B vitamins in particular, as well as all vitamins and minerals, influence the production of mother's milk for continued feeding of the child after birth.

The essential nutrients which promote a smooth pregnancy are interrelated in function. Therefore it is best to achieve proper levels of these nutrients through the diet itself, rather than in supplemented pill form. Recommended levels of nutrient intake are given in the table on page 78, and are designed to meet the needs of the second half of pregnancy. Note that all daily allowances are elevated, and vitamin D, not normally included in the recommendations for adults, is added because of its relation to calcium utilization.

Since the RDA assumes good health at the onset of pregnancy, most nutritionists would regard these as base levels. For some women, however, the recommended calorie intake may be too high, and must be evaluated in terms of weight before pregnancy. Any weight gain should be gradual, not to exceed 20 to 25 pounds.

To achieve high nutritional standards, diet recommendations include at least one quart of milk daily. Milk or some form of milk is considered the most important source of nourishment during pregnancy since it provides calcium, phosphorous, and magnesium in the ideal ratio, and when fortified is one of the few food sources of vitamin D.

To keep calories down and protein up, organ meats, fish, poultry, and cottage cheese are stressed as the focal points of meals. At least four or five eggs a week are suggested, and grains, vegetables, and fruits must all be plentiful to provide the essential vitamins and minerals.

If salt is restricted, an alternative iodine source must be sought. Iron-rich foods are a more reliable source of this mineral than supplements. However, the recommended iron allowance is not readily met on the average American diet so that most women are advised to add iron from nonfood sources. Supplements containing iron sulfate should be avoided since they destroy vitamin E. Foods which have an acidic effect in the body, like yogurt and citrus fruits, enhance iron absorption. The daily menu should also include 2 tablespoons of unsaturated oil to provide the essential fatty acids.

In addition to the nutritional value of the diet, at least 2 quarts of liquid are needed daily to eliminate the double waste build-up, and the roughage of vegetables, fruits, and whole grains is helpful for its laxative action. Yogurt and B vitamins also enhance food movement in the intestine. These foods decrease the need for artificial laxatives which are inadvisable during pregnancy since they push foods through the system too rapidly to permit maximum nutrient absorption.

What Are the Possible Pitfalls?

Many women, unwilling to pay the price of obesity, starve themselves during pregnancy, sacrificing the nutrients needed for a healthy baby. By making educated choices you can, however, limit calorie intake and still achieve adequate levels of all the necessary nutrients.

Many women enter pregnancy with depleted nutrient reserves. If they have been taking oral contraceptives, folacin and pantothenic acid levels are likely to be low, and, additionally, women experiencing morning sickness, which inhibits food retention, often do not meet the high standards this period demands, even though they may follow the RDA guidelines. To compensate for any inadequacies, increased intake of protein, vitamins, and minerals can only be helpful.

The RDA makes no mention of the effects of certain food additives and drugs on fetal development. Studies have shown that barbiturates, tranquilizers, caffeine, nitrates, artificial coloring, and certain preservatives may increase the risk of birth defects.

While a change of diet is usually required during pregnancy, it is at such times of emotional adjustment that food habits are most resistant to change. A printed diet that does not appeal to a woman's individual tastes is likely to be rejected.

After Nine Months of Good Nutrition

A well-balanced, high-quality diet during pregnancy affords the best chance for an uncomplicated birth, a healthy child with built-in resistance to early infection, and abundant supplies of milk for nursing.

Using The Tables of Food Content

The advocacy of high nutritional status during pregnancy is universal. The path you follow to this end, however, can be flexible if you have the information you need to make wise choices. Many printed diets are useless since they fail to consider individual variations in food habits. Naturally you must expect and be willing to modify your customary diet somewhat, but by selecting foods you enjoy with an awareness of the nutritional implications you can tailor your food intake to your tastes.

Use THE TABLES OF FOOD CONTENT to help you pick foods that meet and surpass the recommendations for protein, vitamins, and minerals shown on the Table of Recommended Daily Dietary Allowances During Pregnancy (page 78), and keep calories at a minimum. For added insurance you can easily count the number of grams of protein you are getting each day. Then evaluate your daily menu occasionally using the guidelines in the chapter *Learning to Evaluate Your Diet* as a double check.

Representative Readings

Council on Foods and Nutrition. *Nutrition in Pregnancy.* Chicago: The American Medical Association, 1968.
Davis, Adelle. *Let's Have Healthy Children.* New York: Signet, 1972.

Eastman, Nicholson J., and Russell, Keith P. *Expectant Motherhood*. 5th ed., rev. Boston: Little, Brown, 1970.

Lane, Carolyn, and Zapata, Pamela. *The Pregnant Cook's Book*. New York: Tower Publications, 1972.

Larson, Gena. *Fact Book on Better Food for Better Babies and Their Families*. New Canaan, Conn.: Keats Publishing, 1972.

Rodale, J. I., and *Prevention Magazine* staff. *Natural Health and Pregnancy: A Handbook for Mothers-to-Be*. New York: Pyramid Publications, 1968.

Williams, Phyllis. *Nourishing Your Unborn Child: Nutrition and Natural Foods in Pregnancy*. New York: Nash, 1974.

3. DIET FOR
THE NURSING MOTHER

Rewards of Nursing Motherhood

For an infant, no other food is equal in nutritive value to mother's milk. If a mother receives adequate nutrition in pregnancy, nursing can be easy. But as long as nursing continues, a diet high in all the essential nutrients, including calories, must be maintained to insure the quality of this life-supporting food.

Nutrients for milk production are supplied by the food the nursing mother consumes. During lactation, a woman experiences what will most probably be the period of her greatest nutritional need. The increased activity of nursing spurs the consumption of energy—as much as 1,000 additional calories may be utilized daily. These calories must come from food intake or the need for energy will deplete the woman's vital reserves. Since mother's milk must supply complete protein, carbohydrate, and *all* the child's vitamins and minerals, these nutrients must be made available by the mother's diet.

RECOMMENDED DAILY DIETARY ALLOWANCES FOR LACTATING WOMEN* (Seventh edition, 1968.)

	AGE	WEIGHT	HEIGHT	CALORIES	PROTEIN	CALCIUM	PHOSPHORUS	IODINE	MAGNESIUM	IRON	VITAMIN A	VITAMIN D	VITAMIN E	VITAMIN C	NIACIN	RIBOFLAVIN	THIAMINE	VITAMIN B12	VITAMIN B6	FOLACIN	ZINC
	years	pounds	inches		grams	mg	mg	mcg	mg	mg	IU	IU	IU	mg	mg	mg	mg	mcg	mg	mg	mg
Lactating women	18–35			2,600	66	1,200	1,200	150	450	16	7,200	400	15	80	18	1.9	1.4	4	2.5	.6	25
	35–55			2,500	66	1,200	1,200	150	450	16	7,200	400	15	80	17	1.7	1.3	4	2.5	.6	25

*Published by National Academy of Sciences, National Research Council, Food and Nutrition Board.

Good nutrition also permits the flow of milk to continue over the longest possible period.

The Superabundant Diet

The National Research Council has composed recommendations for the lactating woman as well as for the pregnant woman. Nutrient allowances remain inflated; calories, vitamin A, vitamin C, iodine, zinc, and B vitamins are boosted, while protein and folacin are somewhat lessened.

By the time a woman is ready to nurse she will have hopefully experienced nine months of previously good nutrition and these recommendations will suffice; however, unless health and reserves are believed to be excellent, even these nutrient levels can be elevated.

Foods which supply protein and B vitamins should be placed first on the food list. Include two quarts of milk (or equivalent milk nutrients) daily, plus liver and other organ meats high in iron and B vitamins; iodized salt; and ample portions of fresh fruits, vegetables, and grains to meet, and exceed, the RDA.

You Can't Fool Mother Nature

By the time a woman has given birth she is usually eager to lose her big belly. But a woman who intends to nurse cannot let vanity dictate her diet. All food elements, including calories, are essential at this time to promote good growth in the newborn infant. Many people believe that mother's milk is of high quality by nature; this is not true. Mother's milk reflects what is brought to it, and as this may be the infant's single source of nourishment, it must be of the highest quality possible.

Mother's Milk: The Perfect Food

The reward of breast-feeding on a balanced, high-quality diet is a well-nourished infant, usually free from colic and with fewer allergies than a bottle-fed baby. A breast-fed baby will have a higher resistance to infection and lower incidence of illness from inadequate sterilization of feeding equipment or improper formula preparation and storage.

Prepared formula is an artificial concoction which can include sugar, saturated fats, various amounts of vitamin fortification, and chemical additives. Its potential hazards have caused much controversy. A breast-fed child is spared these hazards.

Using The Tables of Food Content

THE TABLES OF FOOD CONTENT can be used during lactation just as they were used during pregnancy to select foods which bring fulfillment of the specifications of the RDA, based on your personal food preferences. In effect they are the alternative to the strictly defined diets offered to women by new mothers' publications or a busy physician. As during pregnancy, take the time to evaluate the menu to be certain you are satisfying both your needs and the needs of your child.

Representative Readings

Davis, Adelle. *Let's Have Healthy Children*. New York: Signet, 1972.

Rodale, J. I., and *Prevention Magazine* staff. *Natural Health and Pregnancy: A Handbook for Mothers-to-Be*. New York: Pyramid Publications, 1968.

Williams, Phyllis. *Nourishing Your Unborn Child: Nutrition and Natural Foods in Pregnancy*. New York: Nash, 1974.

4. FEEDING YOUNG CHILDREN

How Do Your Children Grow

Attitudes toward eating are fostered from the moment a child begins to take food. If you seek to promote healthy food habits in your child it is far better to start early rather than try and change them at a later stage. It is also far more pleasant to encourage good health through proper nutrition than it is to try and reverse illness and the other manifestations of a poor diet.

A baby who does not nurse must receive all its nourishment in the first few months of life from a bottled formula. At this stage of life the infant's food needs in relation to weight are the greatest. Despite its small size, a newborn's calcium requirement is about half the adult woman's, the call for iron greater than the allowance for an adult male, and its need for B vitamins as high as one-third its parents; by the first year recommended allowances for calcium and phosphorous are almost equal for a 12-pound child and a 175-pound man. This high level of nutriment must come from a relatively small quantity of food, food mild enough not to tax the newly formed digestive organs. Since mother's milk is the most suitable food for the newborn, the most nearly comparable substitute must be found. Cow's milk, the most likely replacement, contains twice as much protein and half as much sugar as human milk. While the fat content is the same, the composition of that fat differs somewhat. Cow's milk is much richer in calcium, phosphorous, and riboflavin, while mother's milk contains more niacin, vitamin A, and vitamin C. Neither offer much iron or vitamin D.

Cow's milk must accordingly be altered before it can be considered ideal for infant nutrition. For this reason most mothers obtain a prepared formula from their doctor. Many of these preparations, which dilute the milk to lower the protein concentration, add sugar, and modify the fat, have been criticized as not really answering a child's needs.

Despite the fact that mother's milk is lower in protein, this nutrient is an important growth factor and an excess has never been known to be harmful. Sugar and fat, on the other hand, can have adverse effects on a child's health. Lactose, the sugar in human milk, is not sweet like the dextrose and maltose often included in infant formulas and does not increase the sugar appetite. Lactose supports the growth of intestinal bacteria needed to synthesize vitamin D and the B vitamins (one reason mother's milk may not need to contain vitamin B). Lactose creates an acid environment in the stomach for increased absorption of vitamin C, calcium, phosphorous, and iron. Conversely, other sugars have an alkaline reaction in the body and may actually inhibit vitamin and mineral absorption.

A sound prepared formula will therefore have less sugar than mother's milk, and any added sugar should be in the form of milk sugar, or lactose only. While fat in the formula is important to provide satiety and facilitate vitamin A and D absorption, infant formulas should not contain high levels of saturated fat (for example coconut and palm oils). Slightly diluted fresh cow's milk, evaporated milk diluted with an equal quantity of water, or even yogurt, can all be used successfully as a formula base. However, you might make note that current information concerning overweight and coronary illness traces contributing dietary factors all the way back to childrearing and the high intake of fat-rich milk. Consequently, many nutritionists recommend feeding infants and growing children skim-milk products only.

When should you begin feeding an infant solid foods? The answer to this question varies depending on the current trend. At present, the general belief is that children can be started on cereals and vegetables at about six months. But some authorities feel that introducing solids too early promotes poor eating habits since tongue and throat muscles are underdeveloped and therefore a child cannot cope properly with nonliquid food. In general, if a child cannot tolerate a food, it is too early to introduce it into the diet: Rather than resorting to chemical alteration of the food to make it more digestible (as in manufactured baby food), you should wait until the child's system is more mature.

The fact remains that a young child cannot handle any significant amount of solid food and should be receiving adequate growth substances from milk and other liquids in the diet. The first foods that are administered should be high in iron and B vitamins in particular.

Most children will exhibit a willingness when they are ready to handle solid foods. At this point they can try almost any food, so long as it is a good source of nutrients, is not highly seasoned, and does not have a tough skin or small hard particles (such as nuts and seeds) which can be inhaled into the windpipe. Salt should be limited since too much sodium can damage young kidneys.

All foods should be offered after the child's nutrient requirements have been satisfied with the milk formula. Then he or she can eat as little or as much of other foods as desired without fear of improper nutrition. Healthy children will eat well and enjoy all the foods you enjoy provided they are not pushed or coaxed to a point of anxiety.

Once the toddler stage is reached a doctor's advice is usually no longer required and children's diets become freer. The ages one to three are usually characterized by slower growth than the first twelve months, so calorie needs are not particularly high. At this time, however, the strength of bones and teeth is determined by mineral deposits in them, and protein is required for muscle growth. So, despite a small food or calorie intake, protein, vitamins, and minerals must remain high.

By the time children reach the prekindergarten stage their interest in food will hopefully be a healthy one. As their activity increases their call for energy will increase. It is very difficult to determine just how many calories young children need, since growth comes in spurts and is highly variable at this time. The most reliable path to follow is to choose foods with regard to their primary ability to promote growth, minimizing fat and sugar and adjusting calories according to the individual rate of development. It is better to be generous than sparing, for too little nutriment can stunt a child's progress.

Foods Kids Like
and Foods That Like Kids

As stated earlier, in infancy and through the prekindergarten stage some form of milk is the most important food in a child's diet. In infant feeding, milk can be enriched with brewers' yeast for B vitamins, a small amount of blackstrap molasses for iron, and any vitamin supplements your doctor has recommended. For added vitamin value, vegetable cooking liquid can be used in place of plain water in the formula. A juice source of vitamin C is also suggested beginning in early childhood. Fish-liver oil can supply the recommended quota of vitamin D.

Although milk continues to provide the essential nourishment, solid foods when introduced should be of high nutritional value, with the emphasis on those low in fat and carbohydrate and high in vitamins and minerals. Avoid added salt and sugar. Whole-grain cereals add iron and B vitamins in the correct proportions. Egg yolk and pureed liver are also valuable in supplementing these nutrients. When introducing any food, start with a small amount so that the digestive system will become accustomed to it and you will be able to determine how the baby will tolerate it. Add only one new taste at a time. As long as a food is easily handled it can be offered in any amount the child demands, provided it is high in food value and not just calories. When the diet becomes more varied, milk can be served in the form of creamed soups, creamed vegetables, and lightly sweetened (preferably with molasses or honey) custards. Yogurt and cottage cheese are also excellent milk alternatives. Nonfat dry milk can add inexpensive protein and calcium enrichment to cereals, soups, and other mixed foods.

Offering a child meat during the first year is unique to the last few decades. Tolerance for fat in early childhood is low and it is better to meet protein requirements through milk and egg-rich foods since only tiny amounts of meat can be assimilated. Meat is valued more for taste exposure than nutrition at this time.

If your child is receiving skim milk rather than whole milk, try to offer other fat-rich foods such as meat, butter, or oil at the same meal. Vitamins A and D and calcium depend on fat for optimum absorption.

Even young children enjoy foods with varying textures. Alternate pureed fruits and vegetables with cottage cheese or a mild cereal like wheat germ moistened with milk to initiate the palate. Let children sample any vegetable, fruit, bean, or grain that is not highly seasoned from the family table.

When offering teething foods, consider fresh vegetable sticks (which add vitamins A and C and few calories) before high-carbohydrate crackers, cookies, and toast. If your child refuses vegetables, remember many fruits provide the same nutrients and can be offered instead.

Children Are People Too

In an attempt to enforce good nutrition many parents are overzealous in encouraging children to eat "foods that are good for them." Since in the first year children derive their primary source of nourishment from milk and do not eat large enough quantities of other items for them to be significant, ample nutrients can be obtained in a bottle if your child is not interested in eating. Pushing food on a child too soon actually deters good food habits.

Children grow at different rates and therefore must be treated as individuals. Appetites will not necessarily parallel those of other children, or even be consistent within a child. During growth sprints children will probably demand more food; at a less active stage a child cannot be expected to tolerate so much food and will probably resent coaxing.

Children tend to imitate the actions of their parents. It is unfair to expect a child to eat "the right foods" if you do not.

Everyone Reaps the Benefits

A healthy child who has been raised on a balanced diet can be expected to eat well if tensions are absent. If you have fostered good eating habits from the beginning, by the time your child reaches the prekindergarten stage, feeding should be a simple matter and will probably be much the same as the rest of the family dining. Otherwise, this can be the hardest stage.

If you can get your children to enjoy good food initially, you can expect them to grow into well-built, alert people. Although all children go through a period of negativism in the preschool years, good food habits instilled early will resurface once this stage is past.

By allowing children to experience new foods at their own pace, and introducing these foods from the general family fare, you can expect better adjustment to "real" food and bypass the expense of specially manufactured baby foods.

Using The Tables of Food Content

Most children's diets are supervised by physicians during the first year and by their parents thereafter. But often the food the doctor prescribes and you emphasize may not be accepted by your child. Rather than forcing these foods, THE TABLES OF FOOD CONTENT can help you find other possibilities which match these in nutritive value.

If you wish to increase the food value of your child's diet, the tables will inform you as to which foods to select in each area. Many parents believe their children are better nourished than they may actually be: a child may readily accept many foods, but consider how much of this food is eaten and then check its nutritive value on the tables. It takes six and a half eggs or a half pound of meat to attain the protein value of one quart of milk, and the calcium value is not even comparable. The tables can help you plan so that food variety does not supersede nutrient quantity.

If your child's appetite is small, the tables can help you select foods which offer the greatest returns and can help you avoid those items in the diet that offer little toward good growth.

If you plan to give a child supplementary vitamins you should first know how the daily menu measures up in terms of each nutrient. Only then can you augment vitamins and minerals wisely. Remember, vitamin enrichment should take into consideration all nutrients in the diet since increased levels of one may elevate the need for others. Multiple-vitamin preparations often fail to take this into account. (The interrelationship of nutrients is discussed in greater depth in *Why Eat? The Elements of Food*.)

Representative Readings

Center for Science in the Public Interest. *White Paper on Infant Feeding Practices*. Washington, D.C., 1974.

Coffin, Lewis A. *The Grandmother Conspiracy: Good Nutrition for the Growing Child*. Santa Barbara, Calif. Capra Press, 1974.

Council on Foods and Nutrition. *Infant Nutrition*. Chicago: The American Medical Association, 1959.

Davis, Adelle. *Let's Have Healthy Children*. New York: Signet, 1972.

Kaufman, Eve, and Marguilies, Jane. *The Healthy Family Cookbook*. New York: Harper & Row, 1974.

Ripault, Christine. *Children's Gastronomic*. New York: Crown, 1968.

Rodale, J. I., and *Prevention Magazine* staff. *Natural Health and Pregnancy: A Handbook for Mothers-to-Be*. New York: Pyramid Publications, 1968.

Spock, Benjamin, and Lowenberg, Miriam. *Feeding Your Baby and Child*. New York: Pocket Books, 1968.

Food for Health

—◆—

While the practice of medicine in America is essentially drug-oriented, there are many diseases which respond favorably to dietary measures and can be cured or controlled by the foods you eat. The several diets which are surveyed here are not designed as guidelines for self-healing, but follow the traditional medical counseling for a particular health problem and its accompanying symptoms. With regard to any ailment it is best to heed the advice of your physician. Most doctors, however, have little training in food and nutrition, and when treating illness through diet are likely to hand out a printed menu or express their dietary recommendations in terms of general food components, advising you to cut down on saturated fats, carbohydrates, eat a balanced diet, etc. Few doctors have the background or the time to devise a diet based on your own individual food preferences.

THE TABLES OF FOOD CONTENT *can complement your doctor's suggestions and help you translate medical prescriptions into daily menus. Although the dietary practices that are discussed here may not be related to your particular ailment, they can show you by example how to cope with any food-related treatment to avoid either unnecessary boredom or harmful misunderstanding.*

In order to use the tables effectively, ask your doctor to explain what elements of food in particular you must restrict or include in your diet to improve your condition. Then you can consult the tables for those foods which meet these specifications. At the same time you will be able to count calories where necessary and compose daily meals which not only include ample supplies of unrestricted nutrients but meals which are composed of foods you like.

It may be that your illness has resulted in a decreased ability to digest certain foods; often the case in stomach, kidney, and intestinal disorders. This does not mean that the nutrients commonly associated with these foods are any less important; indeed, your intake of all vitamins and minerals should be kept especially high to speed recovery and build up resistance. It is even possible that the very lack of certain nutrients contributed to your illness in the first place. To compound this, poor health usually decreases the efficiency of nutrient absorption, which means you must have above-average supplies to restore these protective elements to your body. When any food must be eliminated from your diet, the tables will help you find an adequate substitute so your body can receive all its essential nutriment in a form it can tolerate.

1. CONTROL OF HEART AILMENTS

The Disease of Prosperity

While the cause of atherosclerosis—the hardening, thickening, clogging, and narrowing of the arteries which bring blood to the muscle tissues of the heart and oxygen to the brain—is unknown, it is the major cause of death in people over forty in the United States and Canada.

The major factors suspected of leading to atherosclerosis include high blood pressure, high cholesterol levels in the blood, overweight, excessive eating (particularly of certain fats), too little physical activity, diabetes, excessive smoking, stress and tension, and heredity. Among these blood pressure, blood cholesterol levels, weight, and food consumption levels can all be modified by diet.

This "diet-heart theory" applies both to those who have already experienced coronary illness and to all potential victims (which includes everyone). Although dietary testing in this area is not yet complete, or conclusive, preventative and postcoronary dietary measures appear to be significant in reducing the odds against incurring a heart attack and are supported by the American Heart Association and the National Heart and Lung Institute.

The highest incidence of heart ailments occurs in wealthy countries where the average diet is high in calories, animal fats, cholesterol, and empty calories from refined and processed foods—hence the nickname "the disease of prosperity." In countries where the diet is largely vegetarian and total calorie intake and fat consumption are low, the average blood cholesterol level is 125 to 140 (milligrams of cholesterol per 100 milliliters of blood). The average cholesterol level in the American male is 230 to 240.

There are many unknowns relating to fat metabolism and, in particular, cholesterol balance. The cholesterol in the body is both made there and is a result of the cholesterol in the food we eat. It appears that those who exhibit the high cholesterol levels associated with atherosclerosis either lack the means of limiting its internal manufacture or cannot readily dispose of dietary cholesterol to maintain an optimum low level. A diet high in fat and cholesterol can only compound this problem.

It has been demonstrated that saturated fats promote cholesterol retention while polyunsaturated fats can help to lower blood cholesterol levels. Beginning as early as childhood, high fat consumption can lead to a slow, steady rise in fat deposits in the arteries. For those who are overweight, a cut in calories appears to reduce high cholesterol levels. Weight loss is also advisable since excess poundage can put additional unnecessary strain on the body and the heart, particularly when sudden weight gain occurs in adulthood.

Triglycerides (the name given to fat molecules composed of three molecules of fatty acids and one molecule of glycerol) have been the focal point of much recent research into dietary influence on atherosclerosis. Elevation of blood triglyceride levels (common in coronary patients) appears to be related not only to fat consumption, but to excessive sugar and refined starches in the diet.

Hypertension, or high blood pressure, is another contributing factor to heart ailments. Cross-cultural studies indicate that in societies where salt and overall sodium intake is low, in the range of 1.5 to 3 grams per day, incidence of hypertension is much lower than in America where average sodium intake is as high as 4 to 6 grams daily. Additionally, many sufferers of high blood pressure exhibit a diminished ability to excrete ingested sodium. Hypertension can be treated with antihypertensive drugs, but a low-salt diet may act as a prophylactic *and* help lower high blood pressure to normal levels, resulting in less dependence on drugs. An elevated potassium intake is also useful in bringing down high sodium levels.

Although less attention has been paid to the role of certain vitamins and minerals in relation to the prevention of heart ailments, studies have shown that vitamin B_6, inositol, and choline (each part of the B complex) have the ability to reduce blood cholesterol through their role in the formation of lecithin, a substance which helps disperse fat deposits in the body. Magnesium, too, is known to be important to the proper functioning of the heart, and animal experiments have shown that vitamin-E-deficient diets induce fatal heart ailments. Such preliminary findings indicate that the importance of these nutrients for protection of the heart should be more actively explored.

How to Eat for Your Heart

In order to minimize the risk of having a heart attack, or to speed recovery and prevent recurrence in those who have already endured an attack, specific dietary recommendations have been advanced. To begin with, if you are overweight, and particularly more than 20 percent above the desired weight for your height/age group (see Table of Desirable Weights, page 5), a calorie intake adjusted to achieve and maintain ideal body weight, such as one outlined in the section "Low-Calorie Dieting," is in order. It is also important to avoid large meals that demand increased blood flow for digestion.

Blood cholesterol levels should be kept down with *a diet low in total fat and low in saturated fat*. Polyunsaturated fats should be stressed, that is, used *instead of*, not along with, more highly saturated fat. While the average American diet derives 40 to 45 percent of its calories from fat, if only 25 to

30 percent of your calories come from the fat portion of your diet, blood cholesterol can be controlled. Most nutritionists agree no more than 35 percent of a day's calories should come from fat. Calories from saturated fats should represent less than 10 percent of the total fat intake, and *at least* 10 percent of the daily calories from fats should come from an unsaturated fat source. (Directions for computing the percentage of fat in the diet are given on page 139.)

The cholesterol you consume in your food should remain under 300 milligrams daily (while the average American diet contains 650 to 700 milligrams of cholesterol each day).

In terms of specific foods, a diet aimed at saving your heart involves changing the emphasis you place on certain types of food, not giving up these foods completely. Since cholesterol is found in all animal tissue, limits should be placed on rich sources: muscle meats, shellfish, egg yolks, organ meats (particularly liver, kidney, and brain), and dairy fat.

Saturated fats are generally recognized as being solid at room temperature, and include the fat in cream, butter, lard, cheese, meat, coconut oil, and chocolate. Note that much of the fat in meat is invisible, so that merely trimming external fat is only partially effective. Vegetable shortening and margarine contain both saturated and unsaturated fats. Liquid nut and vegetable oils and certain fish fats are high in polyunsaturates. When unrefined these oils also furnish vitamin E, believed to be important to the proper metabolism of unsaturated fat. The third class of fats, monounsaturates such as olive oil, do not appear to affect cholesterol levels in either direction.

In selecting foods, consideration should be given to the manner of preparation (broiling and baking are preferable to frying; cooking oil is preferable to butter). Other important considerations are calorie- and fat-rich incidentals such as sauces, spreads, and dressings; the grade and size of a meat serving, as well as the particular part of the animal used, is also relative to fat levels. This information is available in THE TABLES OF FOOD CONTENT.

Be aware of hidden fats in pastries, baked goods, casseroles, and prepared dinners, since all contribute to your daily fat intake.

In light of recent evidence, *intake of empty or refined car-*

bohydrates (those not abounding in B vitamins and minerals) should be curtailed. Prepared foods and baked goods are popular sources of empty carbohydrates, but since these foods are also loaded with fat, salt, and calories they should have been crossed off the menu long ago. Refined grains (such as white flour and white rice) and pasta also violate the natural association of B vitamins and carbohydrates.

High levels of B vitamins can and should be maintained, especially through the use of whole unrefined grains, wheat germ, and dried legumes. Since eggs, liver, brains, and kidneys are so rich in the B vitamins that participate in fatty-acid metabolism these foods should not be excluded from the diet despite their cholesterol content. Whole grains, dark leafy greens, and nuts provide the recommended magnesium.

Limit the salt in your food. Many prepared foods, such as canned and some frozen vegetables, breakfast cereals, butter, margarine, baking powders, and nitrate preservatives add sodium to the diet unsuspectedly. Meats and cheeses are high in salt. In the highly restricted salt diet these foods should be kept in control so that total sodium intake does not exceed your doctor's recommendation, which will range from 30 to 800 milligrams daily. Unless otherwise counseled, balance sodium intake with foods rich in potassium. (See the tables and *A Summary of Nutrients* in the appendix.)

Heed the Warning

If you have a heart ailment or would like to minimize the probability of one in the future, a diet such as this can possibly help your chances and cannot harm you. At the same time, the eating pattern specified for control of atherosclerosis will help keep your weight down.

With a working knowledge of the fat and cholesterol content of foods, this type of dietary scheme can be varied and does not involve entirely avoiding foods containing cholesterol or saturated fat, merely balancing intake wisely.

Unlike many therapeutic diets, these recommended changes are economical, nutritionally satisfying, practical, and still allow you to enjoy fine-tasting meals. The concerned reader may also be interested in looking at the diets discussed in the chapter *Natural, Whole, and Organic Food Diets*, as they may fit in with both doctor's instructions and personal tastes.

Don't Sacrifice Your Health to Save It

Many of the foods implicated as high in cholesterol are important sources of other essential nutrients. These foods therefore should be controlled but not eliminated from the diet, and alternate sources of their nutrients should be stressed. With a reduction of fat-rich dairy products and other foods of animal origin, care must be taken to keep protein, riboflavin, vitamin A, and calcium levels high. While some synthetic food substitutes (for example egg replacers) have their place for those on a medically advised, restricted diet, they should not be promoted for the general population since they contain chemical additives and do not, despite promotional information, have the same nutritional value.

Also, if salt intake is greatly reduced, intake of iodine may become deficient.

Using The Tables of Food Content

THE TABLES OF FOOD CONTENT have an important use in planning meals low in saturated fat and cholesterol. When you begin such a diet you should calculate your fat and cholesterol intake by recording the foods you eat in terms of total calories and fat, and then compare your daily totals with the recommendations of your doctor or those given here. The chapter *Learning to Evaluate Your Diet* will show you how to do these calculations.

When selecting food you will be able to see from the tables which items offer low fat and cholesterol, and you will be able to compare and mentally estimate the proportion of fats and calories to help make the proper choices. Since the tables list food items before cooking, be sure to add any fats you use in preparation, including sauces, dressings, etc., which alter fat and calorie content.

The sodium listings will guide you toward low-sodium foods and help you pinpoint hidden sources of sodium in your diet. The tables will also help you choose foods for their high potassium content.

Foods which contribute mostly calories and carbohydrates and no appreciable vitamins, minerals, or protein, that is, empty carbohydrates, will be apparent from the tables too.

Although choline, inositol, and vitamin B_6 are not included in the tables, they are associated with other B vitamins in food. Rich sources of thiamine, riboflavin, and niacin—the principal B vitamins—can be selected to ensure adequate amounts of the entire B vitamin complex. Note that when manufacturers add B vitamins (indicated by the word *enriched* on food labels and on the tables), only the three principal B vitamins are included. Therefore, "enriched" carbohydrates (such as enriched white flour, enriched white rice, enriched white bread, and enriched pasta) are still not comparable to their unrefined counterparts (such as whole-wheat flour, brown rice, whole-grain bread, and whole-wheat pasta).

The introductory paragraphs to each food group in the tables will help you in selecting foods that contain magnesium and vitamin E.

Representative Readings

Barnard, Christiaan. *Heart Attack: You Don't Have to Die.* New York: Delacorte Press, 1972.

Blakeslee, Alton, and Stamler, Jeremiah. *Your Heart Has Nine Lives.* Rev. ed. Englewood Cliffs, N.J.: Prentice-Hall, 1974.

Bond, Clara-Beth Y., et al. *The Low Fat, Low Cholesterol Diet.* Rev. ed. New York: Doubleday, 1971.

Keys, Ancel, and Keys, Margaret. *Eat Well and Stay Well.* Rev. ed. New York: Doubleday, 1963.

Lamb, Lawrence E. *Your Heart and How to Live with It.* New York: Signet, 1975.

2. DIABETES

The Diet You Must Deal With

When carbohydrates are digested they are broken down into simple sugars and contained in the body as *glucose*, the sugar in the blood which provides the cells with energy, and *glycogen*, the storage form of energy. In order to store blood sugar for energy, insulin, the hormone produced by the pancreas, must be present. In diabetes, where there is a lack of sufficient usable insulin, carbohydrates cannot be utilized in a normal fashion. As a result, sugar accumulates in the blood and urine rather than being converted into fuel for the body's use.

There are two major types of diabetes: one occurs in early childhood and the other generally develops around middle age. Childhood diabetes is usually treated with insulin therapy, but both forms respond favorably to, and must be accompanied by, dietary control.

In order to control this illness, the diabetic must be aware of the nutritional make-up of foods. Since the difficulty arises from a decreased tolerance for carbohydrates, some restriction must be placed on this food component in the diet.

Protein metabolism provides an easily tolerated, slowly released source of glucose for the body, so while carbohydrates are kept to a minimum, protein is elevated to maintain even levels of blood sugar and prevent insulin shock (and low blood sugar). These high levels of protein may also retard the development of future degenerative diseases associated with diabetes.

It may well be that the diabetic also has an impaired ability to utilize fats, for it now appears that atherosclerosis, or thickening of the arteries, occurs early and progresses faster in diabetics. Since the emphasis on high-protein foods in the diet often includes an excessive intake of animal fats, this food plan can, without careful attention, easily exceed the recommendation that a maximum of 35 percent of your daily calorie intake come from fat. In order to minimize the risk of heart attack, the diabetic must therefore watch consumption of fats as well as carbohydrates, and replace a large percentage of the saturated fats on the menu with unsaturated ones.

Depending on the age at onset and the severity of the illness, other nutritional factors may figure heavily in recovery. Most children suffer from underweight and undernourishment when diabetes is first discovered. Therefore their body stores of vitamins and minerals must be replenished and protein supplied for growth in the initial stages of treatment. In order to insure a diet of restoration, recommended protein intake may initially be as high as 1.5 grams of protein per pound of *desirable* body weight (which in most instances is higher than actual body weight). To reach a more substantial weight level, as many as 35 to 40 calories may be allotted per pound of desired body weight. While all vitamins and minerals should be stressed, additional thiamine, riboflavin, and niacin, the catalysts of carbohydrate metabolism, are especially important and should be from three to five times the Recommended Daily Allowances (see page 291).

Once the body supplies have been rebuilt, the diet can become somewhat less restricted and calories can revert to a more normal level, determined by individual needs and lifestyle. But since growth may be slowed down by this illness, protein intake should remain plentiful throughout childhood, perhaps as high as 1 gram per pound of body weight, or about one-third the total daily calories. As the child reaches adolescence, weight control may become more important since the diabetic is more susceptible to weight gain and diseases of the heart associated with obesity.

Insulin therapy, generally required in childhood diabetes, may be accompanied by guidelines for calorie spacing which specify the total calorie allowance to be consumed at each of the meals throughout the day.

The adult diabetic, on the other hand, is most often overweight at the onset of illness and must shed these extra pounds in order for any treatment to be effective. Often the weight loss itself will improve carbohydrate tolerance. With proper diet, most sufferers from the adult form of diabetes do not need insulin treatment. In general the diet should meet the standards of the Recommended Daily Allowances, but extra care should be taken to insure that no nutrient is lacking in order to protect an already much strained body from other possible damage. For most people, calories should be lowered. If the diabetic is overweight, food intake should be restricted to 9 to 12 calories per pound. Otherwise the general guideline of 12 to 15 calories per pound is suggested.

The adult form of diabetes should also be treated with an increased protein intake; .45 grams of protein per pound of desired body weight (1 gram per kilogram) is a realistic level.

About 40 percent of the daily calories can come from carbohydrates. For a shortcut in figuring carbohydrate value, the total number of grams of carbohydrate in your daily foods should equal no more than one-tenth of the total daily calories, for example, 200 grams of carbohydrate in a 2,000-calorie diet. Regardless of calorie intake at least 125 grams of carbohydrate should be consumed each day. B vitamins, which influence carbohydrate metabolism, should be correspondingly high.

In all forms of diabetes, carbohydrates should be evenly distributed throughout the day. Carbohydrate tolerance is usually least in the morning; in order to increase the span, breakfast can contain smaller amounts of carbohydrates, supplemented by another small meal at bedtime.

High concentrations of sugar in the blood promote growth of bacteria. To increase resistance to infection, the diabetic should include foods rich in vitamin A and vitamin C in the daily diet.

You Can Eat and Enjoy It

A well-controlled diet allows a diabetic, whether on insulin treatment or not, to lead a normal, active life. A conscientious diabetic can deter further complications and other ailments which often are associated with this condition by understanding and supervising food intake.

How Incomplete Information Works Against You

Although exchange lists and preplanned diets are widely available for diabetics to follow, if food interest cannot be sustained, dietary control will slacken and prevent adequate recovery. Since the planned diets are rather repetitive and do not take personal taste into account, food boredom among diabetics is quite frequent. While exchange lists do permit more variety they are often confusing. These problems are even more acute in the adult variety of diabetes as it often follows many years of generally poor food habits which may be difficult to change.

A lack of familiarity with food values makes it very difficult for the diabetic to plan meals with an eye toward proper nutrient balance. The physician's advice to "stay away from starches and sweets" has resulted in many bizarre diets arising from the patient's limited understanding of food composition. Despite the fact that carbohydrates must be regulated, the vitamins and minerals that are frequently associated with foods rich in carbohydrate must still be present in the diet. They are, after all, instrumental in promoting proper food metabolism and general well-being.

Using The Tables of Food Content

Without a working knowledge of food values, the diabetic cannot choose foods wisely and must either follow a highly controlled regimen (with its psychological as well as physical limitations) or suffer the consequences. Once familiarity with the nutritional value of foods is gained, however, the diabetic can plan meals to suit both bodily needs and culinary preferences.

If your doctor has told you to restrict carbohydrates in your diet, you can now determine for yourself just how many grams of carbohydrate a particular food contains. You can find low-carbohydrate foods that supply the food elements which you may be missing because of your restricted diet,

and you can make other selections rich in protective vitamins. If you wish to increase your intake of B vitamins, the
catalysts of carbohydrate metabolism, the tables can provide
food sources and natural food supplements which offer this
opportunity.

In order to avoid too many fats in the diet, consult the
tables for foods rich in polyunsaturates (linoleic acid) and
good sources of protein which do not overload you with
highly saturated fat.

In order to space your calorie and carbohydrate intake in
conjunction with insulin treatments, use the tables to plan
your meals rather than limiting yourself to a dietician's menu.
With conscientious use of the tables, you can eat foods which
please you as long as you tabulate the nutrients and stay
within the recommended limits. With only slight manipulation
you will find the diabetic menu need not be that different from
the rest of the family's fare.

Representative Readings

Bennet, Margaret. *The Peripatetic Diabetic*. New York:
Hawthorn Books, 1969.

Bowen, Angela. *The Diabetic Cookbook*. New York: Harper
& Row, 1970.

Brothers, Milton, M.D. *Diabetes, The New Approach*. New
York: Grosset and Dunlap, 1976.

Danowski, T. S. *Diabetes as a Way of Life*. Rev. ed. New
York: Coward, McCann & Geoghegan, 1974.

Dolger, Henry, and Seeman, Bernard. *How to Live with
Diabetes*. 3rd ed. New York: Norton, 1972.

Gibbons, Euell, and Gibbons, Joe. *Feast on a Diabetic Diet*.
Rev. ed. New York: Fawcett World Library, 1974.

3. HYPOGLYCEMIA

A Disease on the Rise

Hypoglycemia is the term used to describe low levels of blood sugar, a condition just the opposite of diabetes in which sugar accumulates in the bloodstream. Sugar, in the form of glucose, nourishes all the body cells and is the single source of food for the brain. Unlike other organs, the brain cannot store energy and therefore must have a constant supply of glucose. If not enough glucose is delivered to the brain you can become nervous, confused, disoriented. An undersupply of nourishment in the other cells of the body leaves you weak and tired. And, low levels of blood sugar also generate a constant feeling of hunger.

There are two distinct forms of hypoglycemia. One is "organic," caused by an impairment in the body mechanisms which control insulin and glucose regulation. The other is "functional," the result of oversecretion of insulin triggered by an excessive response to glucose in the bloodstream, nervous anxiety, and extreme muscular exertion. This "functional" form of hypoglycemia, or low blood sugar, is becoming increasingly common in America, an outgrowth of a high-carbohydrate diet and in particular a diet which provides little else in conjunction with the carbohydrate. Where the starches and sugars in our foods were formerly associated with vitamin E, B vitamins, and some amount of protein and calcium, the refining of flour, grain, and sugar and the widespread availability of processed foods which depend on these ingredients has made the American diet largely one of foods stripped of their inherent value. The typical morning meal of fruit juice, cereal, toast, jam, and coffee pours sugar into the bloodstream. This quickly absorbed carbohydrate stimulates the production of insulin, the hormone which regulates sugar levels in the blood. But without protein and fat to slow digestion this sugar is quickly passed to the cells, blood sugar levels drop, and hunger is experienced. Coffee and Danish at midmorning break repeat the stimulation of insulin production and there is again a rapid rise and fall in blood sugar. The typical sandwich-lunch only fortifies this high-carbohydrate syndrome and the ensuing afternoon hunger is satisfied at a handy food machine with some more carbohydrate in the form of candy, cookies, or pastry. Eventually the pancreas (which secretes insulin) becomes so sensitive to this constant stimulation that any food intake immediately triggers insulin secretion which culminates in the removal of glucose from the blood. From this point on it is almost impossible to maintain sufficient sugar in the bloodstream with the result that cell starvation, accompanied by constant hunger, chronic fatigue, and nervous irritability, ensues.

Those who do not indulge in a high-carbohydrate breakfast are apt to skip this meal entirely, thereby supplying no sugar or energy to their system. Thus blood sugar never has a chance to rise above the fasting level which is 80 to 120 milligrams of sugar per 100 cubic centimeters of blood. The normal level of blood sugar during the day, however, should be 140 milligrams per 100 cubic centimeters of blood.

Increasing and Controlling Blood Sugar

Since functional hypoglycemia appears to be triggered by excessive anxiety and an unbalanced diet rather than any physical impairment, control (and prevention) must come from improved food habits. A diet designed to increase sugar in the blood without overstimulating the pancreas is required. Experiments have shown that high levels of protein, along with a moderate amount of fat and carbohydrate, slows digestion and allows sugar to trickle slowly into the bloodstream for several hours. Therefore the first step in treating hypoglycemia is to begin each day with a high-protein meal, offering a minimum of 22 grams of protein. This meal should be followed by frequent, small, high-protein meals throughout the day, as many as six if need be. By introducing food into your system every few hours, blood sugar is kept from falling too low; by keeping these meals small, a sudden increase in blood sugar is prevented, thereby decreasing the chance of overproduction of insulin.

Breakfast, lunch, and dinner, plus midmeal snacks follow this high-protein, moderate-fat, moderate-carbohydrate pattern. At the end of the day, total intake of protein may be as high as 120 to 140 grams, carbohydrate should be confined to 80 to 100 grams, and enough fat should be consumed to provide sufficient calories to maintain weight and appease hunger.

In addition to this balance of protein, fat, and carbohydrate, high levels of vitamins and minerals are essential, particularly those related to carbohydrate metabolism and regulation of nervous tension. Since potassium is easily excreted during stress periods, and magnesium is vital for control of muscle tension and irritability, these two minerals must be elevated. B vitamins are also associated with tension reduction, and since they are the catalysts of food metabolism, thiamine, niacin, and riboflavin must be adequate if food is to be converted to glucose. Since your body has been deprived of proper nourishment during your period of low blood sugar, and since poor health and particularly stress decrease nutrient absorption, all other vitamins and minerals are needed in excess of the RDA which applies to "healthy" persons.

Coffee and other caffeine-rich beverages stimulate insulin production and mask fatigue. They should be avoided for they only hide the symptoms of low blood sugar while detracting from its cure.

Those foods which contain concentrated sources of carbohydrates and none of the vitamins and minerals which contribute to good health should be eliminated from the diet. All cereals, flour, and grain products, plus alcohol, ice cream, syrups, dried fruits, and sweetened fruit drinks should be omitted at first. Once the condition improves, those carbohydrate foods which are well endowed with essential nutrients can be returned to the diet. You should not reinstate processed cereals, white flour, or white sugar, which do not offer the complete range of B vitamins necessary to promote adequate food metabolism. Liberal use of meat, fish, poultry, milk and other dairy products, along with fruits, vegetables, beans, and whole grains amounting to the recommended 80 to 100 grams of carbohydrate form the staples of the hypoglycemic diet. In this manner the illness can be reversed. However, a return to meal skipping or a high-carbohydrate, low-protein diet will only instigate a relapse.

Some Necessary Precautions

People who have hypoglycemia (and this can only be verified by a blood test) are counseled to eat as many as six meals a day. This is not an excuse to overeat. Unless you balance food intake properly, you will end up with an unwanted weight gain.

The principle of a high-protein, low-carbohydrate diet does not mean *no* carbohydrate. Without carbohydrates the body cannot convert fat or protein to energy efficiently and you accumulate ketones and fatty acids in the blood rather than the desired sugar. Too few carbohydrates can be as harmful as too many.

When carbohydrates are restricted in the diet, those nutrients which are supplied along with grain foods, dried beans, fruits, and vegetables—namely thiamine, niacin, other B-complex vitamins, vitamin E, phosphorous, potassium, magnesium, trace minerals, and vitamin C—must receive special attention or they will be deficient in your diet.

Your Prospectus for the Future

If you correctly follow the recommendations of the hypoglycemic diet and maintain a high level of protein and other nutrients you will undoubtedly feel better than you have in many years past. Renewed energy, a cheerful disposition, and overall good health should accompany your increased consumption of all the essential vitamins and minerals.

Using The Tables of Food Content

There is no way to determine the ratio of protein, carbohydrate, and fat in your diet unless you are acquainted with
the composition of the foods you eat.

In order to complement these nutrients with appropriate
amounts of vitamins and minerals you must know which
foods contain them.

To avoid weight gain you must calculate your calorie intake on this new eating plan.

This can all be accomplished most easily through THE
TABLES OF FOOD CONTENT.

Representative Readings

Blevin, Margo, and Grinder, Geri. *The Low Blood Sugar
Cookbook.* New York: Doubleday, 1973.

Martin, Clement G. *Low Blood Sugar: The Hidden Menace
of Hypoglycemia.* New York: Arc Books, 1970.

Revell, Dorothy. *Hypoglycemia Control Cookery.* New York:
Berkeley, 1973.

4. GOUT

The "Rich Man's" Disease

Gout is a disease in which foods high in purines (a particular form of protein) are not properly metabolized. As a result, large quantities of uric acid build up in the blood, and
urate salt deposits form in the soft and bony tissues creating
a painful arthritic condition. People who suffer from gout
usually receive specific dietary advice from their physician,

including a list of foods to be avoided in general and during an attack. Most prominent on this list are muscle and organ meats, fish, game, meat extracts and gravies, lentils, and wine. Certain nitrogen-forming vegetables like beans, mushrooms, peas, asparagus, and spinach also may be restricted, along with oatmeal, whole-wheat cereal, coffee, tea, and cocoa. Carbohydrates, which promote uric acid excretion, are likely to be elevated in the diet, while fats, which decrease uric acid elimination, are restrained.

While you are following these guidelines, however, you must still maintain a diet adequate in protein and the vitamins and minerals you normally receive in conjunction with these now restricted foods. In order to include alternate sources of these nutrients on the menu each day, consult THE TABLES OF FOOD CONTENT for those foods approved on your antigout menu to find which ones offer nutrients in similar quantities. You will notice that grains, for instance, can replace beans and meat as a source of iron, thiamine, and niacin, while milk rounds out the B trio with riboflavin. Cheeses, eggs, and nut-grain combinations contribute high-quality protein and potassium to replace meat and the prohibited vegetables. They also offer magnesium and B_{12}. (For other foods plentiful in both these nutrients, see the introductory notes for the food groups.) Carbohydrate and fat content of foods can also be computed from the tables.

5. ALLERGIES

Food Sensitivity

Many people suffer from individual food allergies, or allergies to entire groups of food. Such sensitivity, which is usually diagnosed by a doctor, often encompasses those items which under ordinary circumstances may be the most healthful in the diet. Milk, wheat, eggs, strawberries, pork, apples, nuts, and chocolate are among the most common offenders. Although certain foods might not be handled properly by your body, you will still need those nutrients associated with these foods. If only one or two foods cause adverse reactions this presents no great problem. But when many foods or an entire family of foods must be eliminated from your diet, the practice of maintaining adequate nutrition requires closer attention.

In order to be sure your body is receiving all the elements it needs to function properly, consult THE TABLES OF FOOD CONTENT to determine what nutrients are provided in the foods you cannot eat. Then go through the remaining food categories and calculate which foods among those you can enjoy also contain these nutrients. (Someone with a milk allergy, for example, can select alternate sources of calcium, riboflavin and vitamin A outside the dairy family.) In this manner you can construct a menu which furnishes ample portions of all essential food elements. You can probably expand your food awareness as well and discover many foods you might otherwise have missed out on.

It may turn out that you cannot easily satisfy your daily requirement for a certain nutrient through other foods. Again, suppose you have a sensitivity toward milk which includes all milk products. You may plan meals rich in soybeans, high-calcium nuts, seeds, and greens to take the place of milk foods and find you still cannot always eat enough of these to meet your calcium needs. You will then be able to decide whether additional vitamin supplementation is necessary.

In most cases it will be relatively simple to revise your eating habits with the information provided in the tables.

Representative Readings

Abrams, H. Leon, and Page, Melvin E. *Your Body is Your Best Doctor*. New Canaan, Conn.: Keats Publishing, A Pivot Health Book, 1972.
Banks, Jane, and Dong, Collin H. *The Arthritic's Cookbook*. New York: Thomas Y. Crowell, 1973.

Bieler, Henry G. *Food Is Your Best Medicine.* New York: Vintage Books, 1973.

Clark, Linda. *Get Well Naturally.* New York: Arc Books, 1968.

Conrad, Manon L. *Allergy Cooking.* New York: Pyramid Publications, 1968.

Davis, Adelle. *Let's Get Well.* New York: Signet, 1968.

Jarvis, D. C. *Arthritis and Folk Medicine.* New York: Fawcett World Library, 1974.

Somekh, Emile. *Allergy and Your Child.* New York: Harper & Row, 1974.

Williams, Roger J. *Nutrition Against Disease.* New York: Pitman, 1971.

6. HOW FOOD AFFECTS
MENTAL HEALTH

It's Not All in Your Head

There is a growing core of physicians, psychotherapists, and laypeople who subscribe to the theory that what we eat affects not only physical health, but mental health as well. In a number of cases of severe depression, nervous irritability, mental fatigue, extreme confusion, irrational behavior, even hopeless schizophrenia, all seemingly without cause, an explanation has indeed been found: dietary inadequacies. This certainly is not to imply that all mental illness is nutritionally based, but that many cases treated within traditional boundaries of mental therapy will never improve without concurrent attention to dietary deficiencies.

Often some of the above symptoms accompany menstruation (at which time hormone balance changes), stress (which can alter nutrient absorption), or a restrictive weight-control regimen. It is quite possible that these conditions demand different dietary considerations.

The brain depends on sugar in the form of glucose for its energy. This glucose is transported to the brain through the bloodstream. If blood sugar is inadequate it is logical that brain functioning will be impaired. There are many reasons low blood sugar may occur. As indicated in the section "Hypoglycemia," a diet of concentrated carbohydrates releases high levels of sugar into the blood. This stimulates insulin production which controls the level of blood sugar, drawing excess glucose out of the bloodstream. A diet which repeatedly calls upon the pancreas to send out high levels of insulin eventually distorts the insulin-producing mechanism in such a way that food immediately sets off insulin flow and results in overstimulation, oversecretion, and overcompensation, so that glucose is overdrawn from the bloodstream. Proteins and fat are digested slowly so that glucose trickles rather than pours into the blood, and unless these nutrients are incorporated properly into the diet, overproduction of insulin and low blood sugar cannot be corrected, nor can any of the side effects which relate to mental functioning be controlled.

In addition to an unbalanced diet, an inadequate supply of vitamins can bring about depressed blood sugar. The B vitamins in particular are involved with glucose metabolism. A diet consisting largely of refined carbohydrates lacks B vitamins. This deficiency, possibly coupled with an abnormally high personal requirement, theorists say can trigger emotional instability. Vitamin E, once closely associated with carbohydrates in the diet, is now refined out of most of our foods. This vitamin, too, may play an important role in clearing up mental difficulties, as well as vitamin A which is interrelated with vitamin E in the body.

A variety of other nutrients have also been implicated in proper mental functioning. Magnesium, for example, is known to regulate nervous irritability. If the diet is deficient in this mineral, or the individual has an exaggerated demand for magnesium, mental aberrations are to be expected.

Individual variance in food metabolism and abnormally high requirements in some people for certain nutrients must be given attention within this theory of nutrition and mental well-being. Some of this can be determined by tests measuring sugar, food oxidation rates, and concentration of vitamins and minerals.

Feeding Your Mind

To discover any deviations in your ability to utilize food, only tests by a competent physician or laboratory can suffice. From this point, a diet responding to obvious deficiencies may be prescribed.

In most cases of low blood sugar, a diet similar to that for a hypoglycemic is in order, specifically one of moderate carbohydrate, always taken in combination with high levels of protein and moderate levels of fat. The goal is to decelerate digestion and create a slow, constant release of energy in the form of glucose into the bloodstream. Meals are spaced throughout the day, usually early morning, midmorning, midday, midafternoon, evening, and bedtime so that food is continually being metabolized for the production of energy.

To determine an acceptable level of protein, Dr. George Watson, a pioneer in this field and author of *Nutrition and Your Mind,* finds that the recommended daily allowance of 1 gram of protein for each 2.2 pounds of body weight is adequate to meet most needs. The remainder of the daily calories come from carbohydrates and fat, and this call for carbohydrates is a *must.* Ideally all foods will be chosen with consideration to their vitamin and mineral content. This nutrient balance applies to all forms of psychonutritional therapy.

Along with this treatment, the physician usually administers megadoses of vitamin supplementation including the B vitamins in conjunction with the other elements consistent with your blood analysis.

Can Psychonutritional Therapy Be Beneficial?

Many people who have received psychonutritional therapy have claimed excellent results and have been provided a model for future living. While this form of therapy is not suitable for all cases of mental illness, it is relatively harmless (certainly less risky than other forms of therapy), comparably inexpensive, and corresponds to what we already know about the ability of our diets to affect our overall health.

Unfortunately, self-diagnosis is somewhat unrealistic here. Often people take as gospel what they read, and overlook many salient points in their condition in order to fit themselves into some pattern. Megadoses of vitamins, if not coupled with a physician's care, may undermine your health.

In Nutrition and Your Mind, Dr. Watson emphasizes individual differences in rates of food metabolism; classifying people as fast, slow, and suboxidizers. He even provides a questionnaire to help readers establish their own oxidation rates. Unfortunately our body mechanisms are not so constant or cut and dried as Dr. Watson implies. Only a blood test can accurately determine your metabolic characteristics, and a diet based on supposition can be as potentially harmful as beneficial.

At this time, psychonutritional therapy is limited and not yet widely recognized as a significant form of treatment, meeting with strong resistance from the psychiatric and medical professions. Unless a trained person diagnoses your rate of food utilization and your need for megadoses of vitamins and minerals, you have no reliable way of deciding where to concentrate your efforts.

Using The Tables of Food Content

If you are under a physician's care and receiving megadoses of vitamins, THE TABLES OF FOOD CONTENT provide the most complete, accurate information for establishing your new food habits. With the tables you can obtain the recommended 1 gram of protein per 2.2 pounds body weight from the foods you prefer. You can then compute the number of calories you have received with this protein, and supply the remainder of your calorie allowance through foods providing both fats and carbohydrates. You can space your nutrients and calories evenly throughout the day so that all meals are balanced. You can then detect any overaccentuation of carbohydrates which may impede progress.

Six meals a day might lead to unwanted weight gain unless

you are aware of the energy potential in the foods you choose.

Although you are receiving high levels of all the vitamins and minerals deemed necessary in your particular case through vitamin supplementation, the foods you choose should still stress these nutrients to give rise to improved food habits for the future.

If you are subject to periods of depression, mental confusion, and other emotional deviations for which you find no psychological cause, you might want to experiment with changing your diet. Evaluate the foods you have been consuming lately in terms of their nutritional make-up (see the chapter *Learning to Evaluate Your Diet*). Does your diet differ greatly from the high-protein, moderate-carbohydrate diet recommended for optimum mental stability? Are the vitamins and minerals involved in proper mental operation lacking? If so, use the tables to find foods which may help ease the situation.

Representative Readings

Blaine, Tom R. *Mental Health Through Nutrition.* New York: Citadel Press, 1974.

Brecher, Arline; Cheraskin, E.; and Rinsdorf, W. *Psychodietetics: Food as the Key to Emotional Health.* New York: Stein & Day, 1974.

Wade, Carlson. *Emotional Health and Nutrition.* New York: Award Books, 1971.

Watson, George. *Nutrition and Your Mind: The Psychochemical Response.* New York: Harper & Row, 1972.

PART II

THE DIET SURVEY

Learning to Evaluate
Your Diet

———◆———

Are you curious about how the meals you eat regularly measure up in terms of nutrition?

Understandably, you may prefer to go on eating just the things you enjoy, but while you may consciously choose to ignore your diet, your body cannot. If, on the other hand, you wish to do something positive about the way you eat, you must first take a closer look at what you eat.

Keeping a complete and accurate account of your total food intake over a given period of time is the beginning of a diet survey, a simple way in which you can evaluate your diet in terms of the nutrients it provides and acquire an honest picture as to which of your eating habits are beneficial and which aspects of your diet could stand improvement. The diet survey, if done conscientiously, can provide you with information about yourself that most people never have, even if they have gone through extensive physical examinations. And while this dietary self-analysis may be time-consuming, it will provide you with knowledge that even the layperson can use effectively to map out the finest eating plan for dining pleasure and health.

A diet survey is the first step a trained nutritionist takes in classifying the food habits of a nation, a community, a given household, or an individual. By preparing your own you will become familiar with the contributions various foods make to your diet and the manner in which you have been using these foods to meet your needs. People who have conducted their own diet surveys are fascinated (and often surprised) by the results.

The actual survey consists of four parts. Keeping a record of your diet, of course, is first. The remaining three steps, to be discussed in detail further on, consist of grouping similar foods together and then using THE TABLES OF FOOD CONTENT

121

to convert these foods into their nutritional equivalents. Put another way, conducting a diet survey is no different from counting calories, except that you're also counting proteins, fats, cholesterol, carbohydrates, vitamins, and minerals.

A note here on the human condition may be appropriate. You must realize right from the start that keeping a record of everything you eat is fraught with anxiety. You'll probably become very self-conscious about what you eat and probably either "forget" to list certain foods or, to record their true quantities, or find yourself cutting down on what you normally eat. Strange as it may sound, this is one instance where you should resist the urge to "diet." You are trying to obtain an accurate measure of your normal *food intake—don't vary it or allow it to be influenced until your recording period is over.*

1. HOW YOUR DIET MEASURES UP

Keeping a Record of Your Food Intake: Step One

A diet survey can be kept over any length of time, but for a representative view of what you eat during a typical time span, it is best to record your diet for five to seven consecutive days, with three days the absolute minimum. In this way you allow for any deviations from your normal eating pattern and obtain a broad picture of what you consume without any intentional influence. If possible, include a weekend.

What you must do is keep *a complete list of all the foods you eat for the entire period you have chosen to evaluate.* A small notebook which you can carry with you at all times is convenient and helps remind you to include any snacks you slip in during the day. Be sure to record *everything* you eat at all meals and between meals no matter how insignificant you may feel it is. If you make it a habit to record immediately after eating you will not be deceived by the selectivity of your memory. The only thing you can leave out is water.

After each entry in your daily record estimate the size of the serving, keeping this as accurate as you can. Doing your diet survey will be much simpler if you record your food in the units used in the tables. Therefore, take a look at the tables before you begin, especially those which include foods common to your diet. You will find all foods in the tables listed by one pound of uncooked weight. Most foods are also evaluated in terms of smaller, individual portions or units, by weight where appropriate or measure when more convenient. So, for example, bread appears both as 1 pound of bread and one average slice. For accuracy, use weight whenever possible (as ½ pound of beef); or volume for liquid ingredients (as 1 cup or 8 ounces orange juice). Many packaged, prepared foods give you the weight of the contents on the wrapper. When you do not know the weight of an item, however, estimate the size of the serving in terms of cups, tablespoons, count (as for nuts), slices (as for bread, cold cuts, cheese), or segments (as for pie or cake). Some people find a small scale, a measuring cup, and measuring spoons helpful here. The introductory notes preceding each table will help clear up any questions you may have pertaining to the measurement and evaluation of food in any one particular food group.

Describe each food as carefully as you can, especially combination dishes like soups, stews, and casseroles where several different ingredients may be involved. Don't forget less obvious items such as butter on bread or vegetables, salad dressing, mayonnaise on a sandwich, sugar and cream in coffee.

Here is a sample of one day's record keeping:

THE DAILY RECORD
Day #1

Meal	Food	Measure
Breakfast	apple juice	½ cup (4 ounces)
	oatmeal, with	1 cup cooked
	honey	1 tablespoon
	wheat germ	2 tablespoons

	skim milk	¼ cup
	coffee, with	
	sugar	1 teaspoon
	whole milk	1 tablespoon
Coffee break	orange	1
Lunch	sandwich of:	
	Swiss cheese	1 slice (1 ounce)
	boiled ham	2 slices (2 ounces)
	rye bread	2 slices
	yellow mustard	2 teaspoons
	potato chips	3 ounce bag
	coffee, with	
	sugar	1 teaspoon
	whole milk	1 tablespoon
4 P.M.	milk chocolate	
	with almonds	1.1-ounce bar
Dinner	cream of mush- room soup,	
	made with milk	1 cup
	rye wafers	2
	pot roast	5 ounces cooked
	(no gravy)	chuck (choice)
	potatoes, mashed	1½ (½ pound)
	with butter	1 tablespoon
	whole milk	1 tablespoon
	canned green	
	beans	½ cup
	salad:	
	romaine lettuce	2 leaves
	tomato	½ medium
	green pepper	½ medium
	French dressing	1 tablespoon
	beer	8 ounces
	skim milk	1 cup (8 ounces)
	lemon meringue	
	pie	1 slice, ⅙ of 9″ pie

Evening	tea, with	
	honey	1 teaspoon
	oatmeal cookies	
	with raisins	2 2" cookies
Other additions	light salting of	
	foods	1 teaspoon

Dividing up the Record: Step Two

Once your five- or seven-day record is complete, you are ready to separate all the foods you've eaten into their characteristic food groups. For this purpose we divide foods into the same thirteen categories used in THE TABLES OF FOOD CONTENT, using a separate blank diet survey form* for each group, that is:

Group I. Meat, Poultry, and Fish
Group II. Eggs
Group III. Milk and Dairy Products
Group IV. Fruit and Fruit Products
Group V. Vegetables and Vegetable Products
Group VI. Flour, Cereal Grains, and Grain Products
Group VII. Legumes and Nuts
Group VIII. Fats and Oils
Group IX. Sugars and Sweets
Group X. Alcoholic and Carbonated Beverages
Group XI. Soups
Group XII. Baby Foods
Group XIII. Miscellaneous

Mark down each food consumed in the *Food* column of the appropriate Individual Nutrient Intake Chart. List the food only once and next to it the size of the serving. Each time the food reappears in your daily record, simply place this additional quantity next to the previous listing. In this

*Blank forms for these charts, known as *Individual Nutrient Intake Charts*, follow the Index and can be easily duplicated for additional diet surveys.

INDIVIDUAL NUTRIENT INTAKE CHART: Group 1. Meat, Poultry, and Fish

Food	Measure	Calories	Protein Gm	Total Fat Gm	Satu-rated Fat Gm	Lino-leic Acid Gm	Choles-terol Mg	Car-bohy-drate Gm	Cal-cium Mg	Iron Mg	Sodium Mg	Potas-sium Mg	A IU	Thi-amine Mg	Ribo-flavin Mg	Nia-cin Mg	C Mg
												Minerals		Vitamins			
Ham, boiled	2 slices																
Beef, chuck, choice pot-roasted	5 oz } 2 oz } 7 oz																
Liver, calf	⅓ lb																
Pork, loin, medium fat with bone	¾ lb																

*Linoleic acid is unsaturated fat.

manner all the whole milk, skim milk, ground beef, white bread, etc. will be arranged together. Once all the daily records have been entered you can total the quantities for each item listed under *Measure*. This is illustrated by the chart for Meat, Poultry, and Fish which appears on page 126, and is based on the completed three-day record supplied at the end of this chapter.

Where a recipe includes several ingredients, as would a beef goulash, list the ingredients in the separate groups to which they belong: the beef with Meat, Poultry, and Fish, the carrots with Vegetables and Vegetable Products, and the noodles with Flour, Cereal Grains, and Grain Products. If you are unsure where to place any food, try the food group which contains its predominant ingredients, for example chicken potpie can be considered with Meat, Poultry, and Fish. When all else fails record it under Miscellaneous.

By separating foods into these different categories you will begin to see how each particular type of food contributes to your nutrient intake and how lack of foods in a given area may lead to nutritional inadequacies. You will also get an idea of simply how much of each food you consume.

Picking up on Nutrients: Step Three

Now come the revelations, when the Individual Nutrient Intake Charts are completed and compiled. This important step will require some care and patience. Starting with the first entry on each of your Individual Nutrient Intake Charts, translate the total measure of each food into its constituent nutrients. To do this, look the food up in the corresponding table of food content. Evaluate the quantity you have consumed compared to the amount listed in the table, divide or multiply proportionately, and record the level of each nutrient your quantity of food provided. For example, if you have consumed a total of 1¾ pounds of ground beef during the survey period, multiply the nutrients attributed to one pound of ground beef on Table I, Meat and Poultry, by 1¾ (or 1.75) to compute the food value. A pocket calculator or slide rule can be very helpful here. Use the notes preceding the

INDIVIDUAL NUTRIENT INTAKE CHART: Group 1. Meat, Poultry, and Fish

Food	Measure	Calories	Protein Gm	Total Fat Gm	Saturated Fat Gm	Linoleic* Acid Gm	Cholesterol Mg	Carbohydrate Gm	Minerals				Vitamins				
									Calcium Mg	Iron Mg	Sodium Mg	Potassium Mg	A IU	Thiamine Mg	Riboflavin Mg	Niacin Mg	C Mg
Ham, boiled	2 slices	132	10.8	9.6	4	tr.	0	0	6	1.6	—	—	0	.24	.08	1.4	—
Beef, chuck, choice pot-roasted	5 oz } 7 oz 2 oz }	653	52.0	47.6	21	1	160	0	21	6.5	117	747	70	.09	.40	7.9	—
Liver, calf	1/3 lb	211	29.0	7.7			455	6.2	12	13.3	110	425	34,020	.30	4.11	17.3	54
Pork, loin, medium fat with bone	3/4 lb	799	45.8	66.8	24	6	195	0	27	7.0	195	795	0	2.23	.53	11.9	—
3-day total		1,795	137.6	131.7	49	7	810	6.2	66	28.4	422	1,967	34,090	2.86	5.12	38.5	54

*Linoleic acid is unsaturated fat.

question. They will explain, for example, how to apply the values for fat from one cut of meat to another when it is not given in the tables.

Continue in this manner until all the foods on your Individual Nutrient Intake Charts have been evaluated. Then total the amount of nutrients in each column at the bottom of each chart.

With these individual charts you can see clearly and graphically how significant each food group is to your diet, whether in terms of protein, fats, carbohydrates, vitamins, minerals, or perhaps only calories. You will know which foods play major roles in elevating the value of your diet and which ones are deficient in certain nutrients. You may be in for some big surprises.

The Final Picture: Step Four

Now it's time to add it all up. On the remaining blank diet survey form prepare the Diet Survey Chart by transferring the total value for each nutrient as revealed on the Individual Nutrient Intake Charts onto a master sheet which follows the same format. Now add up each column of nutrients and divide by the number of days you recorded.

This is what you've been waiting for—your average daily intake of each of the nutrients listed. With this Diet Survey Chart you can see at a glance what your total intake was for any given nutrient during the survey period. You will also have, for the first time, a basis for comparing your diet with any of those previously discussed in THE DIET DIGEST. Now you can decide for yourself where you might like to see some changes made; by simply referring to the nutritional contributions of the individual food groups in your Diet Survey Chart you will know where the changes might best come from.

If, for example, your diet survey appears particularly low in calcium compared with other diets and the Recommended Daily Allowance (RDA), you should go back to THE TABLES OF FOOD CONTENT to locate the most available supplies of this mineral. In looking back to your Diet Survey Chart you

DIET SURVEY CHART (Based on the Three-Day Sample Record at the end of this chapter)

Food	Measure	Calories	Protein Gm	Total Fat Gm	Satu-rated Fat Gm	Lino-* leic Acid Gm	Choles-terol Mg	Car-bohy-drate Gm	Minerals Cal-cium Mg	Iron Mg	Sodium Mg	Potas-sium Mg	Vitamins A IU	Thi-amine Mg	Ribo-flavin Mg	Nia-cin Mg	C Mg
1 Meat, Poultry, Fish		1,795	137.6	131.7	49	7	810	6.2	66	28.4	422	1,967	34,090	2.86	5.12	38.5	54
2 Eggs		176	14.0	12.4	4	1	600	1.0	58	2.4	132	140	1,280	.12	.32	.2	0
3 Milk and Dairy Products		877	63.6	30.6	18	—	100	87.8	1,689	1.7	1,196	1,798	1,200	.39	2.35	1.0	8
4 Fruit and Fruit Products		436	4.9	.8				110.0	105	2.7	11	1,523	1,170	.43	.17	.3	202
5 Vegetables and Vegetable Products		916	21.3	35.6	8	17		137.7	311	10.5	1,434	3,994	10,970	.88	.60	12.8	243
6 Flour, Cereal Grains, and Grain Products		2,483	63.2	62.7	5	5	130	428.6	426	15.0	4,204	1,399	670	1.78	.83	11.9	4
7 Legumes and Nuts		639	26.1	47.1	5	10		37.7	129	7.0	198	1,087	130	.48	.09	6.1	0
8 Fats and Oils		692	tr.	75.2	26	17		7.0	18	.3	1,066	55	1,820	.01	.01	.1	1
9 Sugars and Sweets		386	4.3	11.1				77.5	77	.9	28	169	70	.02	.14	.3	tr.
10 Alcoholic and Carbonated Beverages		421	.7	0				66.1	12	tr.	17	61	0	0	.07	1.4	0
11 Soup		309	10.2	16.5	4	5		30.9	240	1.9	1,864	556	3,330	.10	.40	2.0	1
12 Baby Foods	none																
13 Miscellaneous		13	.9	.8				1.1	60	.3	7,187	23	0	0	0	0	0
3-Day Total		9,143	346.8	424.5	119	62	1,640	991.6	3,191	71.1	17,759	12,772	54,730	7.07	10.10	74.6	513
Average Daily Nutrient Intake		3,048	115.6	141.5	40	21	550	330.5	1,064	23.7	5,920	4,257	18,240	2.36	3.37	24.9	171

*Linoleic acid is unsaturated fat.

will undoubtedly find that few foods from Group III (Milk and Dairy Products) were consumed during this time.

If too many fats were your problem you might want to review those food groups which contributed most to this factor and find substitutes that are lower in fat, but which offer the other nutrients obtained in those fat-rich foods and *which you would enjoy eating instead.*

What The Diet Survey Tells You

Do not make the mistake, as both professionals and laypeople often do, of considering a high or low rating on the diet survey as proof of your health status. It is, however, an indication of where your diet is leading you and may confirm many of your outward symptoms: for instance, too generous a supply of calories might back up a recent weight gain, and low levels of B vitamins might be the clue to an overbearing fatigue that has been plaguing you lately. Most important, your diet survey will either serve as a guideline for continuing your present style of eating or, more probably, it will persuade you to change your food habits to take advantage of what you've learned.

It should be stressed here that THE TABLES OF FOOD CONTENT and THE DIET SURVEY can provide only an estimate of the nutrients that have been made available to your body through your diet. This is not always identical to the amount that you received or assimilated. Inherent differences among food samples, and more significantly the length of storage and the method of preparation of a food, may greatly alter nutritive value. In addition, any stress, illness, or individual quirk of metabolism might also affect your utilization of these nutrients. These are factors that the tables cannot predict. You will have, however, a general picture of what you did provide to your body and if you do not seem to be responding you should investigate other factors such as cooking habits and your current health.

How to Use The Diet Survey

Once you have prepared a thorough, honest diet survey and know how your diet measures up you will be able to utilize THE DIET DIGEST effectively to alter your food patterns as you see fit.

HYPOTHETICAL DIET #1: LOW CALORIE

Let us suppose, for example, after reading and evaluating the diets in the section on weight control, you have decided to begin a low-calorie diet. In addition you wish to have a well-balanced supply of nutrients within this limited calorie framework.

From your Diet Survey Chart you will be able to judge how close you currently are to your low calorie goal. Perhaps, after comparing your chart to the RDA, you will find your protein intake far surpasses the RDA; you are consuming 2,500 calories daily (and gaining weight) and a large percentage of these calories is supplied by fats. It will be obvious then that you can forego some of the protein-and-fat-rich foods on the menu. To find them, look back to the Individual Nutrient Intake Charts you composed to track down where most of this protein and fat is coming from. You trace the source of these nutrients to meat and to dairy products. Both beef and whole milk have accounted for a large portion of calories, protein, and saturated fat. But, they also enriched your diet with B vitamins, vitamin A, and calcium. You predict that by reducing your intake of these two foods you can save calories and fat. You know you can afford to lose some of the protein they supplied, but perhaps you have come close to the RDA for the other nutrients these foods offered. Therefore, you also know that when cutting down on beef and whole milk you should find other foods with good supplies of B vitamins, vitamin A, and calcium to avoid any future deficiencies. THE TABLES OF FOOD CONTENT can help you find such foods.

You can observe from the TABLES that by eating whole grains instead of refined breads and cereals you can keep the

B-vitamin content of your diet high. Skim milk and cottage cheese present calcium and protein with little fat and calories. Fish and poultry offer "meat nutrients" with fewer calories, and by choosing broiled liver instead of pork chops (which you like equally as well) you can control your diet while still enjoying your favorite foods.

By studying your Individual Nutrient Intake Charts you will discover where many unwanted calories came from and may be surprised to find that by cutting back or substituting one food you like for another you also enjoy you will be able to diet without loss of pleasure. You may not have really wanted that extra spoonful of salad dressing but never realized before how it added up in terms of calories and (lack of) nutrients. Or, you may see how you can conserve calories by drinking tomato juice instead of orange juice with your meals. Once the facts are available to you, you can plan a meal of cottage cheese and fruit salad instead of a ham sandwich at lunchtime and know whether you can afford to treat yourself to a baked potato with dinner or a few cookies for dessert without interfering with your goal to lose weight on a balanced, low-calorie plan.

HYPOTHETICAL DIET #2: VEGETARIAN

Likewise, if you've decided to follow one of the vegetarian diets you can observe that when you eliminate all the foods from the meat category several columns of nutrients on your Diet Survey Chart are diminished. You can, if you wish, calculate just how great this loss is to your diet and intelligently choose from the other food groups (again using THE TABLES OF FOOD CONTENT) to correct deficiencies.

HYPOTHETICAL DIET #3: DIET FOR HEALTH

In selecting a menu to improve a heart condition you will know how great your intake of saturated fats, calories, sodium, etc., currently is. Once you determine which of the foods *you presently eat* contribute to this situation you can gauge how your eating habits will affect your recovery. Should you decide to eliminate certain foods from the menu you will not have to forego the essential nutrients they contain, for you will be aware of what you are losing and can thus replace it knowingly.

In effect, THE DIET SURVEY enables you to design your own menu within the framework of many established diets. Or, it gives you the tools to create a diet of your own, as *Design Your Own Diet* explains in greater detail.

The Diet Survey: Summary of Basic Instructions and Aids

Before you begin, familiarize yourself with THE TABLES OF FOOD CONTENT. By simply thumbing through and becoming acquainted with the units and seeing how those foods you are accustomed to eating are measured, you will greatly simplify later calculations.

THE DAILY RECORD

Record accurately all foods eaten over the chosen period. Since you're doing this for a limited period of time only, you'd do well to commit yourself to keeping as precise a record as possible. Having a scale, measuring cup, and measuring spoons handy will be a big help.

1. Go out of your way to measure everything you can; you might even ask the people in the sandwich shop to weigh your sandwich filling, etc.

2. If you do not have time to measure the portion of food make a note of how much space it occupied in the bowl, cup, spoon, etc. Then, at a more convenient time, you can measure how much the cup, bowl, or spoon holds to determine what you ate.

3. Try not to overlook anything, be it the butter on your bread, ketchup, salt, sugar, cooking oil, or other ingredients added during preparation, etc. Be conscious of how much you use and try to estimate its weight or volume. Over five or more days it all adds up.

4. Don't forget snacks, nibbles, sips, and so forth, especially if done with any regularity. You can easily consume a

box of bridge mix, or a bag of pretzels handful by handful, or down a whole bottle of soda in sips. It might be hard to record the handfuls or the sips but you can record the bag or bottle when emptied, or the proportion finished. Use package labels to help you determine weight or volume.

5. Describe foods with as much detail as you can to avoid confusion later on. If you add a spoonful of nuts to your ice cream make a note of it. Later when you total up the separate "spoonfuls" you may find the combined amount significant. The same goes for small amounts of salad ingredients, lettuce and tomato on sandwiches, cheese sprinkled on spaghetti, etc.

6. Your accuracy, of course, need not be 100 percent but since you will have to make some guesses and estimates and later on some compromises in doing the calculations you should try to get as precise a picture as possible.

NUTRIENT INTAKE

Enter foods on the appropriate Individual Nutrient Intake Charts and total quantities in the *Measure* column. Convert total amount of each food into nutritional equivalents (multiplying or dividing as necessary). Add up each column of nutrients.

1. Write the name of each appropriate food group at the top of the blank survey sheets (following Index). Go through your daily record, one day at a time, listing each food and the amount you consumed on the proper chart. Where you know you have repeated items such as butter, salad fixings, eggs, sugar, cooking oil, milk, leave enough room beneath the entry to insert additional quantities in the *Measure* column.

2. You will find that the more your diet includes typical American foods—packaged cereals, commercial baked goods, canned soups and vegetables, prepared meats—the easier it will be to locate foods in the tables. If you are a more adventurous eater, however, don't be discouraged. If you have recorded your meals properly you will be able to dissect them when the time comes, for, after all, all foods can be broken down into the basic staples. For homemade soups, stews, or casseroles note quantities for the predominant ingredients. Of course, if you have the recipe available you can calculate

how much you ate from the ingredients used and the size of your portion. The following recipe breakdown of baked macaroni and cheese will show you how to go about this.

Recipe Breakdown: Baked Macaroni and Cheese

Ingredients *(for 4 servings)*	*Measure*	*Individual Serving*
Enriched macaroni	8 ounces	8 ÷ 4 = 2 ounces
Cheddar cheese	2¼ cups	2¼ ÷ 4 = 9/16 cup
Eggs	2	2 ÷ 4 = ½ egg
Milk (whole)	1 cup	1 ÷ 4 = ¼ cup (or 2 ounces)
Salt	1 teaspoon	1 ÷ 4 = ¼ teaspoon
Wheat germ	2 tablespoons	2 ÷ 4 = ½ tablespoon
Butter	2 tablespoons	2 ÷ 4 = ½ tablespoon

---

3. When you cannot locate a particular food you consumed on the tables, pick the item you feel is most like it. For instance, substitute brick cheese for muenster; a combination of oats, nuts, and raisins for granola; or chocolate-coated nougat with caramel for your typical candy bar. If nutritional labeling provides the missing answers, by all means take advantage of it.

4. In inserting the values for nutrients be careful with columns, numbers, and especially decimal points. The values for different nutrients vary from the thousands to two-place decimals. A ruler can assist you in reading columns of figures. Round numbers off to the nearest whole or decimal according to how that particular nutrient appears on the tables. Round values for cholesterol to the nearest 5 and values for vitamin A to the nearest 10.

5. A mechanical aid such as an adding machine, electronic calculator, or slide rule can simplify the calculations.

DIET SURVEY CHART

Transfer the totals for each nutrient on the Individual Nutrient Intake Charts onto one Diet Survey Chart. Add each column of nutrients on this master table and divide by the number of days encompassed by the survey. You now have your average daily nutrient intake.

1. Compare the Diet Survey Chart to the figures of the RDA. This will serve as a quick gauge of accuracy; if any column is dramatically different from the recommended allowance you will have good reason to recheck your work (unless the cause is obvious). Make sure you entered all foods and nutrient values in every place they belong. Go over your mathematical calculations. If you obtain the same answer a second time you can then be sure the gap is in your diet.

Additional Uses of The Diet Survey and the Tables

In addition to supplying you with the figures for each nutrient in your diet, your diet survey can be used to compute the proportion of your calories coming from the various nutrients. If you wish to know the percentage of calories derived from the fats, carbohydrates, and protein you ate you must multiply by the number of calories each gram of these nutrients supplied. As explained in *Why Eat? The Elements of Food,* each gram of carbohydrate and each gram of protein can generate 4 calories, while each gram of fat can furnish 9 calories. So, for example, if your total daily food consumption added up to 3,048 calories, 116 grams of protein, 142 grams of fat, and 331 grams of carbohydrate you could determine the following:

116 grams protein: $116 \times 4 = 464$ calories
142 grams fat: $142 \times 9 = 1278$ calories
331 grams carbohydrate: $331 \times 4 = 1324$ calories

The total number of calories provided by the protein, fat, and carbohydrate portions of your diet should be about the same as your total calorie intake. From the above figures you can derive the *percentage* of calories coming from each of

RECIPE EVALUATION: Baked Macaroni and Cheese

Food	Measure	Calories	Protein Gm	Total Fat Gm	Saturated Fat Gm	Lino-leic Acid* Gm	Choles-terol Mg	Car-bohy-drate Gm	Calcium Mg	Iron Mg	Sodium Mg	Potassium Mg	Vitamins				
													A IU	Thiamine Mg	Ribo-flavin Mg	Niacin Mg	C Mg
Macaroni, enriched	½ lb	837	28.3	2.7				170.5	61	6.5	4	447	0	2.00	.85	13.5	0
Cheddar cheese, grated	2¼ cups	1,017	63.9	81.9	45	tr.	250	5.4	1,917	2.7	1,782	207	3,330	.09	1.17	tr.	0
Eggs	2	176	14.	12.4	4	tr.	600	1.0	58	2.4	132	140	1,280	.12	.32	.2	0
Milk, whole	1 cup	159	8.5	8.5	5	0	25	12.0	288	.1	122	351	340	.07	.41	.2	2
Salt	1 t	0	0	0	0	0	0	0	15	tr.	2,321	tr.	0	0	0	0	0
Wheat germ	2 T	55	4.2	1.6	tr.	1		7.0	6	1.2	tr.	134	10	.23	.03	1.1	
Butter	2 T	200	tr.	23.0	12	tr.	70	tr.	6	0	276	4	940				0
Total value (4 servings)		2,444	118.9	130.1	66	1	945	195.9	2,351	12.9	4,637	1,283	5,900	2.51	2.78	15.0	2
Nutrients per serving		611	29.7	32.5	16.5	tr.	240	49.0	588	3.2	1,159	321	1,470	.63	.69	3.7	tr.

*Linoleic acid is unsaturated fat.

these nutrients by dividing the number of calories they provided by the total number of calories you consumed. Thus:

464 calories protein: 464 ÷ 3084 = 15 percent protein
1278 calories fat: 1278 ÷ 3084 = 42 percent fat
1324 calories carbohydrate: 1324 ÷ 3084 = 43 percent carbohydrate

The tables can also be employed to assess the nutritional value of a recipe and the calorie, protein, fat, carbohydrate, vitamin, and mineral content per serving. This is done in the manner of the Recipe Breakdown for Baked Macaroni and Cheese on page 136.

THREE-DAY SAMPLE DAILY RECORD
Day #1

Meal	Food	Measure
Breakfast	apple juice	½ cup (4 ounces)
	oatmeal, with	1 cup cooked
	honey	1 tablespoon
	wheat germ	2 tablespoons
	skim milk	¼ cup
	coffee, with	
	sugar	1 teaspoon
	whole milk	1 tablespoon
Coffee break	orange	1
Lunch	sandwich of:	
	Swiss cheese	1 slice (1 ounce)
	boiled ham	2 slices (2 ounces)
	rye bread	2 slices
	yellow mustard	2 teaspoons
	potato chips	3 ounce bag
	coffee, with	
	sugar	1 teaspoon
	whole milk	1 tablespoon

4 P.M.	milk chocolate, with almonds	1.1 ounce bar
Dinner	cream of mush-room soup, made with milk	1 cup
	rye wafers	2
	pot roast (no gravy)	5 ounces cooked chuck (choice)
	potatoes, mashed	1½ (½ pound)
	with butter	1 tablespoon
	whole milk	1 tablespoon
	canned green beans	½ cup
	salad:	
	romaine lettuce	2 leaves
	tomato	½ medium
	green pepper	½ medium
	French dressing	1 tablespoon
	beer	8 ounces
	skim milk	1 cup (8 ounces)
	lemon meringue pie	1 slice, ⅙ of 9″ pie
Evening	tea, with honey	1 teaspoon
	oatmeal cookies with raisins	2 2″ cookies
Other additions	light salting of foods	1 teaspoon

Day #2

Meal	*Food*	*Measure*
Breakfast	orange juice	½ cup (4 ounces)
	whole-wheat toast, with	2 slices
	butter	1 tablespoon
	jam	1 tablespoon
	eggs, fried in	2
	butter	1 tablespoon

	coffee, with	
	sugar	1 teaspoon
	whole milk	1 tablespoon
Coffee break	Danish pastry	1 average
Lunch	creamed cottage	
	cheese	½ cup
	banana	1 medium
	saltine crackers	4
	peanut butter	2 tablespoons
	tea, with	
	sugar	1 teaspoon
	lemon juice	2 teaspoons
6 P.M.	whisky (90-proof)	shot glass (1½ ounces)
Dinner	tomato juice	6 ounces
	calf's liver, broiled	⅓ pound raw
	potatoes, fried with	1½ (¼ pound)
	onion, in	½
	corn oil	1 tablespoon
	canned spinach	½ cup
	hard roll, with	1 medium
	butter	1 teaspoon
	chocolate pud-	
	ding	½ cup
Evening	skim milk	1 cup (8 ounces)
	brownies with	
	nuts, from	
	frozen package	1
Other additions	light salting of	
	foods	1 teaspoon

Day #3

Meal	Food	Measure
Breakfast	orange juice	½ cup (4 ounces)
	corn flakes, with	1 cup

	wheat germ	2 tablespoons
	skim milk	½ cup
	sugar	2 teaspoons
	enriched white	
	toast, with	1 slice
	butter	1 teaspoon
	coffee, with	
	sugar	1 teaspoon
	whole milk	1 tablespoon
Lunch	vegetable soup	1 cup
	sandwich of:	
	pot roast	2 ounces cooked meat
	rye bread	2 slices
	lettuce	1 leaf
	Russian dressing	1 tablespoon
	whole milk	1 cup (8 ounces)
4 P.M.	orange soda	8 ounces
	chocolate-iced cup cakes	2
Dinner	loin pork chops, broiled	2 (¾ pound raw with bone)
	enriched rice	1 cup
	red beans, canned	½ cup
	salad, with lettuce	2 leaves
	tomato	1 medium
	cucumber, peeled	6 slices
	French dressing	1 tablespoon
	cola	8 ounces
	fruit cocktail canned in heavy syrup	½ cup
Evening	pistachio nuts, in shell	¼ pound
Other additions	light salting of food	1 teaspoon

Design Your Own Diet

---

1. YOU TOO CAN BE A DIETICIAN

What Are Your Needs?

One logical extension of THE DIET SURVEY is its application in creating your own diet. The great advantage of this approach is that with a little effort you can tailor-make a menu to fit your individual needs.

Designing your own diet consists of three phases: First you must establish your diet objectives. They may have been imposed by a physician or they may be self-imposed, in which case THE DIET DIGEST and the appendix *Why Eat? The Elements of Food* can serve as guidelines. Once you have your goals set, it is to this end that all further food planning should be directed.

Second, you must discover for yourself how you are currently meeting your food needs. THE DIET SURVEY gives you the means to do this.

Third, once you know where you are and where you want to go, you have merely to select the path you wish to take. No matter what you wish to accomplish, be it a diet that is high in vitamins and minerals, high or low in carbohydrate and protein, low in saturated fat, low in sodium, or rich or sparse in calories, your diet survey, coupled with THE TABLES OF FOOD CONTENT, can show you which foods alone and in combination help you meet these aims.

How to Choose Your Food

To begin, compose a list of foods you enjoy most and those you eat with regularity. Using the tables, assess each for its contribution to the diet based on what *you* consider an average serving. For example, you may favor: bacon, shrimp, half and half in your coffee, ice cream, fresh orange juice, canned peaches, spaghetti. If you consult the tables you will find that each serving of these foods has supplied you with the nutritional resources shown on the following table, *The Foods You Prefer.*

You now have an idea of how these items satisfy or detract from your ultimate goal. Those that support your aims should receive prime consideration when you plan your menus. Place these on a list entitled "Essential Foods." Those that limit your success in one way or another (by being too high in fat, too high in calories, devoid of any vitamins and minerals, etc.) should be placed on a separate list entitled "Indulgence Foods" and reserved for those times when all the essentials of your diet have been met.

The Reject List

Now compose another list—a "Reject" list—enumerating those foods that you will not eat due to choice, health, unavailability, or lack of sufficient funds. Consult THE TABLES OF FOOD CONTENT to determine if any food group has been excluded (or almost excluded) from your diet due to this avoidance of particular foods. You might find, for example, that with your doctor's recommendation you have eliminated the entire Group II (Eggs) from your diet; likewise, you may have drastically reduced the quantity of foods you select from Group I (Meat, Poultry, and Fish); or perhaps some childhood habit has convinced you that vegetables and you are at odds, thus eliminating most of the foods in Group V (Vegetables and Vegetable Products). If many foods from any one group appear on this reject list take the time to evaluate them in terms of the contribution they *could* make to your diet. If these foods are good sources of any nutrient you

THE FOODS YOU PREFER

Food	Measure	Calories	Protein Gm	Total Fat Gm	Saturated Fat Gm	Lino-* leic Acid Gm	Cholesterol Mg	Carbohydrate Gm	Minerals				Vitamins				
									Calcium Mg	Iron Mg	Sodium Mg	Potassium Mg	A IU	Thiamine Mg	Riboflavin Mg	Niacin Mg	C Mg
Bacon	4 slices	184	9.6	15.6	.6			1.0	4	1.0	306	70	0	.16	.05	1.6	—
Shrimp, shelled, cooked	3 oz	104	20.6	.9			140	1.7	72	1.8	159	251	—	.02	.04	3.6	—
Half and half	1 T	20	.5	1.8	1	tr.		.7	16	tr.	17	19	70	tr.	.02	tr.	tr.
Ice cream, rich	1 cup	329	3.8	23.8	13	1	65	26.7	115	tr.	49	141	980	.03	.16	.1	1
Orange juice, fresh	1 cup	111	1.7	.5				25.8	27	.5	3	495	500	.22	.06	.9	124
Peaches, canned in heavy syrup	½ cup	100	.5	.1				25.8	5	.4	3	167	550	.01	.03	.7	4
Spaghetti, enriched, cooked	1 cup	155	4.8	.6				32.2	11	1.3	1	85	0	.20	.11	1.5	0

*Linoleic acid is unsaturated fat.

wish to stress you will be aware of the limitations you have imposed on yourself by shunning them and later you can seek out alternate foods from the tables that offer comparable nutrition.

To use the aversion to vegetables as an example, you will note from the tables that a good, low-fat, low-calorie source of potassium, vitamin A, niacin, vitamin C, and some calcium has been stricken from the menu. By scanning the remaining twelve TABLES OF FOOD CONTENT, though, you will find potassium can be replaced with dried fruits, fresh apricots, bananas, peaches, plums, nuts, and dried beans. Vitamin A is alternately supplied by kidneys and liver, cheese, butter, whole-milk products, apricots, melons, mangoes, peaches, pumpkin, and yellow cornmeal. You can look to Group I (Meat, Poultry, and Fish), Group IV (Fruit and Fruit Products), as well as whole and enriched grains, nuts, and beans to elevate niacin intake. You can depend on extra fruits for vitamin C, and you can make up any calcium deficiency with soy products and a greater dependence on milk and dairy products.

In most instances you will be able to find something you enjoy to take the place of rejected foods unless you are extremely finicky or medically limited in your choice. Where there is no apparent way to satisfy your nutritional needs without one of these disliked foods your course of action will be obvious; you can learn to enjoy these foods or disguise them in preparation; you can forego the benefits you feel a better diet could offer; or, you will have the basis for adding the proper supplementary nutrients to your diet.

Menu Planning

You can now take the foods which you placed on your essential foods list and actually map out daily menus which feature them (including the approximate amount you expect to consume), along with other items which you have found in the tables that complement your dietary aspirations and palate. Naturally, the fewer your food dislikes, the more flexible your menu planning can be.

Now evaluate some of these projected menus in terms of food value just as you did in preparing your diet survey.

Compare the results to the quality of nourishment you are striving to attain. Where you fail to meet your self-imposed qualifications consult the tables to find additions (or substitutes) to the menu which will bring it up to par. Once you are on target you can decide for yourself if there is room to add any of the foods on your Indulgence list. While these indulgence foods should never be stressed, their absence could bring frustrations equally as dissatisfying as the setbacks they present to your dietary goals.

Probably no one will want to plan a set menu for every day's eating. Nor is this necessary. In fact, it is precisely what most of us are seeking to avoid by opting for our own diets rather than some prescribed plan. In the beginning, however, when you are first attempting to create your own diet, a few days of formal planned eating are helpful. After these first few days you should know pretty much by rote which foods are compatible with your new food awareness and which foods are not. When you are uncertain, consult the tables, and from time to time resurvey your diet to determine if you are indeed living up to your standards. If you are not, you know now how to remedy the situation.

Design Your Own Diet: Summary

1. Establish your dietary goals, i.e. a balanced 1,800-calorie diet; a diet containing less than 35 percent fat; a large concentration of B vitamins; a diet conforming to a milk allergy, etc.
2. Conduct a diet survey based on your present mode of eating.
3. Make a list of the foods you eat habitually, then assess their nutritional worth using THE TABLES OF FOOD CONTENT. Divide them into two groups: Essential Foods, or those which further your dietary objectives, and Indulgence Foods, or those which impede your progress.
4. Prepare a separate list of foods you "reject" and check to see if your avoidance of these foods limits your potential intake of any nutrients.
5. Construct several daily menus (including approximate serv-

ing sizes) planned around those foods you consider essential and other foods you enjoy which complement your dietary goals. Do not include at this time any foods which are strictly for pleasure (Indulgence Foods).

6. Analyze the menus you have mapped out, as you would in a diet survey, and compare the results to your goals.

7. You can now see what adjustments are needed to conform to your objectives; if there is still room for them, Indulgence Foods can be worked into the menu.

By actually writing out menus and taking the trouble to evaluate them you will gain enough familiarity with foods and their value to continue your own diet without formal guidelines. Whenever you are in doubt you can turn to the tables for help, and when you feel yourself slipping a diet survey will set you back on the right track.

A Homemade Diet (Sample)

Our friend Fred is going to design his own diet. He is in his early thirties, weighs 170 pounds, is 5 feet 10 inches tall and appears to be in good health. With his new awareness of food and nutrition he has decided to initiate a diet which is low in cholesterol and overall fat, and according to the recommendations of leading heart specialists, low in saturated fat in particular. His aim is to put as little stress as possible on his heart and he wishes to take 10 pounds off his present weight, which has been rising slowly, but steadily, for the past few years. In addition, while Fred is not ready to give up prepared foods outright, he would like to limit his intake of food additives and has sworn off hot dogs, bacon, processed meats in general, white bread, soda, and imitation fruit drinks; he is not quite convinced that he wants to give up all sugar, chocolate, and some other less nutritious snack foods just yet. He does hope that his diet will be well balanced and at least meet the Recommended Daily Allowances for all vitamins and minerals as presented in the table on page 291.

You have already seen the results of Fred's diet survey in the chapter *Learning to Evaluate Your Diet*. His current average daily nutrient intake, as the survey revealed, looks like this:

FRED'S ORIGINAL DIET SURVEY CHART

Food	Measure	Calories	Protein Gm	Total Fat Gm	Satu-rated Fat Gm	Lino-leic* Acid Gm	Choles-terol Mg	Carbo-hydrate Gm	Minerals				Vitamins				
									Cal-cium Mg	Iron Mg	Sodium Mg	Potas-sium Mg	A IU	Thi-amine Mg	Ribo-flavin Mg	Nia-cin Mg	C Mg
1 Meat, Poultry, Fish		1,795	137.6	131.7	49	7	810	6.2	66	28.4	422	1,967	34,090	2.86	5.12	38.5	54
2 Eggs		176	14.0	12.4	4	1	600	1.0	58	2.4	132	140	1,280	.12	.32	.2	0
3 Milk and Dairy Products		877	63.6	30.6	18	—	100	87.8	1,689	1.7	1,196	1,798	1,200	.39	2.35	1.0	8
4 Fruit and Fruit Products		436	4.9	.8				110.0	105	2.7	11	1,523	1,170	.43	.17	.3	202
5 Vegetables and Vegetable Products		916	21.3	35.6	8	17		137.7	311	10.5	1,434	3,994	10,970	.88	.60	12.8	243
6 Flour, Cereal Grains, and Grain Products		2,483	63.2	62.7	5	5		428.6	426	15.0	4,204	1,399	670	1.78	.83	11.9	4
7 Legumes and Nuts		639	26.1	47.1	5	10		37.7	129	7.0	198	1,087	130	.48	.09	6.1	0
8 Fats and Oils		692	tr.	75.2	26	17		7.0	18	.3	1,066	55	1,820	.01	.01	.1	1
9 Sugars and Sweets		386	4.3	11.1				77.5	77	.9	28	169	70	.02	.14	.3	tr.
10 Alcoholic and Carbonated Beverages		421	.7	0				66.1	60	.3	7,187	23	0	0	.07	1.4	0
11 Soup	none																
12 Baby Foods		309	10.2	16.5	4	5	130	30.9	240	1.9	1,864	556	3,330	.10	.40	2.0	1
13 Miscellaneous		13	.9	.8				1.1	12	tr.	17	61	0	0	0	0	0
3-Day Total		9,143	346.8	424.5	119	62	1,640	991.6	3,191	71.1	17,759	12,772	54,730	7.07	10.10	74.6	513
Average Daily Nutrient Intake		3,048	115.6	141.5	40	21	550	330.5	1,064	23.7	5,920	4,257	18,240	2.36	3.37	24.9	171

*Linoleic acid is unsaturated fat.

Fred is a moderately active person, and, as he learned in the section on weight control, if he were to allot 15 calories per pound of body weight daily, 2,550 calories would be adequate to keep his 170 pounds in balance. If we look at his present calorie average, 3,048 calories, it is apparent why his weight has been climbing. To lose those extra 10 pounds in a reasonable amount of time (about two and a half months) he will impose an upper limit on himself of 2,050 calories (adding up to a 500-calorie deficit daily and 35,000 calories over seventy days).

On all counts Fred's present diet exceeds the RDA for his sex and age group. In achieving this high level of nutrients not only has he gone overboard with calories, but his total fat intake accounts for 42 percent of them, higher than the upper limit of 35 percent set by nutrition authorities and certainly excessive for a man who wants to minimize the risk of a coronary. Fred's sodium and cholesterol intakes reflect the national trend which is believed to be higher than the ideal. Fred hopes that his new diet will reduce his cholesterol intake to under 300 milligrams, as recommended by the American Heart Association, and his sodium consumption to 4 milligrams, the lower level of the national average.

Luckily Fred does not have too many specific food demands. He is particularly fond of canned tuna, salmon, shellfish, enjoys a thick juicy steak now and then, and includes peanut butter as a favorite between-meal filler. He adores chocolate and is reluctant to give up the teaspoon of sugar and tablespoon of whole milk that he takes in each of his two daily cups of coffee. His list of preferred foods appears on the next page.

Of these foods the tuna and salmon easily fit in with his food goals. But, as the tables reveal, the other seafoods (shrimp, crab, lobster, and similar shellfish), while low in saturated fat and calories, are a considerable source of cholesterol so that they need some regulation in his diet. As for steak, its high saturated fat and cholesterol values place it in the category of indulgence foods. Peanut butter in limited amounts does not violate any of Fred's dietary demands and will offer a good source of B vitamins when steak and similar red meats are relegated to a lower priority position on the menu. Chocolate, high in both calories and fat, will also have to settle for placement on the indulgence foods list, and al-

FRED'S PREFERRED FOODS

Food	Measure	Calories	Protein Gm	Total Fat Gm	Satu-rated Fat Gm	Lino-leic* Acid Gm	Choles-terol Mg	Carbo-hydrate Gm	Minerals				Vitamins				
									Cal-cium Mg	Iron Mg	Sodium Mg	Potas-sium Mg	A IU	Thi-amine Mg	Ribo-flavin Mg	Nia-cin Mg	C Mg
Tuna, canned in oil, drained	3 oz	169	24.7	7.0	2	tr		0	7	1.6		—	70	.04	.10	10.2	—
Salmon, pink, canned	3½ oz	141	20.5	5.9				0	196	.8	387	361	70	.03	.18	8.0	—
Seafood, i.e., shrimp, shelled, cooked	3 oz	104	20.6	.9			140	1.7	72	1.8	159	251	—	.02	.03	3.6	—
Beef, sirloin, choice, broiled	6 oz	700	38.0	59.4	26	1	135	0	18	5.0	100	640	100	.10	.30	7.8	—
Peanut butter	1 T	93	4.4	7.9	1	2		2.7	10	.3	97	107	—	.02	.02	2.5	0
Milk chocolate	1 oz	147	2.2	9.2	6	tr.		16.1	65	.3	27	109	80	.02	.10	.1	tr.
Sugar	2 t	28	0	0				7.3	0	tr.	tr.	tr.	—	0	0	tr.	tr.
Milk, whole	2 T	20	1	1	1	tr.	5	1.5	36	tr.	15	44	40	.01	.05	tr.	tr.

*Linoleic acid is unsaturated fat.

though the sugar and whole milk belong on this list as well, with Fred's insistence they appear in the essential foods category. Thus, when further analyzed, Fred's preferred foods can be grouped as:

Essential Foods—canned tuna
canned salmon
peanut butter
sugar and whole milk for coffee

Indulgence Foods—shellfish
steak
chocolate

Along with processed meats, white bread, soda, and imitation fruit drinks which additive-conscious Fred eliminates from his menus, his personal dislikes add cabbage, brussel sprouts, beets, and margarine to his reject list. As the tables indicate, cabbage and brussel sprouts are an excellent source of vitamin C and all three vegetables are rich in potassium, however, there are many other foods Fred enjoys which provide these nutrients. Margarine, while lower in cholesterol and saturated fats than butter, can be completely bypassed by using smaller amounts of butter supplemented with unsaturated nut and vegetable oils.

Fred is now ready to plan his menu. To do this he keeps THE TABLES OF FOOD CONTENT by his side, carefully reviewing each of the foods he may want to include to see how it fares in terms of calories, total fat, saturated fat, cholesterol, and vitamins and minerals. He finds that certain foods like eggs, whole-milk products (including cheese), and red and organ meats limit his progress by being high in calories, fat, or cholesterol, so that while he may not eliminate these otherwise nutritious foods, neither will he stress them. He does see, however, that in restricting these items he also reduces his protein, vitamin A, B vitamins, iron, and calcium potential—so he will seek out rich sources of these in other foods as he makes up his menu.

Fish and chicken he finds fit comfortably into his dietary scheme as they offer excellent protein plus B vitamins. Whole grains will add to his B-vitamin intake without adding unwanted fats. Green leafy vegetables are shown to be a potent

low-calorie source for vitamin A, iron, and calcium. Cottage
cheese and skim milk also offer calcium and low-fat protein.
Fred will feature all these foods on his menu.

Since most canned vegetables have added salt, by switching
from canned to fresh and frozen vegetables and easing up on
the salt shaker in general, Fred can reduce his sodium consumption as desired.

If he has any calorie allowance after his nutritional needs
have been satisfied, Fred hopes to add some sweets to his
meals. His first love, chocolate, will be saved for low-fat
days. From the tables he observes that angel food cake and
cookies offer sweet treats that conserve fats. And, to satisfy
his "snack tooth" he will look to fresh fruits, dried fruits
(which offer iron, potassium, and vitamin enrichment), nuts
(rich in protein, magnesium, potassium, and B vitamins), and
milk-based puddings so that he will at least receive something
in return for these indulgences.

With all these findings fresh in his mind Fred designed the
following three-day menu. This menu is simply a modification
of the Three-Day Sample Menu used as the basis for the diet
survey presented in *Learning to Evaluate Your Diet*.

FRED'S PROPOSED THREE-DAY MENU

Day #1

Meal	*Food*	*Measure*
Breakfast	apple juice	½ cup (4 ounces)
	oatmeal, with	1 cup cooked
	honey	1 tablespoon
	wheat germ	2 tablespoons
	skim milk	¼ cup
	coffee, with	
	sugar	1 teaspoon
	whole milk	1 tablespoon
Coffee break	orange	1
Lunch	sandwich of:	
	Swiss cheese	2 slices (2 ounces)
	whole-wheat bread	2 slices

	tomato	2 slices (⅓ tomato)
	lettuce	2 leaves
	mustard	2 teaspoons
	sunflower seeds	½ cup
	coffee, with	
	sugar	1 teaspoon
	whole milk	1 tablespoon
Dinner	minestrone	1 cup
	rye wafers	2
	flounder, broiled	6 ounces raw
	with corn oil	1 tablespoon
	baked potato,	1 (⅓ pound)
	with skim-milk	
	yogurt	2 tablespoons
	fresh green beans	¼ pound
	salad, with	
	lettuce	2 leaves
	tomato	½ medium
	green pepper	½ medium
	lemon juice	½ tablespoon
	corn oil	1 tablespoon
	angel food cake	1/12 cake
	skim milk	1 cup (8 ounces)
Other additions	salting of food	½ teaspoon

Day #2

Breakfast	orange juice	½ cup (4 ounces)
	whole-wheat	
	toast, with	1 slice
	honey	1 teaspoon
	peanut butter	1 tablespoon
	boiled egg	1
	coffee, with	
	sugar	1 teaspoon
	whole milk	1 tablespoon
Coffee break	bran muffin	1

Lunch	uncreamed	
	cottage cheese	½ cup
	banana	1 medium
	peach	1 small
	pitted dates	¼ cup
	pumpkin seeds	2 tablespoons
	whole-wheat	
	crackers	4
	tea, with	
	sugar	1 teaspoon
	lemon	2 teaspoons
Dinner	tomato juice	6 ounces
	veal (boneless	6 ounces raw
	round), sauted	
	with fresh	
	mushrooms	1 cup
	corn oil	2 tablespoons
	lemon	½
	fresh spinach,	¼ pound (½ cup
	with Parmesan	cooked)
	cheese	1 tablespoon
	carrot	1
	celery	2 stalks
	spaghetti,	1 cup cooked
	enriched	
	ice milk	½ cup
Evening	skim milk	1 cup (8 ounces)
	graham crackers	
	(sugar-honey)	2
Other additions	salting of food	½ teaspoon

Day #3

Breakfast	orange juice	½ cup (4 ounces)
	corn flakes, with	1 cup
	wheat germ	2 tablespoons
	skim milk	½ cup
	canned	
	peaches,	
	water pack	¼ cup

	coffee, with	
	sugar	1 teaspoon
	whole milk	1 tablespoon
Lunch	vegetable soup	1 cup
	sandwich of:	
	tuna, in oil	3 ounces meat
	rye bread	2 slices
	mayonnaise	1 tablespoon
	tomato	½
	lettuce	1 leaf
	coffee, with	
	sugar	1 teaspoon
	whole milk	1 tablespoon
Afternoon	skim milk	½ cup (4 ounces)
	vanilla wafers	2
Dinner	chicken breast, baked	1 whole (9½ ounces raw)
	brown rice	1 cup
	red beans, canned	½ cup
	salad, with	
	lettuce	2 leaves
	tomato	1 medium
	cucumber, peeled	6 slices
	Russian dressing	1 tablespoon
	apple juice	1 cup (8 ounces)
	pear	1 medium
Evening	pistachio nuts, in shell	¼ pound
Other additions	salting of food	½ teaspoon

A diet survey based on his new three-day meal plan gave Fred a positive outlook for success. His projected Diet Survey Chart appears on page 158. All nutrients meet and surpass the Recommended Daily Allowance for Fred's age group and his calorie cutback should be sufficient to sustain the desired loss. The fat portion of Fred's diet now accounts for 34 percent of his total calories with twice as much unsaturated fat (linoleic acid) as saturated fat. As the Diet Survey Chart reflects, Group VII (Legumes and Nuts), and Group VIII (Fats and Oils) were the principal contributants of this fat, while most of his saturated fats came from Group III (Milk and Dairy Products). If Fred wishes to further reduce his fat consumption he can consider these alternatives:

1. Eliminating his snack of pistachio nuts. The tables show this will also reduce his intake of iron, but as his diet survey reflects iron well above the RDA this is not crucial.

2. Reducing his snack of sunflower seeds, but this is less advisable since sunflower seeds provide a valuable source of B vitamins and unsaturated fat.

3. Using less oil in food preparation.

4. Cutting down on the size of his servings of meat, poultry and cheese and switching from oil- to water-packed tuna. In this manner he will be able to reduce the quantity of saturated fats in his diet most effectively. While smaller portions would mean the simultaneous loss of some protein this will not be significant since Fred's supply of protein far surpasses his needs and the additional calories coming from this protein are used only as energy, or fuel. He must, however, consider how this will affect his iron, calcium, and particularly his B-vitamin levels. This potential loss could be made up with a vitamin-B-rich supplement of wheat germ or brewers' yeast.

When Fred has reached his desired weight of 160 pounds he can add about 400 calories to the daily menu and on 2,400 calories daily (15 calories per pound of body weight at 160 pounds) he should be able to afford a nice juicy steak and a chocolate bar now and then without too much concern.

FRED'S PROJECTED DIET SURVEY CHART

Food	Measure	Calories	Protein Gm	Total Fat Gm	Saturated Fat Gm	Lino-* leic Acid Gm	Cholesterol Mg	Carbohydrate Gm	Calcium Mg	Iron Mg	Sodium Mg	Potassium Mg	A IU	Thiamine Mg	Riboflavin Mg	Niacin Mg	C Mg
1 Meat, Poultry, and Fish		816	130.5	28.9	7	tr.	150	0	69	10.5	287	1,111	230	.48	.97	40.9	0
2 Eggs		88	7.0	6.2	2	tr.	300	.5	29	1.2	66	70	640	.06	.16	.1	0
3 Milk and Dairy Products		766	69.7	24.5	12	tr.	85	64.2	1,862	1.3	1,239	1,574	1,000	.36	2.29	.8	7
4 Fruit and Fruit Products		836	9.0	1.9				214.6	189	7.5	21	2,667	2,640	.60	.39	4.9	253
5 Vegetables and Vegetable Products		331	17.7	2.1				70.2	325	9.2	208	3,372	18,180	.78	1.07	10.5	270
6 Flour, Cereal Grains, and Grain Products		1,386	47.1	18.3	2	2		270.7	282	11.5	2,490	1,265	140	1.54	.61	11.8	tr.
7 Legumes and Nuts		989	42.4	76.4	9	30		49.8	205	13.0	120	1,581	170	1.75	.25	7.9	0
8 Fats and Oils		665	tr.	74.0	7	38		1	6	.2	280	27	140	.01	.02	.1	1
9 Sugars and Sweets		169	0	0	0			44.7	1	.1	1	15	0	tr.	.01	.1	tr.
10 Alcoholic and Carbonated Beverages	none																
11 Soups		182	7.5	5.0				27.2	56	1.7	1,809	543	5,320	.11	.08	2.3	—
12 Baby Foods	none																
13 Miscellaneous		13	.9	.8				1.1	37	.3	3,706	23					—
3-Day Total		6,241	331.8	238.1	39	70	535	744.0	3,061	56.5	10,227	12,248	28,460	5.69	5.85	79.4	531
Average Daily Nutrient Intake		2,080	110.6	79.4	13	23	180	248.0	1,020	18.8	3,409	4,083	9,490	1.90	1.95	26.5	177

*Linoleic acid is unsaturated fat.

PART III

THE TABLES
OF FOOD CONTENT

The Nutritive Value
of Foods

————◆————

You have before you THE TABLES OF FOOD CONTENT, *which have been referred to throughout this book. The basic information in each table has been furnished by the United States Department of Agriculture and is based on* Agriculture Handbook No. 8, Composition of Foods, *and* Home and Garden Bulletin No. 72, Nutritive Value of Foods. THE TABLES OF FOOD CONTENT *are greatly expanded versions of these tables in order to make them more useful.*

To facilitate use of the tables, similar foods are grouped together into the following categories:

1. *Meat, Poultry, and Fish*
2. *Eggs*
3. *Milk and Dairy Products*
4. *Fruit and Fruit Products*
5. *Vegetables and Vegetable Products*
6. *Flour, Cereal Grains, and Grain Products*
7. *Legumes and Nuts*
8. *Fats and Oils*
9. *Sugars and Sweets*
10. *Alcoholic and Carbonated Beverages*
11. *Soups*
12. *Baby Foods*
13. *Miscellaneous*

For the most part, foods are evaluated in the form in which they are purchased, that is, raw meat trimmed of thick outer fat; fresh vegetables and fruits with skins and ends intact; grains and legumes in their dry, uncooked state. Many of the items which are evaluated are the basic products of food preparation such as flour, sugar, shortening, etc. Foods which are purchased ready-to-serve, as canned fruits and vegetables, prepared dinners, and baked goods are also evaluated and will have less waste than untrimmed raw ingredients.

It is important to keep in mind that storage, handling, and cooking may decrease the nutrient content of a food so you may not always receive the full value expressed in the table. Where these losses could be significant they are discussed prior to the table for each food group. Remember, the tables cannot offer an exact account of the nutrients in a specific food item, and are rather, the reflection of the nutritive content of a representative sampling. No two foods can be expected to have the identical food value; not even oranges from the same tree, eggs from the same chicken, or hamburgers ground from the same cut of beef.

For the purposes of comparison it is convenient to have one standard measure of foods. Therefore, where foods are normally purchased or weighed by the pound, 1 pound of the item is tabulated in the tables. But sometimes a pound is so much more than you might normally use that this amount becomes unwieldy. Thus, for your convenience, as many items as possible are computed in smaller measures—in general, an average serving size. Since liquid foods are generally measured by volume rather than weight, one cup (8 fluid ounces) is used as the constant measure for beverages, oils, and certain dairy products. Although canned soups list weight on the label, it is easiest to evaluate this commodity "by the can," thus both weight and cup measures are given to take care of any variation between brands. Consequently, you must be sure to check the Measure *column before you assess the nutritive value of the foods you are concerned about. A table of standard measures precedes the nutrient tables to help you make any necessary conversions.*

THE TABLES OF FOOD CONTENT *give you the breakdown of foods in terms of calories, protein, total fat, carbohydrate, calcium, iron, sodium, potassium, vitamin A, thiamine, riboflavin, niacin, and vitamin C. For some foods, cholesterol and fatty-acid content are also available. In the computation of fatty-acid content both the amount of saturated fat and that of linoleic acid, the principal polyunsaturated fat, have been calculated. Any discrepancy between their combined amount and the total fat figure is largely a reflection of monounsaturated fats. Additional nutrients that can be found within a food group but for which no data has been compiled are mentioned in the introduction to each table.*

The nutritive value of any prepared foods presented in the tables is based on popular commercial brands and standard recipes. With the onset of nutritional labeling much more information about these items will become available to you. It is, of course, impossible to list here the food value of dishes you prepare at home, but you can compute these yourself from the ingredients in the recipe you use. (See illustration on page 138.)

Most foods are subject to some alteration before eating. Any added sweetening, seasoning, or fat becomes part of its final composition. Be sure to add the food value for these seemingly insignificant items. In addition, if you salt your foods you greatly change the sodium content of your diet. The average consumption of salt in America is estimated to be one to five teaspoons per person daily. If you are heavy-handed with the salt shaker you can expect to add as much as one tablespoon of salt to your diet each day. A light to average salting may increase the salt content by about one teaspoon.

TABLE OF STANDARD MEASURES

Equivalents by Volume
(All measurements level)

1 gallon	= 4 quarts	= 128 fluid ounces
1 quart	{ = 2 pints	= 32 fluid ounces
	= 4 cups	
1 pint	= 2 cups	= 16 fluid ounces
1 cup	{ = 8 fluid ounces	
	= 16 tablespoons	
2 tablespoons	= 1 fluid ounce	
1 tablespoon	= 3 teaspoons	

Equivalents by Weight

1 pound	{ = 16 ounces
	= 453.6 grams
1 ounce	= 28.35 grams
3½ ounces	= 100 grams
1 gram	= .035 ounces

Key to The Tables of Food Content

Zero (0) indicates a lack of the nutrient or a quantity too small to measure.

Dash (—) indicates lack of data for a nutrient possibly present in measurable amounts.

A blank beneath *Saturated Fat, Linoleic Acid,* or *Cholesterol* reflects the absence of this information in the original USDA tables.

1. MEAT, POULTRY, AND FISH

Meat, poultry, and fish are the primary sources of protein in the American diet. This high yield of protein comes from the lean portions of the flesh.

Most muscle meats are also a valuable source of iron and a fair to good source of the B vitamins thiamine and riboflavin—with pork particularly high in thiamine. Although meat contains a good supply of potassium it also has a high natural sodium content; this, plus the addition of salt in seasoning means meat eating simultaneously raises the level of both these minerals rather than contributing to the balance of one against the other.

As the fat content of meat increases, the protein content rapidly diminishes. A higher fat content also means more calories and a lower proportion of vitamins and minerals. Choice grades will have more fat than good grades of meat. Despite variations among animals and cuts, most meat is relatively high in saturated fat, although both poultry and fish contain unsaturated fatty acids as well.

In America, the meat that is most favored comes from muscle tissues. In most other nations, however, none of the animal goes to waste. Organ meats contain far more nutriment than muscle meats and can be expected to provide excellent supplies of B vitamins and iron. Unlike most other meats, liver and other glandular meats are particularly rich in vitamins A and C. Organ meats, however, also contain high levels of cholesterol.

Other nutrients not included in the table which are common to meat, fish, and poultry include vitamin B_{12}, pantothenic acid, and phosphorous. Organ meats, fish liver, and roe are extremely rich sources of most other B vitamins. Salt-water fish provide iodine and fluorine.

Animal flesh is low in carbohydrates, calcium, and with the exception of the organ meats mentioned above, provides no significant amount of vitamins A or C.

Cooking does not greatly alter the nutritive value of meat, although exposure to heat will cause some destruction of thiamine. Organ meats subject to high temperatures will suffer loss of vitamin C. In addition, the extreme heat of pressure-cooking may denature certain amino acids, thereby lowering the protein value of meat, poultry, and fish cooked in this manner. When cooked in liquid (as in stewing and braising), much of the B-vitamin content may be transferred to the cooking medium; to retain these vitamins you should serve the liquid along with the meat as a sauce or gravy.

How to Use the Table

MEAT AND POULTRY

• Since meat is purchased "by the pound," food values are expressed per pound of raw, ready-to-cook meat. To obtain the most accurate record of what you eat, weigh each serving of meat before cooking, or divide the number of servings you obtain into the total weight of the uncooked meat.

• If you cannot actually determine the weight of your portion (for example, when eating meat prepared by others or when dining out) the following guidelines can assist you:

  1 pound boneless meat yields three to four servings
  1 pound meat with moderate bone yields
      two to three servings
  1 pound meat with substantial fat and bone yields
      one to two servings

A serving is defined as 3 ounces cooked lean meat. Although most values in the table are for raw meat, when information is available the table also gives the nutritional breakdown of 3 ounces cooked meat.

• Prepared meats which are more commonly consumed by the unit, as frankfurters, sausages and luncheon meats, bacon, TV dinners, potpies, etc., are listed in terms of individual units based on typical samples.

• To determine fatty-acid and cholesterol content of meat cuts which are not listed, use the values for another cut with similar overall fat content. To determine fatty-acid and cholesterol content of cooked meats use the figures for an equal quantity of the meat when raw.

• Poultry, like meat, is most accurately measured when the number of actual servings per pound of raw meat is calculated. To make your job easier, however, the bird has been broken down into parts when possible (breast, leg, white meat, dark meat, etc.). When using the table for cooked poultry be sure the cooking method corresponds to the one you used.

• Don't forget: Anything you add in cooking—salt, fat, breading, gravy—alters the food value of the meat and should be added into the record when you compute your nutrient intake.

1. MEAT AND POULTRY

Food	Measure	Calories	Protein Gm	Total Fat Gm	Satu-rated Fat Gm	Lino-* leic Acid Gm	Choles-terol Mg	Car-bohy-drate Gm	Minerals				Vitamins				
									Cal-cium Mg	Iron Mg	Sodium Mg	Potas-sium Mg	A IU	Thi-amine Mg	Ribo-flavin Mg	Nia-cin Mg	C Mg
Bacon																	
broiled or fried	1 lb (20 slices)	3,016	38.1	314.3	101	28		4.5	59	5.4	3,084	590	0	1.64	.52	8.3	—
broiled or fried	2 slices	92	4.6	7.8				.5	2	.5	153	35	0	.08	.05	.8	—
Bacon, Canadian																	
broiled or fried	1 lb	980	90.7	65.3	23	6		1.4	54	13.6	8,578	1,778	0	3.75	1.01	21.2	—
broiled or fried	1 oz	79	7.8	5.0				.1	5	1.2	726	123	0	.26	.05	1.4	—
Beef																	
Chuck, choice																	
with bone	1 lb	984	71.6	75.0	36	1	270	0	42	10.7	250	1,370	150	.31	.64	17.2	—
boneless	1 lb	1,166	84.8	88.9	43	2	320	0	50	12.7	295	1,610	180	.36	.75	20.4	—
braised or pot-roasted																	
lean and fat†	3 oz	280	22.3	20.4				0	9	2.8	50	320	30	.04	.17	3.4	—
lean only‡	3 oz	183	25.7	8.1				0	11	3.3	50	320	20	.04	.20	3.9	—
Arm, choice																	
with bone	1 lb	905	78.8	62.9			270	0	49	11.8	250	1,370	130	.34	.70	18.7	—
boneless	1 lb	1,012	88.0	70.3			320	0	54	13.2	295	1,610	140	.38	.78	21.1	—
braised or pot-roasted																	
lean and fat†	3 oz	248	23.3	16.4				0	10	2.9	50	320	30	.04	.18	3.6	—
lean only‡	3 oz	165	26.1	6.0				0	12	3.3	50	320	10	.05	.20	3.9	—
Arm, good																	
with bone	1 lb	768	81.7	46.7			270	0	48	12.5	250	1,370	90	.35	.72	19.5	—
boneless	1 lb	866	92.1	52.6			320	0	54	14.1	295	1,610	100	.39	.82	22.0	—
braised or pot-roasted																	
lean and fat†	3 oz	217	24.3	12.5				0	11	3.2	50	320	10	.04	.18	3.7	—
lean only†	3 oz	153	26.5	4.5				0	12	3.3	50	320	10	.05	.20	4.0	—
Flank steak, choice	1 lb	653	98.0	25.9			320	0	59	14.5	295	1,610	50	.42	.87	23.5	—
braised, lean only	3 oz	168	26.1	6.3				0	12	3.3	50	320	10	.05	.20	3.9	—
Flank steak, good	1 lb	631	98.9	23.1			320	0	59	15.0	295	1,610	50	.43	.88	23.7	—
braised, lean only	3 oz	164	26.4	5.7				0	12	3.3	50	320	10	.05	.20	4.0	—

*Linoleic acid is unsaturated fat.
†Outer layer of fat removed to within ½ inch of lean.
‡All visible fat removed.

1. MEAT AND POULTRY (cont.)

Food	Measure	Calories	Protein Gm	Total Fat Gm	Saturated Fat Gm	Lino-* leic Acid Gm	Cholesterol Mg	Carbohydrate Gm	Calcium Mg	Iron Mg	Sodium Mg	Potassium Mg	A IU	Thiamine Mg	Riboflavin Mg	Niacin Mg	C Mg
Beef (cont.)																	
Hindshank, choice																	
with bone	1 lb	604	38.1	48.9			270	0	50	5.9	135	740	100	.16	.34	9.1	—
boneless	1 lb	1,311	82.6	106.1			320	0		12.7	295	1,610	210	.35	.73	19.8	—
simmered																	
lean and fat†	3 oz	309	21.5	24.1				0	9	2.8	50	320	40	.04	.16	3.3	—
lean only‡	3 oz	158	26.3	5.1				0	12	3.3	50	320	10	.05	.20	4.0	—
Hindshank, good																	
with bone	1 lb	478	39.4	34.4			270	0	24	6.0	135	740	70	.17	.35	9.5	—
boneless	1 lb	1,084	89.4	78.0			320	0	54	13.6	295	1,610	150	.39	.79	21.5	—
simmered																	
lean and fat†	3 oz	263	23.3	18.1				0	10	3.1	50	320	30	.04	.18	3.6	—
lean only‡	3 oz	151	26.6	4.1				0	12	3.3	50	320	10	.05	.20	4.0	—
Porterhouse steak, choice																	
with bone	1 lb	1,603	60.8	148.8	71	3	270	0	33	9.0	250	1,370	300	.26	.55	14.6	—
broiled																	
lean and fat†	3 oz	399	16.9	36.2				0	8	2.2	50	320	60	.05	.14	3.6	—
lean only‡	3 oz	192	25.9	9.0				0	10	3.2	50	320	20	.07	.20	5.1	—
Porterhouse steak, good																	
with bone	1 lb	1,521	62.9	138.9			270	0	33	9.5	250	1,370	280	.27	.56	15.1	—
broiled																	
lean and fat†	3 oz	382	17.6	34.0				0	8	2.2	50	320	60	.05	.15	3.7	—
lean only‡	3 oz	169	26.7	6.1				0	10	3.2	50	320	10	.07	.21	5.1	—
T-Bone steak, choice																	
with bone	1 lb	1,596	59.1	149.1			270	0	32	8.8	250	1,370	300	.25	.53	14.2	—
broiled																	
lean and fat†	3 oz	405	16.7	37.0				0	7	2.2	50	320	70	.05	.14	3.5	—
lean only‡	3 oz	191	26.1	8.8				0	10	3.2	50	320	20	.07	.20	5.1	—

*Linoleic acid is unsaturated fat.
†Outer layer of fat removed to within ½ inch of lean.
‡All visible fat removed.

1. MEAT AND POULTRY (cont.)

Food	Measure	Calories	Protein Gm	Total Fat Gm	Saturated Fat Gm	Lino-leic* Acid Gm	Choles-terol Mg	Carbohydrate Gm	Calcium Mg	Iron Mg	Sodium Mg	Potassium Mg	A IU	Thiamine Mg	Ribo-flavin Mg	Niacin Mg	C Mg
Beef (cont.)																	
T-Bone steak, good																	
with bone	1 lb	1,466	61.7	133.4				0	36	9.2	250	1,370	260	.27	.55	14.9	—
broiled																	
lean and fat†	3 oz	379	17.7	33.6				0	8	2.3	50	320	60	.05	.15	3.7	—
lean only‡	3 oz	171	26.7	6.3				0	10	3.2	50	320	10	.07	.21	5.1	—
Club steak, choice																	
with bone	1 lb	1,443	58.9	132.1			270	0	34	8.7	250	1,370	260	.25	.52	14.1	—
broiled																	
lean and fat†	3 oz	389	17.7	34.8				0	8	2.3	50	320	60	.05	.15	3.7	—
lean only‡	3 oz	209	25.4	11.1				0	10	3.1	50	320	20	.07	.20	5.0	—
Club steak, good																	
with bone	1 lb	1,210	63.1	104.2			270	0	37	9.7	250	1,370	210	.27	.56	15.1	—
broiled																	
lean and fat†	3 oz	341	19.6	28.5				0	9	2.6	50	320	50	.05	.15	4.0	—
lean only‡	3 oz	186	26.1	8.2				0	10	3.2	50	320	20	.07	.20	5.1	—
Round bone sirloin, choice																	
with bone	1 lb	1,316	71.1	112.3			270	0	42	10.5	250	1,370	220	.30	.63	17.1	—
boneless	1 lb	1,420	76.1	121.1			320	0	45	11.3	295	1,610	240	.33	.68	18.4	—
broiled																	
lean and fat†	3 oz	332	19.7	27.4				0	9	2.5	50	320	40	.05	.15	4.0	—
lean only‡	3 oz	177	27.6	6.6				0	11	3.3	50	320	10	.08	.21	5.5	—
Round bone sirloin, good																	
with bone	1 lb	1,175	74.4	94.9			270	0	42	11.3	250	1,370	190	.32	.66	17.9	—
boneless	1 lb	1,275	80.7	103.0			320	0	45	12.2	295	1,610	210	.35	.72	19.4	—
broiled																	
lean and fat†	3 oz	303	21.0	23.6				0	9	2.7	50	320	40	.06	.16	4.3	—
lean only‡	3 oz	157	27.1	4.5				0	11	3.3	50	320	10	.07	.21	5.2	—

*Linoleic acid is unsaturated fat.
†Outer layer of fat removed to within ½ inch of lean.
‡All visible fat removed.

1. MEAT AND POULTRY (cont.)

Food	Measure	Calories	Protein Gm	Total Fat Gm	Saturated Fat Gm	Lino-leic* Acid Gm	Cholesterol Mg	Carbohydrate Gm	Calcium Mg	Iron Mg	Sodium Mg	Potassium Mg	Vitamins A IU	Thiamine Mg	Riboflavin Mg	Niacin Mg	C Mg
Beef (cont.)																	
Double bone sirloin, choice																	
with bone	1 lb	1,240	61.1	108.4	52	2	270	0	34	9.3	135	740	220	.26	.54	14.7	—
boneless broiled	1 lb	1,510	74.4	132.0			320	0	41	11.3	295	1,610	260	.32	.66	17.9	—
lean and fat†	3 oz	350	19.0	29.7				0	9	2.5	50	320	50	.05	.15	3.9	—
lean only‡	3 oz	185	26.2	8.1				0	10	3.2	50	320	20	.07	.20	5.1	—
Double bone sirloin, good																	
with bone	1 lb	1,075	64.6	88.4			270	0	37	9.9	135	740	180	.28	.57	15.4	—
boneless broiled	1 lb	1,329	79.8	109.3			320	0	45	12.2	295	1,610	220	.34	.71	19.1	—
lean and fat†	3 oz	313	20.7	24.9				0	9	2.7	50	320	40	.06	.16	4.2	—
lean only‡	3 oz	163	27.0	5.2				0		3.3	50	320	10	.07	.21	5.2	—
Hipbone sirloin, choice																	
with bone	1 lb	1,585	55.8	149.3			270	0	31	8.5	250	1,370	300	.24	.50	13.3	—
boneless broiled	1 lb	1,869	65.8	176.0			320	0	36	10.0	295	1,610	350	.28	.59	15.7	—
lean and fat†	3 oz	417	16.4	38.5				0	8	2.1	50	320	70	.05	.14	3.4	—
lean only‡	3 oz	206	25.5	10.7				0	10	3.1	50	320	20	.07	.20	5.0	—
Hipbone sirloin, good																	
with bone	1 lb	1,402	60.0	126.8			270	0	34	8.8	250	1,370	250	.26	.53	14.4	—
boneless broiled	1 lb	1,665	71.2	150.6			320	0	41	10.4	295	1,610	300	.31	.63	17.1	—
lean and fat†	3 oz	378	18.0	33.4				0	8	2.3	50	320	60	.05	.15	3.8	—
lean only‡	3 oz	179	26.4	7.4				0	10	3.2	50	320	10	.07	.20	5.1	—
Short plate, choice																	
with bone	1 lb	1,615	59.7	150.6			270	0	32	8.9	250	1,370	300	.25	.53	14.4	—
boneless simmered	1 lb	1,814	67.1	169.2			320	0	36	10.0	295	1,610	340	.29	.59	16.1	—
lean and fat†	3 oz	406	17.7	36.7				0	8	2.3	50	320	70	.03	.14	2.7	—
lean only‡	3 oz	190	25.5	9.0				0	11	3.3	50	320	20	.04	.19	3.9	—

*Linoleic acid is unsaturated fat.   †Outer layer of fat removed to within ½ inch of lean.   ‡All visible fat removed.

1. MEAT AND POULTRY (cont.)

Food	Measure	Calories	Pro-tein Gm	Total Fat Gm	Satu-rated Fat Gm	Lino-leic* Acid Gm	Choles-terol Mg	Car-bohy-drate Gm	Cal-cium Mg	Iron Mg	Sodium Mg	Potas-sium Mg	A IU	Thi-amine Mg	Ribo-flavin Mg	Nia-cin Mg	C Mg
Beef (cont.)																	
Short plate, good																	
with bone	1 lb	1,413	63.9	126.6				0	36	9.5	250	1,370	250	.27	.57	15.3	—
boneless	1 lb	1,615	73.0	144.7				0	41	10.9	295	1,610	290	.31	.65	17.5	—
simmered																	
lean and fat†	3 oz	370	19.1	32.0				0	8	2.5	50	320	60	.03	.15	2.9	—
lean only‡	3 oz	171	26.0	6.6				0	11	3.3	50	320	10	.04	.20	3.9	—
Rib, choice																	
with bone	1 lb	1,673	61.8	156.1	75	3	270	0	38	9.2	250	1,370	310	.27	.55	14.8	—
boneless	1 lb	1,819	67.1	169.6	81	3	320	0	41	10.0	295	1,610	340	.29	.60	16.1	—
roasted																	
lean and fat†	3 oz	377	17.1	33.8				0	8	2.2	50	320	70	.04	.13	3.1	—
lean only‡	3 oz	207	24.2	11.5				0	10	3.1	50	320	20	.06	.18	4.4	—
Round, choice																	
with bone	1 lb	863	88.5	53.9	26	1	270	0	53	13.1	250	1,370	110	.38	.79	21.3	—
boneless	1 lb	894	91.6	55.8	27	1	320	0	54	13.6	295	1,610	110	.39	.82	22.0	—
broiled																	
lean and fat†	3 oz	224	24.5	13.2				0	10	3.0	50	320	30	.07	.19	4.8	—
lean only‡	3 oz	162	26.8	5.2				0	11	3.2	50	320	10	.07	.21	5.1	—
Rump, choice																	
with bone	1 lb	1,167	67.0	94.0	47	2	270	0	39	10.0	250	1,370	190	.29	.60	16.1	—
boneless	1 lb	1,374	78.9	114.8	55	2	320	0	45	11.8	295	1,610	230	.34	.70	19.0	—
roasted																	
lean and fat†	3 oz	297	20.2	23.4				0	9	2.7	50	320	40	.05	.15	3.7	—
lean only‡	3 oz	178	24.9	8.0				0	10	3.2	50	320	20	.06	.19	4.5	—
Rump, good																	
with bone	1 lb	1,037	70.1	81.9				0	42	10.3	250	1,370	160	.30	.62	16.8	—
boneless	1 lb	1,229	83.0	97.1				0	50	12.2	295	1,610	200	.36	.73	19.9	—
roasted																	
lean and fat†	3 oz	272	21.3	20.1				0	9	2.7	50	320	30	.05	.16	3.9	—
lean only‡	3 oz	163	25.4	6.1				0	11	3.2	50	320	10	.07	.19	4.5	—

*Linoleic acid is unsaturated fat.   †Outer layer of fat removed to within ½ inch of lean.   ‡All visible fat removed.

1. MEAT AND POULTRY (cont.)

Food	Measure	Calories	Protein Gm	Total Fat Gm	Satu-rated Fat Gm	Lino-leic* Acid Gm	Choles-terol Mg	Carbo-hydrate Gm	Cal-cium Mg	Iron Mg	Sodium Mg	Potas-sium Mg	A IU	Thi-amine Mg	Ribo-flavin Mg	Nia-cin Mg	C Mg
Beef (cont.)																	
Ground (hamburger),																	
lean																	
broiled	1 lb	812	93.9	45.4	22	1		0	54	14.1			90	.40	.83	22.5	—
	3 oz	188	23.5	9.7				0	10	3.0	41	478	20	.08	.20	5.1	—
regular																	
broiled	1 lb	1,216	81.2	96.2	48	2		0	45	12.2		1,070	160	.35	.72	19.5	—
	3 oz	245	20.7	19.4				0	9	2.7	40	386	30	.08	.18	4.6	—
Beef and vegetable stew, canned	1 lb	358	26.3	14.1				32.2	54	4.1	1,864	789	4,400	.13	.23	4.4	15
	1 cup	185	13.6	7.3				16.7	28	2.1	964	408	2,280	.07	.12	2.3	8
Beef, corned																	
cooked	1 lb	1,329	71.7	113.0	54	2		0	41	10.9	5,897	272		.14	.68	7.7	0
	3 oz	319	19.6	26.1				0	8	2.5	1,491	129		.02	.15	1.3	0
Beef, corned, canned	1 lb	980	114.8	54.0	26	tr.		0	17	19.5		907		.09	1.09	15.4	0
	3 oz	184	21.5	10.1				0		3.7				.02	.20	2.9	0
Corned-beef hash, canned	1 lb	821	39.9	51.3	25	1		48.5	59	9.1	2,449	495		.05	.42	9.6	0
	1 cup	448	21.8	28.0				26.5	32	5.0	1,337			.03	.23	5.2	
Beef, dried, chipped	1 lb	921	155.6	28.6	14	1		0	91	23.1	19,505	907		.32	1.45	17.2	
	1 cup	167	28.2	5.2				0	16	4.2	3,536	164		.06	.26	3.1	
cooked, creamed	½ cup	377	20.1	25.2	14	tr.		17.4	257	2.0	1,754	375	880	.15	.47	1.5	tr.
Beef potpie, frozen	1 pie; 8 oz	436	16.6	22.5				40.8	23	2.3	830	211	930	.08	.14	2.6	tr.
Brains (beef, calf, hog, sheep)	1 lb	567	47.2	39.0	7	2	9,000+	3.6	45	10.9	567	993	0	1.05	1.18	20.1	82
Chicken																	
Fryers, ready-to-cook																	
whole or cut-up	1 lb	382	57.4	15.1	5	3		0	37	5.9		327	2,260	.20	1.17	17.1	—
fried, meat only	3 oz	179	26.7	6.7				0	11	1.4	67	372	80	.05	.30	8.3	—
fried, light meat	3 oz	169	27.5	5.2				1.0	10	1.1	58	283	40	.04	.21	11.1	—
fried, dark meat	3 oz	189	26.1	8.0	3	1		1.1	12	1.5	75		60	.06	.39	5.8	—
Back	1 lb	385	40.4	23.5				0	29	4.2			760	.13	.55	10.5	—
Breast	1 lb	394	74.5	8.6				0	39	4.3			270	.18	.57	28.3	—
fried	½ breast (9½ oz)	234	44.2	5.1				1.2	23	2.6			160	.11	.34	16.8	—
fried		156	24.9	4.9				0	9	1.3			70	.04	.17	11.3	—
Drumstick	1 lb	313	51.2	10.6				0	35	4.4			340	.18	.87	11.7	—
fried	1 avg (4 oz)	78	12.8	2.7				0	9	1.1			80	.04	.22	2.9	—
fried	1 avg	87	12.0	3.8				.4	6	.8			50	.03	.15	2.6	—

*Linoleic acid is unsaturated fat.

1. MEAT AND POULTRY (cont.)

Food	Measure	Calories	Protein Gm	Total Fat Gm	Saturated Fat Gm	Linoleic Acid Gm*	Cholesterol Mg	Carbohydrate Gm	Calcium Mg	Iron Mg	Sodium Mg	Potassium Mg	A IU	Thiamine Mg	Riboflavin Mg	Niacin Mg	C Mg
Chicken (cont.)																	
Neck	1 lb	329	33.7	20.5				0	24	4.1	—	—	660	.10	.53	6.5	—
Thigh	1 lb	435	61.6	19.1				0	41	5.4	—	—	620	.20	1.13	19.3	—
fried	1 avg	109	13.4	5.3				1.2	6	1.1	—	—	90	.03	.22	3.1	—
Wing	1 lb	325	41.1	16.5				0	22	3.3	—	—	530	.09	.32	9.1	—
fried	1 avg	62	6.7	3.4				.6	2	.5	—	—	60	.01	.06	1.6	—
Roasters, ready-to-cook																	
whole or cut up	1 lb	791	60.3	59.3	26	16		0	33	5.3	66	322	3,050	.25	.63	22.1	—
roasted, meat only	3 oz	157	25.2	5.4				0	10	1.3	66	322	130	.09	.13	7.3	—
roasted, light meat	3 oz	156	27.7	4.2				0	9	1.1	57	362	90	.07	.09	10.1	—
roasted, dark meat	3 oz	158	25.1	5.6				0	12	1.5	75	283	140	.10	.16	4.5	—
Hens and cocks, ready-to-cook																	
whole or cut up	1 lb	987	57.6	82.1				0	33	4.6	—	—	3,570	.20	.62	27.1	—
stewed, meat only	3 oz	178	25.7	7.6				0	10	1.3	47	244	210	.03	.13	8.2	—
Capon, ready-to-cook																	
whole or cut up	1 lb	937	70.9	70.2				0									
Chicken, canned, boned	1 lb	898	98.4	53.1	17	11		0	95	6.8	932	626	1,060	.17	.56	19.7	17
	½ cup	168	18.4	10.0	3	2			18	1.3	—	117	200	.03	.10	3.7	3
Chicken potpie, frozen	1 pie; 8 oz	497	15.2	26.1	7	3		50.4	25	2.3	—	347	2,060	.22	.31	3.2	10
Chili con carne, canned with beans	1 lb	603	34.0	27.7	13	1		55.3	145	7.7	2,409	1,057	270	.14	.32	5.7	—
	1 cup	332	18.7	15.2	3	1		30.4	80	4.2	1,325	582	150	.08	.18	3.1	—
Chili con carne, canned without beans	1 lb	907	46.7	67.1	32	1		26.3	172	6.4	—	—	680	.08	.54	10.2	—
	1 cup	509	26.2	37.7	18	1		14.8	97	3.6	—	—	380	.04	.30	5.7	—
Chop suey with meat—see Vegetables and Vegetable Products																	
Chow mein with chicken—see Vegetables and Vegetable Products																	
Duck, ready-to-cook	1 lb	1,213	59.5	106.4				0	37	6.0	—	—	—	.29	.71	24.8	—
Gizzards, chicken simmered	1 lb	513	91.2	12.2				3.2	45	13.2	295	1,089	—	.12	.89	20.3	—
	3 oz	127	23.1	2.8				.6	8	2.7	49	181	—	.02	.18	4.4	—

*Linoleic Acid is Unsaturated Fat.

1. MEAT AND POULTRY (cont.)

Food	Measure	Calories	Protein Gm	Total Fat Gm	Saturated Fat Gm	Lino-lete* Acid Gm	Choles-terol Mg	Carbohydrate Gm	Minerals				Vitamins				
									Calcium Mg	Iron Mg	Sodium Mg	Potassium Mg	A IU	Thiamine Mg	Riboflavin Mg	Niacin Mg	C Mg
Gizzards, goose	1 lb	631	97.1	24.0				0	—	—	—	—	—	—	—	—	—
Gizzards, turkey	1 lb	712	92.1	33.1				5.0	—	—	—	—	—	.22	.58	22.9	—
simmered	3 oz	168	23.0	7.4				.9	—	—	—	—	—	.03	.12	5.0	—
Goose, ready-to-cook	1 lb	1,172	54.3	104.3				0	33	5.3	263	771	—	.53	.63	22.1	—
roasted, meat only	3 oz	200	29.1	8.4				0	12	1.5	44	128	—	.09	.14	8.0	—
Guinea hen, ready-to-cook	1 lb	594	88.0	24.4				0	—	—	106	519	—	—	—	—	—
Ham—see Pork																	
Hamburger—see Beef																	
Heart, beef	1 lb	490	77.6	16.3				3.2	23	18.1	390	875	90	2.42	3.98	34.1	9
braised	3 oz	161	26.8	4.9			680	.6	5	5.1	89	199	30	.21	1.05	6.5	1
Heart, calf	1 lb	562	68.0	26.8				8.2	14	13.6	426	943	140	2.86	4.76	36.7	5
braised	3 oz	178	23.8	7.8			680	1.5	3	3.8	97	214	30	.05	.79	6.9	tr.
Heart, chicken	1 lb	608	84.4	27.2				.5	18	15.0	358	721	140	.26	3.63	20.8	18
simmered	3 oz	148	21.7	6.2			680	.1	3	3.1	59	120	30	.05	.79	4.5	3
Heart, hog	1 lb	513	76.2	20.0				1.8	14	15.0	245	481	140	1.94	5.62	29.8	14
braised	3 oz	167	26.4	5.9			680	.5	4	4.2	56	110	30	.17	1.47	5.7	1
Heart, lamb	1 lb	735	76.2	43.5				4.5	50	—	—	—	320	2.04	3.36	28.6	5
braised	3 oz	223	25.3	12.3			680	.9	12	—	—	—	90	.18	.88	5.5	tr.
Heart, turkey	1 lb	776	69.9	50.8				.9	—	—	313	1,089	140	1.04	3.88	22.5	18
simmered	3 oz	185	28.3	11.3			680	.2	—	—	52	181	30	.21	.84	4.9	3
Kidneys, beef	1 lb	590	75.3	30.4				4.1	50	33.6	798	1,021	3,130	1.61	11.57	29.2	68
braised	3 oz	216		10.3			1,700	.7	15	11.2	217	278	990	.44	4.13	9.2	27
Kidneys, calf	1 lb	513	73.9	20.9			1,700	.5	18	18.1	522	807	600	2.65	7.85	44.6	54
Kidneys, hog	1 lb	481	76.2	16.3			1,700	5.0	50	30.4	907	1,043	3,130	2.32	10.98	33.6	68
Kidneys, lamb	1 lb	476		15.0			1,700	4.1	59	34.5	—	—	—	—	—	—	—
Lamb																	
Leg, choice																	
with bone	1 lb	845	67.7	61.7	35	2	265	0	38	5.3	280	1,110	—	.61	.84	19.6	—
boneless	1 lb	1,007	80.7	73.5	41	2	320	0	45	6.4	340	1,340	—	.72	1.00	23.4	—

*Linoleic acid is unsaturated fat.

1. MEAT AND POULTRY (cont.)

Food	Measure	Calories	Pro-tein Gm	Total Fat Gm	Satu-rated Fat Gm	Lino-leic* Acid Gm	Choles-terol Mg	Car-bohy-drate Gm	Cal-cium Mg	Iron Mg	Sodium Mg	Potas-sium Mg	A IU	Thi-amine Mg	Ribo-flavin Mg	Nia-cin Mg	C Mg
Lamb (cont.)																	
roasted																	
lean and fat†	3 oz	239	21.7	16.2				0	9	1.5	60	250	--	.13	.23	4.7	--
lean only‡	3 oz	159	24.6	6.0				0	11	1.9	60	250	--	.14	.26	5.3	--
Leg, good																	
with bone	1 lb	790	68.4	55.2			265	0	33	5.7	280	1,110	--	.61	.85	19.7	--
boneless	1 lb	948	82.1	66.2			320	0	45	6.8	340	1,340	--	.73	1.02	23.7	--
roasted																	
lean and fat†	3 oz	228	22.1	14.8			265	0	9	1.5	60	250	--	.13	.23	4.8	--
lean only‡	3 oz	157	24.6	5.7			320	0	10	1.9	60	250	--	.14	.26	5.3	--
Loin, choice																	
with bone	1 lb	1,146	63.7	97.0			265	0	35	4.7	280	1,110	--	.57	.79	18.5	--
boneless	1 lb	1,329	73.9	112.5			320	0	41	5.4	340	1,340	--	.66	.92	21.4	--
broiled																	
chops, lean and fat†	3 oz	308	18.9	25.2			265	0	8	1.1	60	250	--	.10	.20	4.3	--
lean only‡	3 oz	161	24.2	6.4			320	0	10	1.7	60	250	--	.13	.24	5.2	--
Loin, good																	
with bone	1 lb	1,068	65.0	87.4			265	0	39	5.0	280	1,110	--	.58	.80	18.8	--
boneless	1 lb	1,252	76.2	102.5			320	0	45	5.9	340	1,340	--	.68	.94	22.0	--
broiled																	
chops, lean and fat†	3 oz	292	19.5	23.1			265	0	9	1.3	60	250	--	.11	.20	4.4	--
lean only‡	3 oz	158	24.2	6.1			320	0	9	1.7	60	250	--	.13	.24	5.2	--
Rib, choice																	
with bone	1 lb	1,229	54.7	110.2	62	3	265	0	33	3.6	280	1,110	--	.49	.68	15.8	--
boneless	1 lb	1,538	68.5	137.9	77	4	320	0	41	4.5	340	1,340	--	.61	.85	19.8	--
broiled																	
chops, lean and fat†	3 oz	349	17.2	30.5			265	0	8	.9	60	250	--	.10	.18	3.9	--
lean only‡	3 oz	181	23.3	9.0			320	0	9	1.6	60	250	--	.13	.23	5.1	--

*Linoleic acid is unsaturated fat.
†Outer layer of fat removed to within ½ inch of lean.
‡All visible fat removed.

1. MEAT AND POULTRY (cont.)

Food	Measure	Calories	Protein Gm	Total Fat Gm	Saturated Fat Gm	Lino-leic Acid Gm	Choles-terol Mg	Car-bohy-drate Gm	Cal-cium Mg	Iron Mg	Sodium Mg	Potas-sium Mg	A IU	Thi-amine Mg	Ribo-flavin Mg	Nia-cin Mg	C Mg
Lamb (cont.)																	
Rib, good																	
with bone	1 lb	1,108	56.1	96.3	52	3	265	0	32	3.9	280	1,110	—	.50	.70	16.2	—
boneless	1 lb	1,415	71.7	122.9	60	3	320	0	41	5.0	340	1,340	—	.64	.89	20.7	—
broiled																	
chops, choice, lean and fat†	3 oz	324	18.2	27.3				0	8	1.0	60	250	—	.10	.19	4.1	—
lean only‡	3 oz	177	23.5	8.5				0	9	1.6	60	250	—	.13	.23	5.1	—
Shoulder, choice																	
with bone	1 lb	1,082	58.9	92.0			265	0	35	3.9	280	1,110	—	.53	.73	17.1	—
boneless	1 lb	1,275	69.4	108.4			320	0	41	4.5	340	1,340	—	.62	.86	20.1	—
roasted																	
lean and fat†	3 oz	290	18.6	23.3				0	9	1.0	60	250	—	.11	.20	4.0	—
lean only‡	3 oz	176	23.0	8.6				0	10	1.6	60	250	—	.13	.24	4.9	—
Shoulder, good																	
with bone	1 lb	1,010	59.1	83.8			265	0	34	4.2	280	1,110	—	.53	.74	17.2	—
boneless	1 lb	1,202	70.3	99.8			320	0	41	5.0	340	1,340	—	.63	.88	20.5	—
roasted																	
lean and fat†	3 oz	276	18.9	21.6				0	9	1.1	60	250	—	.11	.20	4.2	—
lean only‡	3 oz	172	23.0	8.2				0	9	1.1	60	250	—	.13	.24	4.9	—
Liver, beef	1 lb	635	90.3	17.2			1,360	24.0	36	29.5	617	1,275	199,130	1.16	14.79	61.6	140
fried	3 oz	196	22.6	9.1				4.5	9	7.5	158	326	45,770	.22	3.59	14.1	23
Liver, calf	1 lb	635	87.1	21.3			1,360	18.6	36	39.9	331	1,275	102,060	.90	12.32	51.8	161
fried	3 oz	224	25.3	11.3				3.4	11	12.2	101	388	28,030	.21	3.57	14.1	32
Liver, chicken	1 lb	585	89.4	16.8	6	1	1,360	13.2	54	35.8	318	780	54,890	.86	11.29	49.0	79
simmered	3 oz	141	22.7	3.8				2.7	9	7.3	52	129	10,540	.15	2.31	10.0	14
Liver, goose	1 lb	826	74.8	45.4				24.5			635	1,043					
Liver, hog	1 lb	594	93.4	16.8			1,360	11.8	45	87.1	331	1,184	49,440	1.36	13.76	74.2	103
fried	3 oz	207	25.6	9.9				2.1	13	24.9	95	339	12,770	.29	3.74	19.1	19
Liver, lamb	1 lb	617	95.3	17.7			1,360	13.2	45	49.4	236	916	229,070	1.81	14.89	76.5	152
broiled	3 oz	224	27.7	10.6				2.4	14	15.3	73	284	63,850	.42	4.38	21.3	31

*Linoleic Acid is Unsaturated Fat.   †Outer layer of fat removed to within ½ inch of lean.   ‡All visible fat removed.

1. MEAT AND POULTRY (cont.)

Food	Measure	Calories	Protein Gm	Total Fat Gm	Saturated Fat Gm	Lino-leic* Acid Gm	Cholesterol Mg	Carbohydrate Gm	Calcium Mg	Iron Mg	Sodium Mg	Potassium Mg	A IU	Thiamine Mg	Riboflavin Mg	Niacin Mg	C Mg
Liver, turkey	1 lb	626	96.2	18.1			1,360	13.2			286	726	80,290	.81	8.75	59.9	—
simmered	3 oz	149	23.9	4.1				2.7			47	121	15,000	.14	1.79	12.3	—
Lungs, beef	1 lb	435	79.8	10.4				0								28.1	—
Lungs, calf	1 lb	481	76.2	17.2				0									—
Lungs, lamb	1 lb	467	87.5	10.4				0									—
Pancreas, beef, medium fat	1 lb	1,284	61.2	113.4				0									—
Pancreas, beef, lean	1 lb	640	79.8	33.1				0									—
Pancreas, calf	1 lb	730	87.1	39.9				0	36	12.7	304	1,252					—
Pancreas, hog	1 lb	1,098	66.7	90.3				0	50	4.5	200	984					—
Paté de foie gras,	1 lb	2,096	51.7	198.7	24	6		21.8						.40	1.36	11.4	—
canned	1 T	66	1.6	6.2				.7						.01	.04	.4	—
Pheasant, ready-to-cook	1 lb	596	95.9	20.5				0									—
Pig's feet, pickled	1 lb	903	75.8	67.1				0									—
Pork																	
Ham, medium-fat																	
with bone and skin	1 lb	1,188	61.3	102.6	37	9	260	0	35	9.3	260	1,060	0	2.98	.72	16.0	—
skinless, boneless	1 lb	1,397	72.1	120.7	43	11	320	0	41	10.9	320	1,295	0	3.51	.84	18.8	—
roasted																	
lean and fat†	3 oz	321	19.7	26.2				0	9	2.6	55	334	0	.44	.20	3.9	—
lean only‡	3 oz	186	25.5	8.6				0	11	3.3	55	334	0	.55	.25	4.9	—
Ham, thin																	
with bone and skin	1 lb	1,077	64.0	88.9			260	0	38	9.6	260	1,060	0	3.13	.76	16.7	—
skinless, boneless	1 lb	1,275	75.8	105.2			320	0	45	11.3	320	1,295	0	3.70	.89	19.8	—
roasted																	
lean and fat†	3 oz	297	20.7	23.1				0	9	2.7	55	334	0	.46	.21	4.1	—
lean only‡	3 oz	180	25.9	7.7				0	11	3.3	55	334	0	.57	.26	5.0	—
Loin, medium fat																	
with bone	1 lb	1,065	61.1	89.0	32	8	260	0	36	9.3	260	1,060	0	2.97	.71	15.9	—

*Linoleic acid is unsaturated fat.
†Outer layer of fat removed to within ½ inch of lean.
‡All visible fat removed.

1. MEAT AND POULTRY (cont.)

Food	Measure	Calories	Protein Gm	Total Fat Gm	Satu-rated Fat Gm	Lino-leic* Acid Gm	Chole-terol Mg	Car-bohy-drate Gm	Cal-cium Mg	Iron Mg	Sodium Mg	Potas-sium Mg	A IU	Thi-amine Mg	Ribo-flavin Mg	Nia-cin Mg	C Mg
Pork (cont.)																	
boneless																	
roasted	1 lb	1,352	77.6	112.9	41	10	320	0	45	11.8	320	1,295	0	3.76	.90	20.1	—
lean and fat†	3 oz	310	21.0	24.4				0	9	2.7	55	334	0	.79	.22	4.8	—
lean only‡	3 oz	218	25.2	12.2				0	11	3.3	55	334	0	.93	.27	5.6	—
broiled																	
lean and fat†	3 oz	335	21.2	27.2				0	10	2.9	55	334	0	.82	.24	5.0	—
lean only‡	3 oz	231	26.2	13.2				0	11	3.3	55	334	0	.97	.28	5.8	—
Loin, thin																	
with bone	1 lb	953	63.7	75.4			260	0	36	9.6	260	1,060	0	3.09	.74	16.6	—
boneless	1 lb	1,216	81.2	96.2			320	0	45	12.2	320	1,295	0	3.95	.95	21.1	—
roasted																	
lean and fat†	3 oz	285	22.1	21.2				0	9	2.9	55	334	0	.82	.24	5.0	—
lean only‡	3 oz	218	25.2	12.2				0	11	3.3	55	334	0	.93	.27	5.6	—
broiled																	
lean and fat†	3 oz	308	22.5	23.5				0	10	3.0	55	334	0	.86	.25	5.2	—
lean only‡	3 oz	231	26.2	13.2				0	11	3.3	55	334	0	.97	.28	5.8	—
Boston Butt, medium fat																	
with bone and skin	1 lb	1,220	65.9	104.1	37	9	260	0	38	9.8	260	1,060	0	3.20	.77	17.1	—
skinless, boneless	1 lb	1,302	70.3	111.1	40	10	320	0	41	10.4	320	1,295	0	3.42	.82	18.3	—
roasted																	
lean and fat†	3 oz	303	19.3	24.4				0	9	2.5	55	334	0	.43	.20	3.8	—
lean only‡	3 oz	209	23.1	12.3				0	10	2.9	55	334	0	.51	.23	4.5	—
Boston Butt, thin																	
with bone and skin	1 lb	1,067	70.1	85.0			260	0	42	10.6	260	1,060	0	3.42	.82	18.3	—
skinless, boneless	1 lb	1,139	74.8	90.7			320	0	45	11.3	320	1,295	0	3.65	.88	19.8	—
roasted																	
lean and fat†	3 oz	272	20.7	20.3				0	9	2.7	55	334	0	.45	.21	4.0	—
lean only‡	3 oz	197	23.8	10.5				0	10	3.0	55	334	0	.51	.23	4.6	—
Picnic, medium fat																	
with bone and skin	1 lb	1,083	59.0	92.2	33	8	260	0	34	9.0	260	1,060	0	2.87	.69	15.4	—
skinless, boneless	1 lb	1,315	71.7	112.0	40	10	320	0	41	10.9	320	1,295	0	3.49	.84	13.6	—

*Linoleic acid is unsaturated fat.   †Outer layer of fat removed to within ½ inch of lean.   ‡All visible fat removed.

1. MEAT AND POULTRY (cont.)

Food	Measure	Calories	Protein Gm	Total Fat Gm	Saturated Fat Gm	Lino-leic* Acid Gm	Cholesterol Mg	Carbohydrate Gm	Calcium Mg	Iron Mg	Sodium Mg	Potassium Mg	Vitamins A IU	Thiamine Mg	Riboflavin Mg	Niacin Mg	C Mg
Pork (cont.)																	
simmered																	
lean and fat†	3 oz	321	19.9	26.1				0	9	2.6	55	334	0	.46	.21	4.1	—
lean only‡	3 oz	182	24.9	8.4				0	10	3.1	55	334	0	.57	.26	5.1	—
Picnic, thin																	
with bone and skin	1 lb	932	63.2	73.3				0	37	9.4	260	1,060	0	3.06	.74	16.4	—
skinless, boneless	1 lb	1,129	76.7	88.9				0	45	11.3	320	1,295	0	3.71	.89	19.9	—
simmered																	
lean and fat†	3 oz	282	21.3	21.2	32	8	260	0	9	2.7	55	334	0	.50	.22	4.5	—
lean only‡	3 oz	166	25.5	6.4				0	11	3.2	55	334	0	.58	.27	5.1	—
Spareribs, medium fat	1 lb	976	39.2	89.7				0	22	5.9	190	775	0	1.91	.46	10.2	—
braised, edible part	3 oz	377	17.8	33.3				0	8	2.2	55	334	0	.37	.18	2.9	—
Spareribs, thin	1 lb	857	39.6	76.4			260	0	23	6.0	190	775	0	1.93	.46	10.3	—
braised, edible part	3 oz	351	18.8	30.1				0	8	2.4	55	334	0	.39	.19	3.1	—
Pork, cured																	
Country style, long-cure																	
Ham, medium fat																	
with skin and bone	1 lb	1,535	66.7	138.0	50	12		1.2	—	—	—	—	0	—	—	—	—
skinless, boneless	1 lb	1,765	76.7	159.0	57	14		1.4	—	—	—	—	0	—	—	—	—
Ham, lean																	
with bone and skin	1 lb	1,209	76.1	98.0				1.2	—	—	—	—	0	—	—	—	—
skinless, boneless	1 lb	1,406	88.5	113.0				1.4	—	—	—	—	0	—	—	—	—
Commercial, light cure																	
Ham, medium fat																	
with bone and skin	1 lb	1,100	68.3	89.7	32	8		0	39	10.1			0	2.82	.76	16.0	—
skinless, boneless	1 lb	1,279	79.4	104.3	38	9		0	45	11.8			0	3.28	.88	18.6	—
roasted																	
lean and fat†	3 oz	248	17.9	18.9				0	8	2.2	797	279	0	.40	.15	3.1	—
lean only‡	3 oz	160	21.7	7.5				0	9	2.7			0	.50	.20	3.9	—
Boston Butt, medium fat																	
with bone and skin	1 lb	1,227	72.5	101.7	37	9		0	42	11.0	279	—	0	2.99	.81	17.0	—

*Linoleic acid is unsaturated fat. †Outer layer of fat removed to within ½ inch of lean. ‡All visible fat removed.

1. MEAT AND POULTRY (cont.)

Food	Measure	Calories	Protein Gm	Total Fat Gm	Saturated Fat Gm	Linoleic Acid Gm	Cholesterol Mg	Carbohydrate Gm	Calcium Mg	Iron Mg	Sodium Mg	Potassium Mg	A IU	Thiamine Mg	Riboflavin Mg	Niacin Mg	C Mg
Pork, cured (cont.), skinless, boneless, roasted	1 lb	1,320	78.0	109.3	39	10		0	45	11.8	—	—	0	3.22	.87	18.2	—
lean and fat†	3 oz	283	19.6	22.0				0	9	2.6	797	279	0	.45	.18	3.5	—
lean only‡	3 oz	208	23.8	11.8				0	10	3.1			0	.55	.21	4.3	—
Commercial, light cure, Picnic, medium fat, with bone and skin, roasted	1 lb	1,060	62.5	87.8	32	8		0	37	9.3			0	2.58	.69	14.6	—
skinless, boneless, roasted	1 lb	1,293	76.2	107.0	39	10		0	45	11.3			0	3.15	.84	17.8	—
lean and fat†	3 oz	277	19.2	21.6				0	9	2.5	797	279	0	.45	.17	3.4	—
lean only‡	3 oz	181	24.3	8.5				0	11	3.2			0	.56	.22	4.3	—
Canned ham	1 lb	875	83.0	55.8	20	5		4.1	50	12.2	4,990	1,542	0	2.42	.87	17.3	—
Canned ham	3 oz	164	15.6	10.5	4	1		.8	9	2.3	936	289	0	.45	.16	3.2	—
Pork and gravy, canned	1 lb	1,161	74.4	80.7	29	7		28.6	59	10.9	154	1,379	0	2.22	.77	15.9	—
Rabbit, ready-to-cook	1 lb	581	75.0	29.0	11	3		0	72	4.7	35	315		.29	.20	45.9	—
stewed	3 oz	185	25.1	8.7				0	18	1.3				.04	.06	9.7	—
Raccoon, roasted	3 oz	219	25.0	12.4				0						.51	.45		—
Sausage, cold cuts, and luncheon meats																	
Blood sausage or pudding	1 lb	1,787	64.0	167.4				1.4									—
	1 oz	112	4.0	10.5				tr.									—
Bockwurst	1 lb	1,198	51.3	107.5				2.7									—
	1 (10/lb)	120	5.1	10.8				.3									—
Bologna, all meat	1 lb	1,256	60.3	103.4				16.8									—
	1 slice (3" diam. x 1/8")	36	1.7	3.0				.5									—
	1 slice (4" diam.)	63	3.0	5.2				.8									—
Bologna, with cereal	1 lb	1,188	64.4	93.4				17.7									—
	1 slice (4" diam.)	59	3.2	4.7				.9									—
Braunschweiger	1 lb	1,447	67.1	124.3	45	11		10.4	45	26.8			29,620	.78	6.55	37.0	—
	1 slice (2" diam. x 1/4")	32	1.5	2.7	1	tr.		.2	1	.6			650	.02	.14	.8	—

*Linoleic acid is unsaturated fat. †Outer layer of fat removed to within 1/2 inch of lean. ‡All visible fat removed.

1. MEAT AND POULTRY (cont.)

Food	Measure	Calories	Protein Gm	Total Fat Gm	Saturated Fat Gm	Lino-* leic Acid Gm	Cholesterol Mg	Carbohydrate Gm	Calcium Mg	Iron Mg	Sodium Mg	Potassium Mg	A IU	Thiamine Mg	Riboflavin Mg	Niacin Mg	C Mg
Sausage, cold cuts, and luncheon meats (cont.)																	
Brown-and-serve sausage	1 lb	1,783	61.2	163.3				12.2	—	—	—	—	—	—	—	—	—
Capicola	1 (20/lb)	89	3.1	8.2				.6	—	—	—	—	—	—	—	—	—
	1 lb	2,263	91.6	207.7	75	19		0	—	—	—	—	—	—	—	—	—
Cervelat, dry	1 slice (2½" diam. x ⅛")	71	2.9	6.5				0	—	—	—	—	0	—	—	—	—
	1 lb	2,046	111.6	170.6	2	1		7.7	64	12.2	—	—	0	1.22	1.04	24.9	—
	1 oz	128	7.0	10.7				.5	4	.8	—	—	0	.08	.06	1.6	—
Cervelat, soft	1 lb	1,393	84.4	111.1				7.3	50	12.7	—	—	—	.51	1.17	19.2	—
	1 oz	87	5.3	6.9				.5	3	.8	—	—	—	.03	.07	1.2	—
Country-style sausage (smoked)	1 lb	1,565	68.5	141.1	51	13		0	41	10.4	—	—	—	1.00	.87	14.0	—
	1 oz	98	4.3	8.8	3	1		0	3	.7	—	—	—	.06	.05	.9	—
Deviled ham	1 lb	1,592	63.1	146.5	53	13		0	36	9.5	—	—	0	.64	.45	7.3	—
	1 T	46	1.8	4.2	2	tr.		0	1	.3	—	—	0	.02	.01	.2	—
Frankfurter all types	1 lb	1,402	56.7	125.2				8.2	32	8.6	4,990	998	0	.71	.90	12.2	—
all meat	1 lb	1,343	59.4	115.7				11.3	—	—	—	—	—	—	—	—	—
	1 (10/lb)	134	5.9	11.6				1.1	—	—	—	—	—	—	—	—	—
with nonfat dry milk	1 lb	1,361	59.4	116.1				15.4	—	—	—	—	—	—	—	—	—
	1 (10/lb)	136	5.9	11.6				1.5	—	—	—	—	—	—	—	—	—
with cereal	1 lb	1,125	65.3	93.4				.9	—	—	—	—	—	—	—	—	—
	1 (10/lb)	113	6.5	9.3				.1	—	—	—	—	—	—	—	—	—
canned	1 lb	1,002	68.8	82.1				.9	41	10.0	—	—	—	.15	.56	10.7	—
	1 cocktail frank	111	.8	.9				tr.	tr.	.1	—	—	—	tr.	.01	.1	—
Headcheese	1 lb	1,216	70.3	99.8	36	9		4.5	41	10.4	—	—	0	.18	.45	4.0	—
	1 slice (4"x4"x⅛")	76	4.4	6.2	2	tr.		.3	3	.7	—	—	0	.01	.03	.3	—
Knockwurst	1 lb	1,261	64.0	105.2				10.0	36	9.5	—	—	—	.77	.85	11.8	—
	1 (3 oz)	236	12.0	19.7				1.9	7	1.8	—	—	—	.14	.16	2.2	—

*Linoleic acid is unsaturated fat.

1. MEAT AND POULTRY (cont.)

Food	Measure	Calories	Protein Gm	Total Fat Gm	Saturated Fat Gm	Lino-leic* Acid Gm	Cholesterol Mg	Carbohydrate Gm	Calcium Mg	Iron Mg	Sodium Mg	Potassium Mg	A IU	Thiamine Mg	Riboflavin Mg	Niacin Mg	C Mg
Sausage, cold cuts, and luncheon meats (cont.)																	
Liverwurst, fresh	1 lb	1,393	73.5	116.1				8.2	41	24.5	—	—	28,800	.91	5.90	25.9	—
	1 slice (4" diam. x ⅜")	65	3.4	5.4				.4	2	1.1	—	—	1,350	.04	.28	1.2	—
Liverwurst, smoked	1 lb	1,447	67.1	124.3				10.4	45	26.8	—	—	29,620	.78	6.55	37.0	—
	1 oz	90	4.2	7.8				.7	3	1.7	—	—	1,850	.05	.41	2.3	—
Luncheon meat boiled ham	1 lb	1,061	86.2	77.1	28	7		0	50	12.7	—	—	0	2.00	.68	11.8	—
	1 slice (6"x3½")	66	5.4	4.8	2	tr.		0	3	.8	—	—	0	.12	.04	.7	—
chopped, cured pork, canned	1 lb	1,334	68.0	112.9	41	8		5.9	41	10.0	5,597	1,007	0	1.41	.95	13.6	—
	1 oz	83	4.2	7.1	3	tr.		.4	3	.6	350	63	0	.09	.06	.9	—
Minced ham	1 lb	1,034	62.1	76.7	28	7		20.0	36	9.5	—	—	0	1.68	1.00	15.4	—
	1 slice (4"x4"x⅛")	65	3.9	4.8	2	tr.		1.2	3	.6	—	—	0	.10	.06	1.0	—
Mortadella	1 lb	1,429	92.5	113.4				2.7	54	14.1	—	—	—	—	—	—	—
	1 slice (3½" diam. x ⅛")	45	2.9	3.5				.1	2	.4	—	—	—	—	—	—	—
Polish-style sausage	1 lb	2,259	42.6	117.0				5.4	41	10.9	—	—	—	—	—	—	—
	1 oz	141	2.7	7.3				.3	3	.7	—	—	—	—	—	—	—
Pork and beef (chopped together)	1 lb	1,524	70.8	135.6				0	41	10.4	—	—	0	1.54	.86	14.1	—
	1 oz	95	4.4	8.5				0	3	.7	—	—	0	.10	.05	.9	—
Pork sausage	1 lb	2,259	42.6	230.4	83	21		tr.	23	6.4	3,357	635	0	1.95	.76	10.4	—
	1 oz	141	2.7	14.4	5	1		tr.	1	.4	210	40	0	.12	.05	.6	—
	1 link (8/12 oz pkg)	212	4.0	21.6	8	2		tr.	2	.6	315	60	0	.18	.07	1.0	—
Salami, dry	1 patty (8/lb)	282	5.3	28.8	10	3		tr.	3	.8	420	79	0	.24	.09	1.3	—
	1 lb	2,041	108.0	172.8				5.4	64	16.3	—	—	0	1.68	1.13	24.0	—
	1 slice (3½" diam.)	42	2.2	3.6				.1	1	.3	—	—	—	.03	.02	.5	—

*Linoleic acid is unsaturated fat.

1. MEAT AND POULTRY (cont.)

Food	Measure	Calories	Protein Gm	Total Fat Gm	Saturated Fat Gm	Linoleic Acid Gm	Cholesterol Mg	Carbohydrate Gm	Calcium Mg	Iron Mg	Sodium Mg	Potassium Mg	A IU	Thiamine Mg	Riboflavin Mg	Niacin Mg	C Mg
Sausage, cold cuts, and luncheon meats (cont.)																	
Salami, cooked	1 lb	1,411	79.4	116.1				6.4	45	11.8				1.13	1.09	18.6	
	1 slice (4" diam.)	71	4.0	5.8				.3	2	.6				.06	.05	.9	
Scrapple	1 slice (2¼" diam. x ¼")	41	2.3	3.3				.2	1	.3				.03	.03	.5	
	1 lb	975	39.9	61.7				66.2	23	5.4				.86	.41	8.2	
	3½ oz	215	8.8	13.6				14.6	5	1.2				.19	.09	1.8	
Vienna sausage, canned	1 lb	1,089	63.5	89.8				1.4	36	9.5				.39	.58	11.9	
	1 sausage (7/5 oz can)	38	2.2	3.2				tr.	1					.01	.02	.4	
Squab	1 lb	569	38.0	45.1				0	35	.3	435	1,633					
Sweetbreads, beef braised	1 lb	939	66.2	72.6			1,135	0			99	371					
	3 oz	274	22.2	19.9				0									
Sweetbreads, calf braised	1 lb	426	80.7	9.1			1,135	0						.37	.76	11.7	
	3 oz	144	27.9	2.7				0						.05	.14	2.5	
Sweetbreads, lamb braised	1 lb	426	64.0	17.2			1,135	0									
	3 oz	150	24.1	5.2				0									
Sweetbreads, hog, see Pancreas																	
Tongue, beef braised	1 lb	714	56.5	52.0				1.4	28	7.2	252	679		.42	.99	17.2	
	3 oz	209	18.4	14.3				.3	6	1.9	52	140		.04	.25	3.0	
smoked	1 oz	—	4.9	8.2										.01	.06	.9	
Tongue, calf braised	1 lb	454	64.6	18.5				3.1	100	4.8							
	3 oz	137	20.5	5.1				.9	22	1.2							
Tongue, hog braised	1 lb	741	57.9	53.8				1.7						.59	.99	17.2	0
	3 oz	217	18.9	14.9				.4						.06	.25	3.0	
Tongue, lamb braised	1 lb	659	46.0	50.7				1.7									
	3 oz	218	17.6	15.6				.4									
Tongue, sheep braised	1 lb	877	45.4	72.2				7.9									
	3 oz	277	17.0	21.7				2.1									

*Linoleic acid is unsaturated fat.

1. MEAT AND POULTRY (cont.)

Food	Measure	Calories	Protein Gm	Total Fat Gm	Saturated Fat Gm	Lino-leic Acid Gm	Cholesterol Mg	Carbohydrate Gm	Calcium Mg	Iron Mg	Sodium Mg	Potassium Mg	A IU	Thiamine Mg	Riboflavin Mg	Niacin Mg	C Mg
Tongue, canned, pickled	1 lb	1,211	87.5	92.1	—	—	—	1.4	—	—	—	—	—	—	—	—	—
Tongue, potted or deviled	1 oz	76	5.5	5.8	—	—	—	tr.	—	—	—	—	—	—	—	—	—
	1 lb	1,315	84.4	104.3	—	—	—	3.2	—	—	—	—	—	—	—	—	—
Tripe, beef, pickled	1 oz	82	5.3	6.5	—	—	—	.2	—	—	209	86	—	—	—	—	—
Turkey, ready-to-cook roasted	1 lb	281	53.5	5.9	—	—	—	0	—	—	—	—	—	.16	.50	5.9	—
	1 lb	722	66.6	48.7	—	—	—	0	—	—	—	—	—	.01	.03	.4	—
meat only	3 oz	163	27.0	5.2	—	—	—	0	7	1.5	111	315	—	.04	.15	6.6	—
light meat	3 oz	151	28.2	3.8	—	—	—	0	—	1.0	70	352	—	.04	.12	9.5	—
dark meat	3 oz	174	25.7	7.1	—	—	—	0	—	2.0	85	341	—	.03	.20	3.6	—
Turkey potpie	1 pie; 8 oz	447	13.2	23.6	—	—	—	45.6	27	2.0	837	259	2,020	.20	.18	3.6	—
"TV" dinners																	
Beef pot roast, oven-browned potatoes, peas, and corn	11 oz	331	40.8	10.0	6	tr.	—	19.0	31	5.0	808	761	340	.19	.30	6.5	16
Fried chicken, mashed potatoes, mixed vegetables	11 oz	506	37.5	24.9	9	4	—	33.1	120	3.5	1,006	328	1,730	.19	.54	15.3	12
Meat loaf with tomato sauce, mashed potatoes, peas	11 oz	408	25.0	20.9	3	tr.	—	30.6	59	4.1	1,226	359	1,340	.33	.44	5.4	14
Sliced turkey, mashed potatoes, peas	11 oz	349	26.2	9.4	—	—	—	39.6	81	3.4	1,247	549	410	.21	.28	7.1	12
Veal																	
Chuck, with bone	1 lb	628	70.4	36.0	17	1	320	0	40	10.5	320	1,150	—	.52	.94	23.6	—
boneless	1 lb	785	88.0	45.0	—	—	410	0	50	13.2	410	1,450	—	.64	1.17	29.5	—
braised	3 oz	201	23.9	11.0	—	—	—	0	10	3.0	70	430	—	.08	.25	5.5	—
Flank with bone	1 lb	1,410	74.1	121.0	—	—	410	0	45	11.2	410	1,450	—	.54	.98	24.8	—
boneless	1 lb	1,424	74.8	122.0	—	—	410	0	45	11.3	410	1,450	—	.54	.99	25.1	—
stewed	3 oz	334	19.9	27.7	—	—	—	0	9	2.6	70	430	—	.04	.19	3.6	—

*Linoleic acid is unsaturated fat.

1. MEAT AND POULTRY (cont.)

Food	Measure	Calories	Protein Gm	Total Fat Gm	Saturated Fat Gm	Lino-leic* Acid Gm	Cholesterol Mg	Carbohydrate Gm	Calcium Mg	Iron Mg	Sodium Mg	Potassium Mg	A IU	Thiamine Mg	Riboflavin Mg	Niacin Mg	C Mg
Veal (cont.)																	
Foreshank																	
with bone	1 lb	368	46.5	19.0	—	—	—	0	26	7.1	210	755	—	.34	.62	15.6	—
boneless	1 lb	708	89.4	36.0	—	—	320	0	50	13.6	410	1,450	—	.65	1.19	29.9	—
stewed	3 oz	185	24.6	8.9	—	—	410	0	10	3.1	70	430	—	.04	.22	4.3	—
Loin																	
with bone	1 lb	681	72.3	41.0	—	—	—	0	41	10.9	320	1,150	—	.53	.96	24.2	—
boneless	1 lb	821	87.1	50.0	—	—	320	0	50	13.2	410	1,450	—	.64	1.16	29.2	—
broiled	3 oz	201	22.6	11.5	—	—	410	0	9	2.7	70	430	—	.06	.21	4.6	—
Plate																	
with bone	1 lb	828	65.6	61.0	—	—	—	0	39	9.7	320	1,150	—	.48	.87	22.0	—
boneless	1 lb	1,048	83.0	77.0	—	—	320	0	50	12.2	410	1,450	—	.61	1.10	27.8	—
stewed	3 oz	260	22.4	18.2	—	—	410	0	10	2.8	70	430	—	.04	.21	3.9	—
Rib																	
with bone	1 lb	723	65.7	49.0	23	1	—	0	38	9.8	210	755	—	.48	.87	22.0	—
boneless	1 lb	939	85.3	64.0	—	—	320	0	50	12.7	410	1,450	—	.62	1.13	28.6	—
roasted	3 oz	231	23.3	14.5	—	—	410	0	10	2.9	70	430	—	.11	.27	6.7	—
Round with rump																	
with bone	1 lb	573	68.1	31.0	—	—	—	0	38	10.1	210	755	—	.50	.90	22.8	—
boneless	1 lb	744	88.5	41.0	11	1	320	0	50	13.2	410	1,450	—	.64	1.17	29.6	—
broiled	3 oz	185	23.2	9.5	—	—	410	0	9	2.7	70	430	—	.06	.21	4.6	—
Venison, meat only	1 lb	572	95.0	18.0	—	—	—	0	45	—	—	—	—	1.03	2.19	28.6	—

*Linoleic acid is unsaturated fat.

FISH

● Fish is evaluated in terms of "whole fish" (including head, tail, fins, entrails, and bones; unless marked *dressed*) or "flesh only." If you cannot weigh your serving before it is cooked you can estimate with the following guidelines. A standard-size serving of fish is 3 ounces, cooked weight.

    1 serving dressed whole fish = 6½ ounces raw
    1 serving fish fillets = 4½ ounces raw
    1 serving fish steaks = 5⅓ ounces raw

When the figures are available, 3 ounces cooked fish is shown on the table.

● Prepared fish, such as canned tuna, canned salmon, sardines, anchovies, frozen fish sticks, fried shrimp, etc., are evaluated in terms of a standard serving size or by the individual piece.

● Specific values for cholesterol in fish are not available, however an average value of 320 milligrams per pound has been assigned to fish fillets and 265 milligrams per pound to fish steaks.

1. FISH

Food	Measure	Calories	Pro-tein Gm	Total Fat Gm	Satu-rated Fat Gm	Lino-* leic Acid Gm	Choles-terol Mg	Car-bohy-drate Gm	Cal-cium Mg	Iron Mg	Sodium Mg	Potas-sium Mg	A IU	Thi-amine Mg	Ribo-flavin Mg	Nia-cin Mg	C Mg
Abalone																	
in shell	1 lb	187	35.6	1.0				6.5	70	4.6	—	—	—	.35	.26	—	—
flesh only	1 lb	445	84.8	2.3				15.4	168	10.9	—	—	—	.83	.62	—	—
	4½ oz	125	23.9	.6				4.3	47	3.1	—	—	—	.23	.17	—	—
canned	1 lb	363	72.6	1.4				10.4	64	—	—	—	—	.54	—	—	—
	3 oz	68	13.6	.3				2.0	12	—	—	—	—	.10	—	—	—
Anchovy	1 can (2 oz)	100	10.9	5.8				.2	95	—	—	—	—	—	—	—	—
Bass, black sea																	
whole	1 lb	165	34.0	2.1				0	—	—	120	453	—	—	—	—	—
baked, stuffed (with bacon, butter, onion, celery, bread cubes)	3 oz	222	13.9	13.5				9.8	—	—	—	—	—	—	—	—	—
flesh only	1 lb	422	87.1	5.4				0	—	—	308	1,161	—	—	—	—	—
	4½ oz	119	24.5	1.5				0	—	—	87	327	—	—	—	—	—
Bass, small- and large-mouth																	
whole	1 lb	146	26.6	3.7				0	—	—	—	—	—	.14	.04	3.0	—
flesh only	1 lb	472	85.7	11.8				0	—	—	—	—	—	.46	.13	9.6	—
	4½ oz	133	24.1	3.3				0	—	—	—	—	—	.13	.04	2.7	—
Bass, striped																	
whole	1 lb	205	36.9	5.3				0	—	—	—	—	—	—	—	—	—
flesh only	1 lb	476	85.7	12.2				0	—	—	—	—	—	—	—	—	—
oven-fried (with milk, breadcrumbs, butter, salt)	3 oz	168	18.4	7.3				5.7	—	—	—	—	—	—	—	—	—
Bluefish																	
whole	1 lb	271	47.4	7.6				0	53	1.4	171	—	—	.27	.22	4.5	—
flesh only	1 lb	531	93.0	15.0				0	104	2.7	336	—	—	.52	.43	8.8	—
baked or broiled (with butter or margarine)	3 oz	136	22.5	4.5				0	25	.6	89	—	40	.09	.09	1.6	—
fried (with egg, milk or water, breadcrumbs)	3 oz	176	19.5	8.4				4.0	30	.8	125	—	—	.09	.09	1.5	—

*Linoleic acid is unsaturated fat.

1. FISH (cont.)

The columns below are grouped: **Minerals** spans Calcium, Iron, Sodium, Potassium; **Vitamins** spans A, Thiamine, Riboflavin, Niacin, C.

Food	Measure	Calories	Protein Gm	Total Fat Gm	Saturated Fat Gm	Linoleic Acid* Gm	Cholesterol Mg	Carbohydrate Gm	Calcium Mg	Iron Mg	Sodium Mg	Potassium Mg	A IU	Thiamine Mg	Riboflavin Mg	Niacin Mg	C Mg
Bonito, flesh only	1 lb	762	108.9	33.1				0									
	4½ oz	214	30.6	9.3				0									
Carp, whole	1 lb	156	24.5	5.7				0	68	1.2	68	389	230	.01	.05	2.0	2
flesh	1 lb	522	81.6	19.1				0	227	4.1	227	1,297	770	.04	.18	6.7	5
	4½ oz	147	23.0	5.4				0	64	1.2	64	365	217	.01	.05	1.9	1
Catfish, fillets	1 lb	467	79.8	14.1				0		1.8	272	1,497		.18	.13	7.7	
	4½ oz	131	22.4	4.0				0		.5	77	421		.05	.04	2.2	
Caviar, granular	1 lb	1,188	122.0	68.0			1,300+	15.0	1,252	53.5	9,979	816					
	1 oz	74	7.6	4.2			80+	.9	78	3.3	623	51					
	1 T	42	4.4				50+	.5	45	1.9	356	29					
Caviar, pressed	1 lb	1,433	156.0	75.8			1,300+	22.2									
	1 oz	90	9.8	4.7			80+	1.4									
	1 T	51	5.6	2.7			50+	.8									
Chub, whole	1 lb	217	22.9	13.2				0									
flesh	1 lb	658	69.4	39.9				0									
	4½ oz	185	19.5	11.2				0									
Clams, soft in shell	1 lb	130	22.2	3.0				2.1		5.4	57	373					
shucked	1 lb	372	63.5	8.6				5.9		15.4	163	1,066					
	1 serving (2½/lb)	149	25.4	3.4				2.4									
Clams, hard or round in shell	1 lb	62	8.6	.7				4.5	53	6.2	65	426					
shucked	1 lb	363	50.3	4.1				26.8	313	5.8	158	240					
	1 serving (2½/lb)	145	20.1	1.6				10.7	125	34.0	930	1,411					
Clams, canned solids and liquid	1 lb	236	35.8	3.2				12.7	249	13.6	372	564		.04	.48	4.6	
drained solids	½ cup	78	12.6	2.0				1.5		18.6		635					

*Linoleic acid is unsaturated fat.

1. FISH (cont.)

Food	Measure	Calories	Protein Gm	Total Fat Gm	Saturated Fat Gm	Lino-leic* Acid Gm	Cholesterol Mg	Carbohydrate Gm	Calcium Mg	Iron Mg	Sodium Mg	Potassium Mg	A IU	Thiamine Mg	Riboflavin Mg	Niacin Mg	C Mg
Clam broth	1 cup	45	5.4	.3				4.9	45								9
Cod, flesh only broiled	1 lb	354	79.8	1.4				0	27	1.8	318	1,733	0	.27	.33	10.0	9
Cod, canned	3 oz	146	24.4	4.5				0		.9	94	349	150	.07	.09	2.6	
Cod, dried, salted	1 lb	386	87.1	1.4				0	1,021						.34		
	1 piece 5½"x 1½"x½"x	590	131.5	3.2				0									
Crab, in shell, steamed	1 lb	103	23.0	.6			270	0	179	1.7			4,720	.35	.18	6.1	4
Crab meat, steamed	1 lb	202	37.7	4.1			106	1.1	94	.7			1,860	.14	.07	2.4	2
Crab, canned	3 oz	80	14.8	1.6				.4	37					.35	.38	8.7	
	1 lb	458	78.9	11.3				5.0	204	3.6	4,536	499		.14	.15	3.5	
	1 can, 6½ oz	186	32.1	4.6				2.0	83	1.5	1,843	203					
Crayfish in shell	1 lb	39	7.9	.3				.7	42	6.8				.01	.02	1.0	
flesh	1 lb	327	66.2	2.3				5.4	349	1.9				.05	.19	8.8	
	4½ oz	92	18.6	.6				1.5	98					.01	.05	2.5	
Dogfish (grayfish)	1 lb	708	79.8	40.8	19				82					.23			
	4½ oz	199	22.4	11.5	5				23					1.06			
Eel	1 lb	1,057	72.1	83.0	29					3.2			7,300	1.00	1.66	6.2	
	4½ oz	297	20.3	23.3	8					.9			2,050	.28	.47	1.7	
Eel, smoked	1 lb	1,497	84.4	126.1													
	4½ oz	421	23.7	35.5										.16	.20		
Eulachon (smelt)	4½ oz	150	18.6	7.9										.04	.06		
Finnan haddie (smoked haddock)	1 lb	467	105.2	1.8				0						.28	.24	9.6	
Fish cakes, frozen	4½ oz	131	29.6	.5				0						.08	.07	2.7	
	1 cake, 2 oz	153	5.3	10.1				9.8									
Fish flakes, canned	1 lb	503	112.0	2.7				0	222	3.6							
	3 oz	94	21.0	.5				0	42	.7							

*Linoleic acid is unsaturated fat.

1. FISH (cont.)

Food	Measure	Calories	Protein Gm	Total Fat Gm	Saturated Fat Gm	Lino-leic* Acid Gm	Cholesterol Mg	Carbohydrate Gm	Calcium Mg	Iron Mg	Sodium Mg	Potassium Mg	A IU	Thiamine Mg	Riboflavin Mg	Niacin Mg	C Mg
Fish sticks, frozen	1 lb	799	75.0	40.0				30.0	50	1.8			0	.18	.32	7.3	
	10 sticks (one 8-oz pkg)	400	37.5	20.0				15.0	25	.9			0	.09	.16	3.6	
Flounder																	
whole	1 lb	118	25.0	1.2				0	18	1.2	117	512		.08	.08	2.5	
flesh	1 lb	358	75.8	3.6				0	54	3.6	354	1,551		.24	.23	7.6	
baked	3 oz	173	25.7	7.0				0	20	1.2	203	503	0	.06	.07	2.1	2
Frog's legs	1 lb	215	48.3	.9				0	53	4.4				.41	.74	3.4	
Grouper																	
whole	1 lb	170	37.6	1.0				0						.33			
flesh	1 lb	395	87.5	2.3				0						.77			
Haddock	4½ oz	111	24.6	.6				0						.22			
fried (dipped in egg, milk, breadcrumbs)	1 lb	358	83.0					5.0	104	3.2	277	1,379	0	.19	.29	13.6	2
Hake	3 oz	141	16.8	5.5				0	34	1.0	152	298		.03	.06	2.7	
	3 lb	336	74.8	1.8				0	186		336	1,647		.43	.91		
	4½ oz	95	21.0	.5				0	52		95	462		.12	.26		
Halibut broiled	1 lb	454	94.8	5.4				0	59	3.2	245	2,037	2,200	.29	.30	37.8	
	3 oz	147	21.6	6.0				0	14	.7	115	450	580	.04	.06	7.1	
Herring																	
Atlantic	1 lb	798	78.5	51.3	10	10		0		5.0			520	.10	.68	16.4	12
Pacific	1 lb	445	79.4	11.8	2	2		0		5.9	336	1,905	450	.10	.74	16.0	
canned, plain	3 oz	178	17.1	11.7	2	2		0	126	1.5				.15	.15	3.0	
canned in tomato sauce	3 oz	151	13.5	9.0	2	2		3.2						.09			
pickled, Bismarck	3 oz	191	17.5	12.9	2	2		0							.09		
salted or brined	1 lb	989	86.2	68.9	10	10		0						.86			
smoked, bloaters	1 lb	889	88.9	56.2	10	10		0									
smoked, kippers	1 lb	957	100.7	58.5	10	10		0	299	6.4			110		1.26	15.0	
Lake trout																	
dressed, whole	1 lb	282	30.7	16.8				0		1.3				.15	.20	4.6	
	6½ oz	115	12.5	6.8				0		.5				.06	.08	1.9	

*Linoleic acid is unsaturated fat.

1. FISH (cont.)

Food	Measure	Calories	Protein Gm	Total Fat Gm	Saturated Fat Gm	Lino-leic Acid* Gm	Cholesterol Mg	Carbohydrate Gm	Calcium Mg	Iron Mg	Sodium Mg	Potassium Mg	A IU	Thiamine Mg	Riboflavin Mg	Niacin Mg	C Mg
Lake trout (cont.) fillets	1 lb	762	83.0	45.4				0		3.6				.41	.54	12.4	—
	4½ oz	214	23.3	12.7				0		1.0				.12	.15	3.5	—
Lobster whole	1 lb	107	19.9	2.2			235	.6	34	.7				.48	.06	1.7	—
meat only	1 lb	413	76.7	8.6			900	2.3	132	2.7				1.84	.23	6.6	—
canned	1 lb	431	84.8	6.8				1.4	295	3.6	953	816		.46	.31	—	—
Lobster Newburg	3 oz	81	15.9	1.3				.3	55	.7	179	153		.09	.06	—	—
	4 oz	220	21.0	12.0				5.8	99	3.5	260	194		.08	.12	—	—
Lobster paste	1 oz	51	5.9	2.7				.4							.07	—	—
	1 t	13	1.5	.7				.1							.02	—	—
Lobster salad	1 lb	499	45.9	29.0				10.4	163	4.1	563	1,199		.41	.36	—	82
	4 oz	125	11.5	7.2				2.6	41	1.0	141	300		.10	.09	—	20
Mackerel, Atlantic whole	1 lb	468	46.5	29.9				0	12	2.4			1,100	.36	.80	20.0	—
flesh	1 lb	866	86.2	55.3				0	23	4.5			2,040	.66	1.49	37.1	—
broiled	3 oz	202	18.7	13.5				0	5	1.0			450	.13	.23	6.5	—
canned, solids and liquid	1 lb	830	87.5	50.3				0	839	9.5			1,950	.26	.96	26.3	—
	3½ oz (about 3 oz meat)	183	19.3	11.1				0	185	2.1			430	.06	.21	5.8	—
Mackerel, Pacific dressed, whole	1 lb	519	71.5	23.8				0	26	6.9			390				—
flesh	1 lb	721	99.3	33.1				0	36	9.5			540				—
	4½ oz	203	27.9	9.3				0	10	2.7			150				—
canned, solids and liquid	1 lb	816	95.7	45.4				0	1,179	10.0			120	.12	1.50	39.7	—
	3½ oz (about 3 oz meat)	180	21.1	10.0				0	260	2.2			30	.03	.33	8.8	—
Mackerel, smoked	1 lb	993	108.0	59.0				0	—	—							—

*Linoleic acid is unsaturated fat.

1. FISH (cont.)

Food	Measure	Calories	Protein Gm	Total Fat Gm	Saturated Fat Gm	Linoleic Acid* Gm	Cholesterol Mg	Carbohydrate Gm	Calcium Mg	Iron Mg	Sodium Mg	Potassium Mg	A IU	Thiamine Mg	Riboflavin Mg	Niacin Mg	C Mg
Mullet																	
whole	1 lb	351	47.1	16.6				0	63	4.3	195	702	—	.16	.19	12.4	—
flesh	1 lb	662	88.9	31.3				0	118	8.2	367	1,325	—	.30	.36	23.4	—
	4½ oz	186	25.0	8.8				0	33	2.3	103	372	—	.08	.10	6.6	—
Mussels																	
in shell	1 lb (12–14)	125	18.9	2.9				4.3	116	4.5	380	414	—	.21	.28	—	—
meat only	1 lb	431	65.3	10.0				15.0	399	15.4	1,311	1,429	—	.73	.96	—	—
Ocean perch (redfish), Atlantic																	
fillet	1 lb	399	81.6	5.4				0	91	4.5	358	1,220	—	.46	.38	8.4	—
fried (dipped in egg, milk, breadcrumbs)	3 oz	195	16.3	11.4				5.8	28	1.1	131	243	—	.09	.09	1.5	—
Ocean perch, Pacific																	
flesh	1 lb	431	86.2	6.8				0	—	—	286	1,769	—	—	—	—	—
	4½ oz	121	24.2	1.9				0	—	—	80	498	—	—	—	—	—
Octopus	1 lb	331	69.4	3.6				0	132	—	—	—	—	.11	.28	7.9	—
Oysters, Eastern																	
in shell	1 lb	30	3.8	.8				1.5	43	2.5	33	55	140	.06	.08	1.1	—
meat only	1 lb	299	38.1	8.2				15.4	426	24.9	331	549	1,390	.63	.82	11.2	—
	1 cup (13–19)	158	20.1	4.3				8.1	225	13.1	175	290	730	.33	.43	5.9	—
Oysters, Western meat only	1 lb	413	48.1	10.0				29.0	386	32.7	—	—	—	.56	—	5.9	137
Oysters, fried (dipped in egg, milk, breadcrumbs)	3 oz	205	7.4	11.9				15.9	130	6.9	177	174	380	.15	.25	2.7	—
Oysters, canned	1 lb	345	38.6	10.0				22.2	127	25.4	—	318	—	.09	.91	3.8	—
	3½ oz	76	8.5	2.2				4.9	28	5.6	—	70	—	.02	.20	.8	—
Oyster stew frozen, condensed	1 can, 15 oz	434	19.6	26.8				29.3	557	4.7	2,891	872	800	.25	.68	1.3	—
prepared with milk	1 cup	192	9.3	11.7				13.8	282	1.6	1,060	408	380	.10	.37	.5	—

*Linoleic acid is unsaturated fat.

1. FISH (cont.)

Food	Measure	Calories	Protein Gm	Total Fat Gm	Satu-rated Fat Gm	Lino-leic* Acid Gm	Choles-terol Mg	Carbo-hydrate Gm	Cal-cium Mg	Iron Mg	Sodium Mg	Potas-sium Mg	A IU	Thi-amine Mg	Ribo-flavin Mg	Nia-cin Mg	C Mg
Perch, white whole	1 lb	193	31.5	6.5				0	—	—	—	—	—	—	—	—	—
flesh	1 lb	535	87.5	18.1				0	—	—	—	—	—	—	—	—	—
flesh	4½ oz	150	24.6	5.1				0	—	—	—	—	—	—	—	—	—
Perch, yellow whole	1 lb	161	34.5	1.6				0	—	1.1	120	407	—	.11	.30	3.1	—
whole	1 lb	413	88.5	4.1				0	—	2.7	308	1,043	—	.27	.77	7.9	—
flesh	4½ oz	116	24.9	1.2				0	—	.8	87	293	—	.08	.22	2.2	—
Pike, blue whole	1 lb	180	38.1	1.8				0	—	—	—	—	—	—	—	—	—
whole	1 lb	408	86.6	4.1				0	—	—	—	—	—	—	—	—	—
flesh	4½ oz	115	24.4	1.2				0	—	—	—	—	—	—	—	—	—
Pike, Northern whole	1 lb	104	21.6	1.3				0	—	—	—	—	—	—	—	—	—
whole	1 lb	399	83.0	5.0				0	—	—	—	—	—	—	—	—	—
flesh	4½ oz	112	23.3	1.4				0	—	—	—	—	—	—	—	—	—
Pollack dressed, whole	1 lb	194	41.6	1.8				0		—	98	714	—	.10	.21	3.2	—
fillets	1 lb	431	92.5	4.1				0		—	218	1,588	—	.23	.46	7.1	—
	4½ oz	121	26.0	1.2				0		—	61	447	—	.06	.13	2.0	—
Pompano, flesh	1 lb	753	85.3	43.1				0		—	213	866	—				
	4½ oz	212	24.0	12.1				0		—	60	244	—				
Porgy, flesh	1 lb	508	86.2	15.4				0	245		286	1,302	—	1.87	1.00		
	4½ oz	143	24.2	4.3				0	69		80	366	—	.53	.28		
Red and gray snapper	1 lb	422	89.8	4.3				0	73	3.6	304	1,465	—	.78	.11		
	4½ oz	119	25.3	1.2				0	21	1.0	86	412	—	.22	.03		
Roe—cod, carp, herring, haddock, pike, shad baked or broiled	1 lb	590	110.7	10.4			1,300+	6.8	11	2.7	—	—	—	.45	3.45	6.3	64
	3 oz	108	18.9	2.4				1.6		2.0	63	113	—	—	—	—	—

*Linoleic acid is unsaturated fat.

1. FISH (cont.)

Food	Measure	Calories	Protein Gm	Total Fat Gm	Saturated Fat Gm	Linoleic* Acid Gm	Cholesterol Mg	Carbohydrate Gm	Calcium Mg	Iron Mg	Sodium Mg	Potassium Mg	A IU	Thiamine Mg	Riboflavin Mg	Niacin Mg	C Mg
Roe—salmon, turbot, sturgeon	1 lb	939	114.3	47.2			1,300+	6.4	—	—	—	—	—	1.71	3.28	10.4	82
Roe, canned—cod, haddock, herring	1 lb	535	97.5	12.7			1,300+	1.4	68	5.4	—	—	—	—	—	—	10
	3½ oz	118	21.5	2.8			300+	.3	15	1.2	—	—	—	—	—	—	2
Sablefish, flesh only	1 lb	862	59.0	67.6				0	—	—	254	1,624	—	.51	.40	—	—
	4½ oz	242	16.6	19.0				0	—	—	71	457	—	.14	.11	—	—
Salmon, Atlantic flesh only	1 lb	984	102.1	60.8				0	358	4.1	—	—	—	—	.36	32.6	41
	4½ oz	277	28.7	17.1				0	101	1.2	—	—	—	—	.10	9.2	12
canned	1 lb	921	98.4	55.3				0	—	—	—	—	—	—	—	—	—
	3½ oz	203	21.7	12.2				0	—	—	—	—	—	—	—	—	—
Salmon, Chinook (King) steak	1 lb	886	76.2	62.3	19	1		0	—	—	180	1,593	1,240	.40	.92	—	—
	5⅓ oz	294	25.2	20.6	6	tr.		0	—	—	60	528	410	.13	.30	—	—
canned	1 lb	953	88.9	63.5	20	1		0	699†	—	—	1,660	1,040	.12	.64	33.1	—
	3½ oz	210	19.6	14.0	4	tr.		0	154†	—	—	366	230	.03	.14	7.3	—
Salmon, Coho, canned	1 lb	694	94.3	32.2				0	1,107†	4.1	1,592‡	1,538	360	.03	.79	33.7	0
	3½ oz	153	20.8	7.1				0	244†	.9	351‡	339	80	—	.18	7.4	—
Salmon, pink steak	1 lb	475	79.8	14.8	4	tr.		0	—	—	255	1,222	—	.57	.18	—	—
	5⅓ oz	158	26.6	4.9				0	—	—	85	407	—	.19	.06	—	—
canned	1 lb	640	93.0	26.8	7	tr.		0	889†	3.6	1,755‡	1,637	320	.15	.83	36.2	—
	3½ oz	141	20.5	5.9				0	196†	—	387‡	361	70	.03	.18	8.0	—
Salmon, Sockeye, canned	1 lb	776	92.3	42.2	2	tr.		0	1,175†	5.4	2,368‡	1,560	1,040	.19	.74	33.2	—
	3½ oz	171	20.3	9.3				0	259†	2.3	522‡	344	230	.04	.16	7.3	—
Salmon, baked or broiled	3 oz	156	23.1	6.3				0	64	1.2	99	380	140	.14	.05	8.4	—
	1 lb	798	98.0	42.2				0	—	—	—	—	—	—	—	—	—
Salmon, smoked	3 oz	151	18.5	8.0				0	12	1.0	—	—	—	—	—	—	—

*Linoleic acid is unsaturated fat.
†Based on total contents of can. If bones are discarded value is greatly reduced.
‡Salt added.

1. FISH (cont.)

Food	Measure	Calories	Pro-tein Gm	Total Fat Gm	Satu-rated Fat Gm	Lino-leic* Acid Gm	Choles-terol Mg	Car-bohy-drate Gm	Cal-cium Mg	Iron Mg	Sodium Mg	Potas-sium Mg	Vitamins A IU	Thi-amine Mg	Ribo-flavin Mg	Nia-cin Mg	C Mg
Sardines, Atlantic canned in oil	1 lb	1,411	93.4	110.7				2.7	1,606	15.9	2,313	2,540	820	.10	.74	20.1	—
	3½ oz	311	20.6	24.4				.6	354	3.5	510	560	180	.02	.16	4.4	—
drained solids, with skin and bones	3 oz	174	20.6	9.5					374	2.5	705	506	190	.03	.17	4.6	—
skinless, boneless	3 oz	174	20.6	9.5					46	2.5	705	506	190	.03	.17	4.6	—
Sardines, Pacific canned in brine or mustard	1 lb	889	85.3	54.4				7.7	1,374	23.6	3,447	1,179	120				—
	3½ oz	196	18.8	12.0				1.7	303	5.2	760	260	30				—
canned in tomato sauce	1 lb	894	84.8	55.3				7.7	2,037	18.6	1,814	1,452	120	.05	1.22	24.1	—
	3½ oz	197	18.7	12.2				1.7	449	4.1	400	320	30	.01	.27	5.3	—
Scallops	1 lb	367	82.0	1.2				15.0	118	8.2	227	408			.29	5.8	—
steamed	3 oz	96	19.9						99	2.6							—
Scallops, breaded, fried, frozen	1 lb	880		38.0				48.0									—
	3 oz	166	15.4	7.2				9.0									—
Sea bass	1 lb	435	97.1	2.3				0									—
	4½ oz	122	27.3	.6				0									—
Shad	1 lb	771	84.4	45.4				0		2.3	245	1,497		.68	1.09	38.1	—
baked (with butter or margarine & bacon)	3 oz	172	19.9	9.7				0	21	.5	68	323	30	.11	.22	7.4	—
Shrimp in shell	1 lb	285	56.7	2.5			390	4.7	197	5.0	438	689		.06	.09	10.0	—
	5.8 oz (yields ap. 3 oz cooked meat)	104	20.6	.9			140	1.7	72	1.8	159	251		.02	.03	3.6	—
Shrimp shelled	1 lb	413	82.1	3.6			565	6.8	286	7.3	635	998		.09	.14	14.5	—
	4½ oz	116	23.1				160	1.9	80	2.1	179	281		.03	.04	4.1	—
French fried	3 oz	193	17.4	9.3				8.6	62	1.7	159	196		.03	.07	2.3	—

*Linoleic acid is unsaturated fat.

1. FISH (cont.)

Food	Measure	Calories	Protein Gm	Total Fat Gm	Saturated Fat Gm	Linoleic Acid Gm	Cholesterol Mg	Carbohydrate Gm	Calcium Mg	Iron Mg	Sodium Mg	Potassium Mg	A IU	Thiamine Mg	Riboflavin Mg	Niacin Mg	C Mg
Shrimp (cont.)																	
canned, wet pack	1 lb	363	73.5	3.6				3.6	268	8.2			220	.03	.12	6.6	—
canned, dry pack	1 lb	526	109.8	5.0				3.2	522	14.1		553	270	.04	.15	8.2	—
canned, solids only	3 oz	99	20.7	.2				.6	99	2.7		105	50	.01	.03	1.5	—
frozen, breaded	1 lb	631	55.8	3.2				90.3	172	4.5				.12	.13	9.0	—
Shrimp paste	1 oz	119	10.5	.6				17.1	33	.9				.03	.03	1.7	—
	1 t	13	1.5	.7				.4							.07		—
Skate	1 lb	51	5.9	2.7				.1							.02		—
Smelt, flesh only	1 lb	445	97.5	3.2				0		1.8				.11	.56	6.1	—
	4½ oz	125	27.4	.9				0		.5				.03	.16	1.7	—
canned	1 lb	445	84.4	9.5				0						.04			—
	4½ oz	125	23.7	2.7				0						.01			—
Snail	1 lb	907	83.5	61.2				9.1	1,624	7.7		1,551		.24	.23	7.6	—
	3½ oz	171	15.8	11.6					307	1.5		436		.07	.06	2.1	—
Snail, giant African	1 lb	408	73.0	6.4				20.0	54	15.9	354			.09	.54		—
Sole, flesh only	1 lb	331	44.9	6.4				0	15	3.6	100						—
	4½ oz	358	75.8	3.6				0	54	1.0							—
Squid	1 lb	101	21.3	1.0				0		2.3							—
Sturgeon	1 lb	381	74.4	4.1				6.8									—
with skin and bones	1 lb	362	69.8	7.3				0									—
flesh only	1 lb	426	82.1	8.9				0									—
steamed	3 oz	137	21.8	4.9				0	34	1.7	93	201					—
smoked	1 lb	676	141.5	8.2				0									—
Swordfish, flesh only	3 oz	126	26.5	1.5				0	86	4.1							—
broiled (with butter or margarine)	1 lb	535	87.1	18.1				0					7,170	.24	.23	36.4	—
	3 oz	149	24.0	5.1				0	23	1.1			1,760	.03	.04	9.3	—
Trout, brook																	
whole	1 lb	224	42.7	4.7				0						.03	.16		—
flesh	1 lb	458	87.1	9.5				0						.16	.33		—
	4½ oz	129	24.5	2.7				0						.09	.09		—

*Linoleic acid is unsaturated fat.

1. FISH (cont.)

							Vitamins										
											Minerals						
Food	Measure	Calories	Protein Gm	Total Fat Gm	Satu-rated Fat Gm	Lino-leic* Acid Gm	Choles-terol Mg	Car-bohy-drate Gm	Cal-cium Mg	Iron Mg	Sodium Mg	Potas-sium Mg	A IU	Thi-amine Mg	Ribo-flavin Mg	Nia-cin Mg	C Mg
Trout, lake—see lake trout																	
Trout, rainbow																	
flesh with skin	1 lb	885	97.5	51.7	11	2		0						.34	.92	38.0	—
	4½ oz	249	27.4	14.5	3	tr.		0						.10	.26	10.7	—
Tuna																	
bluefin, flesh	1 lb	658	114.3	18.6	6	tr.		0		5.9				—	—	—	—
	4½ oz	185	32.2	5.2	2	tr.		0		1.7				—	—	—	—
yellowfin, flesh	1 lb	603	112.0	13.6	5	tr.		0			168			—	—	—	—
	4½ oz	170	31.5	3.8	1	tr.		0			47			—	—	—	—
canned in oil	1 lb	1,306	109.8	93.0	25	38		0	27	5.0	3,629	1,365	410	.18	.39	46.0	—
	1 can, 6½ oz	531	44.6	37.8	10	15		0	11	2.0	1,474	555	170	.07	.16	18.7	—
drained solids	3 oz	169	24.7	7.0				0	7	1.6			170	.04	.10	10.2	—
canned in water	1 lb	576	127.0	3.6				0	73	7.3	186	1,266			.45	60.3	—
	1 can, 6½ oz	234	51.6	1.5				0	30	3.0	76	514			.18	24.5	—
Tuna salad	4 oz	771	66.3	47.7				15.9	91	5.9			1,320	.18	.50	22.7	5
	1 lb	193	16.6	11.9				4.0	23	1.5			330	.04	.12	5.7	1
Turtle, green, meat	1 lb	404	89.8	2.3				0						—	—	—	—
canned	3½ oz	106	23.4	.7				0						—	—	—	—
Whale meat	1 lb	708	93.4	34.0	5	—		0	54		354	100	8,440	.39	.35	—	29
Whitefish																	
whole	1 lb	330	40.3	17.5				0		.9	111	637	4,820	.30	.26	6.4	—
flesh	1 lb	703	85.7	37.2				0		1.8	236	1,356	10,250	.64	.54	13.6	—
baked, stuffed (with bacon, butter, onion, celery, bread)	3 oz	184	13.0	12.0				5.0	100	.4	167	249	1,710	.09	.09	2.0	tr.
smoked	1 lb	703	94.8	33.1				0	19						—	—	—	—
Whiting, flesh only	3 oz	133	17.9	6.3				0									
	1 lb	330	40.3	17.5				0		.9	111	637	4,820	.30	.26	6.4	—
	4½ oz	93	11.3	4.9				0		.3	31	179	1,360	.08	.07	1.8	—

*Linoleic acid is unsaturated fat.

2. EGGS

Although this food group is composed of only one item, it deserves individual attention. Eggs, eaten alone or combined with other foods in casseroles, custards, meat loaves, baked goods, and a wide range of prepared products, comprise a major part of the American diet. They are different from all other foods in nutritional composition.

Eggs are an excellent source of high-quality protein, contain only a trace of carbohydrate, and possess a moderate amount of fat (largely saturated) concentrated in the yolk. Also in the yolk are: vitamin A, vitamin D (making eggs one of the few food sources of this nutrient), iron, calcium, and most of the B vitamins including, B_6, B_{12}, biotin, and pantothenic acid. With the exception of riboflavin, only small amounts of vitamins and minerals are located in egg whites.

The only vitamin that is noticeably missing from eggs is vitamin C, for apparently the developing chick has no need for this nutrient.

Gentle cooking has no appreciable effect on the nutritive value of eggs, but method of preparation must be considered in terms of added ingredients. If you've consumed a couple of sunny-side-up eggs, don't forget to include the butter they were fried in. Scrambled eggs may mean a few tablespoons of milk as well as the fat used in the frying pan.

How to Use the Table

• Nutritive values in the table are based on one egg and are in accord with government standards for size:

Official regulations specify that:
One dozen large eggs weigh a minimum of 24 ounces.
One dozen medium eggs weigh a minimum of 21 ounces.
One dozen small eggs weigh a minimum of 18 ounces.

2. EGGS

Food	Measure	Calories	Protein Gm	Total Fat Gm	Saturated Fat Gm	Lino-leic Acid Gm	Cholesterol Mg	Carbohydrate Gm	Calcium Mg	Iron Mg	Sodium Mg	Potassium Mg	A IU	Thiamine Mg	Riboflavin Mg	Niacin Mg	C Mg
Chicken eggs																	
whole	1 lge	88	7.0	6.2	2	tr.	300	.5	29	1.2	66	70	640	.06	.16	.1	0
	1 med	78	6.2	5.5	2	tr.	265	.4	26	1.1	59	62	570	.05	.14	tr.	0
	1 sm	65	5.2	4.6	1.6	tr.	220	.4	22	.9	49	52	470	.04	.12	tr.	0
white	1 med	16	3.4	tr.			0	.1	3	tr.	45	43	0	tr.	.07	tr.	0
yolk	2 T	59	2.7	5.8	2	tr.	255	.2	26	1.2	9	17	580	.05	.08	tr.	0
dried, whole	2 T	83	6.6	5.8				.6			60	65	600	.05	.17	.2	0
dried, whole, stabilized	3½ oz	592	47.0	41.2	13	3		4.1	187	8.7	427	463	4,290	.33	1.20	.1	0
dried, white, flakes	3½ oz	609	48.9	42.9	13	3		2.5	194	9.0	444	482	4,460	.34	1.25	.7	0
dried, white, powdered	3½ oz	349	75.1	.2			0	5.3	62	1.0	1,033	937	0	.04	1.87	.7	0
dried, yolk	3½ oz	372	80.2	.2				5.7	66	1.0	1,103	1,000	0	.04	1.99	.1	0
	3½ oz	664	33.2	56.6	18	4	2,950	2.5	275	10.8	1,100	186	5,980	.41	.86	.1	0
Duck eggs	1 lge	172	12.0	13.0				.6	50	2.5	110	116	1,110	.16	.27	.1	—
	1 med	141	9.8	10.7				.5	41	2.1	90	95	910	.13	.22	.1	—
	1 sm	120	8.4	9.1				.4	35	1.8	77	81	770	.11	.19	.1	—
Goose eggs	1 lge	222	16.7	16.0				1.6	—	—	—	—	—	—	—	—	—
	1 med	167	12.5	12.0				1.2	—	—	—	—	—	—	—	—	—
Turkey eggs	1 lge	156	10.5	10.9				1.6	—	—	—	—	—	—	—	—	—
	1 med	136	9.4	9.4				1.4	—	—	—	—	—	—	—	—	—
	1 sm	122	8.5	8.5				1.2	—	—	—	—	—	—	—	—	—

*Linoleic acid is unsaturated fat.

3. MILK AND DAIRY PRODUCTS

While milk per se is often considered children's food, milk appears in various forms on many adult menus. Cheese, yogurt, cottage cheese, sour cream, and ice cream are all milk derivatives, and although their nutritional values vary depending on the amount of butterfat added or removed, milk and dairy products contain the greatest assortment of nutrients of any food group.

First and foremost, milk is the primary source of calcium in most American diets; indeed, those who do not select milk in one of its many forms daily are likely to exhibit eventual signs of calcium deficiency since few other foods possess this mineral in such abundance.

The milk group also provides high-quality protein which is valuable on its own and also as a booster for the protein in cereals and grains, making cereal with milk, rice pudding, bread and cheese, and other familiar milk-and-grain combinations particularly good sources of protein in the diet. Milk is an excellent source of riboflavin and a fair source of thiamine, although certain processing may reduce the thiamine content. Whole milk is noted for its vitamin-A content and skim-milk products frequently have vitamin-A fortification. Vitamin D is also added to liquid milk and many dry-milk powders.

Although the level of iron in milk is not extremely high, the form of iron present is easily utilized by the body, making the milk group a noteworthy source of iron too. Among the vitamins and minerals not represented in the table, phosphorous, vitamin B_{12}, and magnesium are all plentiful in the milk family. Only vitamin C is noticeably absent from dairy products.

The calorie and fat content of milk and dairy products spans a wide range. Those products that have had much of the butterfat removed, such as skim milk and nonfat dry milk, yogurt, buttermilk, and certain cheeses, are low in saturated fat and calories and proportionately higher in other nutrients. As the fat content increases, calories are added and the proportion of most other nutrients diminishes so that cream, ice cream, and sour cream have less nutritional significance than milk. The exception to this rule of diminishing nutrition lies in vitamin A which is found only in the fat portion of foods and is therefore absent from skim-milk products unless it is artificially introduced.

In general, cheese is a concentrated source of most of the nutrients found in whole milk and offers a much better return for your money in terms of food value than meat. Whole-milk products, including cheese, are relatively high in saturated fat and cholesterol, although they tend to be consumed in smaller quantity than meat or eggs and therefore their cholesterol content is considered somewhat less detrimental.

The addition of nonfat milk solids to many foods, including yogurt and liquid milks, can greatly increase the nutritive value of these products. Nonfat milk powder in the dry form can be added to grains in baking or to cream soups, sauces, and puddings to elevate their nutritional value.

Dairy desserts reflect the food value of their basic component (heavy cream, light cream, whole milk, skim milk, etc.) plus added sugar, thickeners, and flavorings. Fat content varies accordingly. While generally high in carbohydrates and calories, they do offer nutritive rewards for this expenditure.

How to Use the Table

• With the exception of cheese, milk products are seldom bought by weight. Therefore the nutritive value of milk and most dairy products is expressed in terms of 1 cup (8 fluid ounces).
• Cheese, however, is commonly purchased in pound units. The weight of a cheese is always given on the package, but when you do not have access to a label use the common measures provided in the table. In general, an average slice of cheese weighs one ounce.

3. MILK AND DAIRY PRODUCTS

Food	Measure	Calories	Protein Gm	Total Fat Gm	Saturated Fat Gm	Linoleic Acid Gm*	Cholesterol Mg	Carbohydrate Gm	Calcium Mg	Iron Mg	Sodium Mg	Potassium Mg	A IU	Thiamine Mg	Riboflavin Mg	Niacin Mg	C Mg
Buttermilk	1 cup	88	8.8	.2				12	296	.1	318	343	10	.10	.44	.2	2
Cheese, natural																	
Bleu or Roquefort	1 lb	1,669	97.5	138.3	80	4		9.1	1,429	2.3	—	—	5,620	.12	2.77	5.4	0
	1 oz	104	6	8.6	5	tr.		1	89	.1	—	—	350	.01	.17	.3	0
	1 cubic inch	62	3.6	5.2	3	tr.		tr.	53	.1	—	—	210	tr.	.10	.2	0
Brick	1 lb	1,678	100.7	138.3	80	4		8.6	3,311	4.1	—	—	5,620		2.06	.5	0
	1 oz	105	6.3	8.6	5	tr.		.5	207	.3	—	—	350		.13	tr.	0
	1 cubic inch	63	3.8	5.2	3	tr.		tr.	124	.2	—	—	210		.08	.1	0
Camembert	1 lb	1,356	79.4	112.0				8.2	476	2.3	—	503	4,580	.18	3.42	3.6	0
	1 oz	85	5	7				.5	30	.1	—	31	290	.01	.21	.2	0
	1 wedge; 3 per 4-oz pkg	113	6.6	9.4				.7	40	.2	—	42	380	.02	.29	.3	0
Cheddar	1 lb	1,805	113.4	146.1	80	4	455	9.5	3,402	4.5	3,175	372	5,940	.02	2.07	.3	0
	1 oz	113	7.1	9.1	5	tr.	30	.6	213	.3	198	23	370	.01	.13	tr.	0
	1 cubic inch	68	4.2	5.5	3	tr.	20	.4	127	.2	119	14	220	tr.	.08	tr.	0
	½ cup grated	226	14.2	18.2			55	1.2	426	.6	396	46	740	.02	.26	.5	0
Cottage, creamed	1 lb	481	61.7	19.1	10	1	70	13.2	426	1.4	1,039	386	770	.13	1.12	.3	0
	1 cup	259	33.3	10.1	5	tr.	40	7.1	230	.8	560	208	420	.07	.60	.2	0
Cottage, uncreamed	1 lb	390	77.1	1.4			50	12.2	408	1.8	1,315	327	50	.14	1.27	.5	0
	1 cup	172	33.9	.6			20	5.4	180	.8	579	144	20	.06	.56	.2	0
Cream	1 lb	1,696	36.3	171.0	94	5	545	9.5	281	.9	1,134	336	6,990	.07	1.10	.5	0
	3-oz pkg	318	6.8	32.0	18	1	100	1.8	53	.2	213	63	1,310	.07	.21	.1	0
	1 T	53	1.1	5.3	3	tr.	20	tr.	2	tr.	7	2	40	tr.	.01	tr.	0

*Linoleic acid is unsaturated fat.

3. MILK AND DAIRY PRODUCTS (cont.)

Food	Measure	Calories	Protein Gm	Total Fat Gm	Satu-rated Fat Gm	Lino-leic* Acid Gm	Choles-terol Mg	Carbo-hydrate Gm	Cal-cium Mg	Iron Mg	Sodium Mg	Potas-sium Mg	A IU	Thi-amine Mg	Ribo-flavin Mg	Nia-cin Mg	C Mg
Cheese, natural																	
Limburger	1 lb	1,565	96.2	127.0				10.0	2,676	2.7	—	—	5,170	.36	2.27	.7	0
	1 oz	98	6.0	7.9				.6	167	.2	—	—	320	.02	.14	tr.	0
Parmesan	1 lb	1,783	163.3	117.9				13.2	5,171	1.8	3,329	676	4,810	.09	3.31	1.0	0
	½ cup grated, packed	275	25.2	18.2				2.0	797	.3	513	104	740	.01	.51	.2	0
	1 T, grated	20	1.8	1.3				tr.	57	tr.	37	7	50	tr.	.04	tr.	0
Swiss	1 lb	1,678	124.7	127.0	70	4	385	7.7	4,196	4.1	3,221	472	5,170	.03	1.81	.2	0
	1 oz	105	7.8	7.9	4	tr.	30	.5	262	.3	201	30	320	tr.	.11	tr.	0
	½ cup grated	210	15.6	15.8	8	tr.	50	1.0	524	.6	402	60	640	tr.	.22	tr.	0
Cheese, pasteurized process																	
American	1 lb	1,678	105.2	136.1	80	4	385	8.6	3,162	4.1	5,153	363	5,530	.07	1.85	.1	0
	1 slice (16/lb)	105	6.6	8.5	5	tr.	30	.5	198	.3	322	23	350	tr.	.12	tr.	0
Swiss	1 lb	1,610	119.8	122.0	70	4	385	7.3	4,023	4.1	5,294	454	4,990	.03	1.81	.2	0
	1 slice (16/lb)	101	7.5	7.6	4	tr.	30	.5	251	.3	331	28	312	tr.	.11	tr.	0
Pasteurized, process cheese food	1 lb	1,465	89.8	108.9				32.2	2,586	3.6	—	—	4,450	.11	2.62	.7	0
	1 oz	92	5.6	6.8				2.0	162	.2	—	—	280	tr.	.16	tr.	0
	1 cubic inch	58	3.6	4.3				1.3	102	.1	—	—	180	tr.	.10	tr.	0
Pasteurized process cheese spread	1 lb	1,306	72.6	97.1			295	37.2	2,563	2.7	7,371	1,089	3,950	.05	2.47	.6	0
	1 oz	82	4.5	6.1			20	2.3	160	.2	461	68	250	tr.	.15	tr.	0
	2 T	100	5.6	7.5			25	2.9	197	.2	568	84	300	tr.	.19	tr.	0
Cream, half and half	1 cup	324	7.7	28.3	15	1		11.1	261	.1	111	312	1,160	.07	.39	.2	2
	1 T	20	.5	1.8	1	tr.		.7	16	tr.	7	19	70	tr.	.02	tr.	tr.

*Linoleic acid is unsaturated fat.

3. MILK AND DAIRY PRODUCTS (cont.)

Food	Measure	Calories	Protein Gm	Total Fat Gm	Saturated Fat Gm	Lino-leic* Acid Gm	Oleic Acid Gm	Choles-terol Mg	Carbo-hydrate Gm	Calcium Mg	Iron Mg	Sodium Mg	Potassium Mg	A IU	Thiamine Mg	Ribo-flavin Mg	Niacin Mg	C Mg
Cream, light	1 cup	506	7.2	49.2	26	1			10.3	245	.1	103	293	2,020	.07	.36	.2	2
	1 T	32	.5	3.1	2	tr.			.6	15	tr.	6	18	130	tr.	.02	tr.	tr.
Cream, heavy (whipping)	1 cup	838	5.2	89.5	50	3			7.4	179	.1	76	212	3,660	.05	.26	.1	2
	1 T	53	.3	5.6	3	tr.			.5	11	tr.	5	13	230	tr.	.02	tr.	tr.
Cream, sour	1 cup	485	7	47	26	1			10	235	.1	—	—	1,930	.07	.35	.1	2
Cream substitute, powdered contains skim milk and lactose	1 t	10	tr.	.6					1.1	10	tr.		—	10	tr.			—
contains skim milk, lactose and sodium hexametaphosphate	1 t	10	tr.	.5					1.2	2	tr.	11	—	20	tr.	.02	tr.	—
Custard, baked	1 cup	305	14.3	14.6	7	1			29.4	297	1.1	209	387	930	.11	.50	.3	1
Ice cream, 10% fat	1 cup	257	6.0	14.1	8	tr.		60	27.6	194	.1	84	248	590	.05	.28	.1	1
Ice cream, 16% fat	1 cup	329	3.8	23.8	13	1		65	29.3	115	tr.	49	141	980	.03	.16	.1	1
Ice milk	1 cup	199	6.3	6.7	4	tr.			26.6	204	.1	89	255	280	.07	.29	.1	1
Milk, whole, 3.5% fat	1 cup	159	8.5	8.5	5	tr.		25	12	288	.1	122	351	340	.07	.41	.2	2
Milk, skim	1 cup	88	8.8	.2					12.5	296	.1	127	355	10	.09	.44	.2	2
Milk, partially skimmed	1 cup	145	10.3	4.9	3	tr.		5	14.8	352	.2	150	430	200	.10	.52	.2	2
Milk, canned, evaporated, undiluted	1 cup	345	17.6	19.9	10	1			24.4	635	.3	297	764	810	.10	.86	.5	3
Milk, canned, condensed, sweetened, undiluted	1 cup	982	24.8	26.6	15	1			166.2	802	.3	343	961	1,100	.24	1.16	.6	3

*Linoleic acid is unsaturated fat.

3. MILK AND DAIRY PRODUCTS (cont.)

Food	Measure	Calories	Protein Gm	Total Fat Gm	Saturated Fat Gm	Linoleic* Acid Gm	Cholesterol Mg	Carbohydrate Gm	Calcium Mg	Iron Mg	Sodium Mg	Potassium Mg	Vitamins A IU	Thiamine Mg	Riboflavin Mg	Niacin Mg	C Mg
Milk, instant, nonfat dry†	3.2 oz (1-qt. envelope)	326	32.5	.6				46.8	1,173	.5	477	1,565	30	.32	1.61	.8	6
low-density, 1⅓ cups per quart	1 cup (dry)	244	24.4	.5				35.1	880	.4	358	1,174	20	.24	1.21	.6	5
	1 T	15	1.5	tr.				2.2	55	tr.	22	73	tr.	.02	.08	tr.	tr.
high-density, ⅞ cup per quart	1 cup (dry)	372	37.1	.7				53.5	1,341	.6	545	1,789	30	.36	1.84	.9	7
	1 T	23	2.3	tr.				3.3	84	tr.	34	112	tr.	.02	.12	.1	tr.
Milk, regular, nonfat dry† ¾ cup per quart	1 cup (dry)	412	40.7	.9				59.3	1,483	.7	603	1,979	30	.40	2.04	1.0	8
	1 T	26	2.5	tr.				3.7	93	tr.	38	124	tr.	.03	.13	.1	tr.
Milk, goat	1 cup	164	7.8	9.8	5	tr.		11.2	315	.2	83	439	390	.10	.27	.7	2
Milk, human	3½ oz	77	1.1	4.0	2	tr.		9.5	33	.1	16	51	240	.01	.04	.2	5
Milk drinks																	
Malted milk, dry powder†	1 oz (3 heaping t)	115	4.1	2.3				19.8	81	.6	123	202	290	.09	.15	.1	0
Malted milk, beverage	1 cup	244	11.0	10.3				27.5	317	.7	214	470	590	.14	.49	.2	2
Chocolate drink (skim-milk)	1 cup	190	8.3	5.8	3	tr.		27.3	270	.5	115	355	200	.10	.40	.3	3
Chocolate drink (whole-milk)	1 cup	213	8.5	8.5	7	tr.		27.5	278	.5	118	365	330	.08	.40	.3	3
Cocoa	1 cup	243	9.5	11.5				27.3	295	1.0	128	363	400	.10	.45	.5	3
Pudding, chocolate, cornstarch	1 cup	385	8.1	12.2	8	tr.		66.8	250	1.3	146	445	390	.05	.36	.3	1
Pudding, vanilla, cornstarch	1 cup	283	8.9	9.9	5	tr.		40.5	298	tr.	166	352	410	.08	.41	.3	2
Pudding mix—see Miscellaneous																	

*Linoleic acid is unsaturated fat.
†Values apply to unfortified product.

3. MILK AND DAIRY PRODUCTS (cont.)

Food	Measure	Calories	Protein Gm	Total Fat Gm	Saturated Fat Gm	Lino-leic* Acid Gm	Choles-terol Mg	Car-bohy-drate Gm	Cal-cium Mg	Iron Mg	Sodium Mg	Potas-sium Mg	Vitamins A IU	Thi-amine Mg	Ribo-flavin Mg	Nia-cin Mg	C Mg
Whey, fluid	1 cup	63	2.2	.8				12.4	124	.3			30	.08	.35	.2	—
Whey, dried	1 lb	1,583	58.5	5.0				333.4	2,930	6.4			230	2.26	11.39	3.6	—
	½ cup	322	11.9	1.0				67.7	595	1.3			50	.46	2.31	.7	—
Yogurt, partially skim-milk (plain)	1 cup	123	8.3	4.2	2	tr.		12.7	294	tr.	125	350	170	.10	.44	.2	2
Yogurt, whole-milk (plain)	1 cup	152	7.4	8.3	5	tr.		12.0	272	tr.	115	323	340	.07	.39	.2	2

*Linoleic acid is unsaturated fat.

4. FRUIT AND FRUIT PRODUCTS

Fruits are among the few food products that need no preparation before they can be eaten; they are most delicious just as they come from the tree or vine. This is not to say that they are always, or even often, consumed in this manner, and the very fact that fruits are frequently stored, canned, frozen, dried, or cooked before they reach us brings many changes in their inherent nutritive value.

The line of demarcation between a fruit and a vegetable is thin, but technically speaking a fruit is considered the "succulent product of a perennial or woody plant, consisting of the ripened seeds and adjacent tissues," while a vegetable is the "stem, leaves, or root of the plant." Following this definition, both avocados and tomatoes fall into the category of fruits, but since most people consider them vegetables, they are evaluated in the next table, Vegetables and Vegetable Products.

The word *fruit* immediately brings to mind vitamin C, and indeed all fruits contain some amount of this vitamin. Oranges, grapefruits, tangerines, lemons, cantaloupes, papayas, and strawberries head the list of vitamin-C-rich fruits, but noteworthy amounts of this vitamin are obtained from most berries, fresh apricots, watermelon, pineapple, and bananas too.

Vitamin A is the second essential vitamin in fruits; actually it exists in the provitamin form, known as carotene, which is later converted to vitamin A in the body. Apricots and cantaloupes are noted for their vitamin-A value, while lesser amounts are found in a variety of other fruits.

Dried fruits are important for their iron content; citrus fruits, cantaloupes, bananas, and apricots provide the highest potential for potassium in the diet; and vitamin B_6 and magnesium (which are not represented in the table) are contributed by bananas and prunes.

Although certain fruits have been cited for their high nutritive content, all fruits offer an assortment of vitamins, minerals, and enzymes which make them important in meal planning. In addition, fruits add water and roughage to the diet making them a great aid in elimination.

You should realize that the vitamin and mineral values expressed here for fruits represent an average sampling. These food values are subject to variation depending on handling, length of storage, exposure to light, heat, even on the soil in which they were grown. Vitamin C in particular is highly unstable and exposure to air and heat rapidly reduces the vitamin-C content in foods. Fruit held for any length of time after cutting will contain much less of this vitamin than the table indicates. Since you can't depend on exact numbers, you should use the table to help pinpoint those fruits with the highest potential for vitamins and minerals. You can maximize your nutrient intake by eating fruit raw, as fresh as possible, and consuming more than the recommended amount of a nutrient to compensate for storage dissipation, cooking loss, and low vitamin content from improper ripening. Cold storage also helps preserve vitamin levels.

Despite the fact that they are rich in natural sugars, most-fruits, when unsweetened, are low in calories. Fruits contain no fat and have little protein significance in our diets.

Prepared fruit products, including canned fruits and many fruit juices, may have sugar added—greatly increasing their calorie content. The heavier the syrup the more sugar (and carbohydrates and calories) in the product. In the case of canned fruits, much of the vitamin-C value is in the liquid rather than the fruit and, of course, the heat of the canning process makes these less reliable as a source of vitamin C than the fresh fruits they are derived from. Natural enzymes are also destroyed by heat processing.

Frozen fruits and fruit juices contain most of the original nutrient value of their fresh form. However, once they begin to defrost, vitamin content dissipates.

How to Use the Table

You will need to know the weight of a piece or a portion of fruit in order to determine its nutritional make-up. Here a small kitchen scale will be a great aid. When you purchase fruit by the pound, dividing by the number of individual units will also give you a fairly good idea of the weight of each portion.

• When you cannot actually weigh out servings, however, use the values in the table for the average fruit portions that are included, making necessary adjustments if obvious differences are noticeable. For example, if you have consumed a particularly large banana you might consider it to be 1½ times the medium-size (6-inch) fruit shown here.

• Canned and frozen fruits always show the weight of contents on the package label and if you know how much of the contents you ate you can figure the value in terms of weight. When you do not know weight, use the figures in the table based on volume (cups). Both the fruit and the accompanying liquid are included in these measures unless otherwise noted, and values are given for water-packed varieties and those canned in heavy syrup. The main difference is in terms of calories and carbohydrates; fruits packed in light or medium syrup lie somewhere in between.

• Dried fruits are calculated in terms of pounds and either individual pieces or cup measures.

• Fruit juices are tabulated by the cup (8 fluid ounces).

• A limited selection of other fruit products is found in this table, i.e., apple sauce, cranberry sauce. Fruit jams and jellies are so dependent on sugar and vitamin-destructive cooking in their preparation that they are included in the table of Sugar and Sweets. Dessert items baked with fruits, like fruit pies and cakes, are listed in the table of Flour, Cereal Grains, and Grain Products.

4. FRUIT AND FRUIT PRODUCTS

Food	Measure	Calories	Protein Gm	Total Fat Gm	Saturated Fat Gm	Linoleic* Acid Gm	Cholesterol Mg	Carbohydrate Gm	Minerals				Vitamins				
									Calcium Mg	Iron Mg	Sodium Mg	Potassium Mg	A IU	Thiamine Mg	Riboflavin Mg	Niacin Mg	C Mg
Apples	1 lb	242	.8	2.5				60.5	29	1.3	4	459	380	.12	.08	.3	16
	1 med (2½")	80	.3	.8				20.0	10	.4	1	152	130	.04	.03	.1	5
Apples, dried	1 lb	1,247	4.5	7.3				325.7	141	7.3	23	2,581	—	.26	.53	2.3	48
	½ cup	136	.5	.8				35.6	15	.8	3	283	—	.03	.06	.3	5
Apple butter	1 T	33	.1	.1				8.3	3	.1	tr.	45	0	tr.	tr.	tr.	tr.
Apple juice	1 cup	117	.3	tr.				29.7	15	1.5	3	252	—	.02	.04	.2	2
Apple sauce, unsweetened	1 lb	186	.9	.3				49.0	18	2.3	9	354	180	.08	.05	.2	5
	½ cup	52	.3	.1				13.7	5	.6	3	99	50	.02	.01	.1	1
Apple sauce, sweetened	1 lb	413	.4	.5				108.0	18	2.3	9	295	180	.08	.05	.2	5
	½ cup	111	.1	.1				29.0	5	.6	2	79	50	.02	.01	.1	1
Apricots	1 lb	217	4.3	.9				54.6	72	2.1	4	1,198	11,510	.14	.16	2.6	42
	1 med (12/lb)	18	.4	.1				4.4	6	.2	tr.	98	940	.01	.01	.2	3
Apricots, canned, water pack	1 lb	172	3.2	.5				43.5	54	1.4	5	1,116	8,310	.09	.10	1.7	18
	½ cup	45	.8	.1				11.5	14	.4	1	295	2,190	.02	.03	.4	5
Apricots, canned, heavy syrup	1 lb	390	2.7	.5				99.8	50	1.4	5	1,061	7,920	.08	.10	1.6	17
	½ cup	111	.8	.1				28.4	14	.4	1	302	2,260	.03	.03	.5	5
Apricots, dried	1 lb	1,179	22.7	2.3				301.6	304	24.9	118	4,441	49,440	.06	.71	14.9	57
	½ cup (20 halves)	195	3.7	.4				49.8	50	4.1	19	733	8,160	.01	.02	2.5	9
Apricot nectar	1 cup	143	.8	.3				36.6	23	.5	tr.	378	2,380	.03	.03	.5	7
Bananas	1 lb	262	3.4	.6				68.5	25	2.2	3	1,141	590	.14	.18	2.2	31
	1 med (8¾")	101	1.3	.2				26.4	10	.6	1	439	230	.05	.07	.8	12
Banana flakes	1 lb	1,542	20.0	3.0				401.9	145	12.7	18	6,700	3,450	.82	1.07	12.7	29
	½ cup	170	2.2	.4				44.2	16	1.4	4	737	380	.09	.12	1.4	3
Blackberries	1 lb	250	5.2	3.9				55.6	138	3.9	4	733	860	.14	.18	1.6	90
	½ cup	40	.8	.6				8.8	22	.6	1	116	140	.02	.03	.3	14
Blackberries, canned, water pack	1 lb	181	3.6	2.7				40.8	100	2.7	5	522	610	.07	.09	1.0	32
	½ cup	48	1.0	.7				10.8	26	.7	1	138	161	.02	.02	.3	8

*Linoleic acid is unsaturated fat.

4. FRUIT AND FRUIT PRODUCTS (cont.)

Food	Measure	Calories	Protein Gm	Total Fat Gm	Saturated Fat Gm	Linoleic* Acid Gm	Cholesterol Mg	Carbohydrate Gm	Calcium Mg	Iron Mg	Sodium Mg	Potassium Mg	A IU	Thiamine Mg	Riboflavin Mg	Niacin Mg	C Mg
Blackberries, canned, heavy syrup	1 lb	413	3.6	2.7				100.7	95	2.7	5	494	580	.06	.09	1.0	30
	½ cup	118	1.0	.8				28.7	27	.8	1	141	170	.02	.03	.3	9
Blueberries	1 lb	259	2.9	2.1				63.8	63	4.2	4	338	420	.13	.25	1.9	58
	½ cup	40	.4	.3				9.8	10	.6	1	52	60	.02	.04	.3	9
Blueberries, canned, water pack	1 lb	177	2.3	.9				44.5	45	3.2	5	272	180	.06	.07	.9	30
	½ cup	44	.6	.2				11.0	11	.8	1	67	44	.01	.02	.2	7
Blueberries, frozen, unsweetened	1 lb	249	3.2	2.3				61.7	45	3.6	5	367	320	.14	.27	2.1	33
	½ cup	44	.6	.4				10.9	8	.6	5	65	60	.02	.05	.4	6
Breadfruit	1 lb	360	5.9	1.0				91.5	115	4.2	52	1,533	150	.39	.12	3.1	101
Cherries, sour	1 lb	213	4.4	1.1				52.5	81	1.5	7	702	3,670	.18	.22	1.5	37
	½ cup	40	.8	.2				9.8	15	.3	1	131	690	.03	.04	.3	7
Cherries, sour, pitted, canned, water pack	1 lb	196	3.6	.9				48.5	68	1.4	9	590	3,090	.13	.11	.8	23
	½ cup	53	1.0	.2				13.0	18	.4	2	158	830	.03	.03	.2	6
Cherries, sour, pitted, canned, heavy syrup	1 lb	404	3.6	.9				103.0	64	1.4	5	562	2,940	.13	.10	.7	22
	½ cup	107	1.0	.2				27.2	17	.4	1	148	780	.03	.03	.2	6
Cherries, sweet	1 lb	286	5.3	1.2				71.0	90	1.6	8	780	450	.20	.24	1.7	41
	½ cup	54	1.0	.2				13.3	17	.3	1	146	80	.04	.04	.3	8
Cherries, sweet, canned, pitted, water pack	1 lb	218	4.1	.9				54.0	68	1.4	5	590	260	.09	.11	.8	15
	½ cup	60	1.1	.2				14.9	19	.4	1	162	70	.02	.03	.2	4
Cherries, sweet, canned, pitted, heavy syrup	1 lb	367	4.1	.9				93.0	59	1.4	5	572	250	.09	.11	.7	15
	½ cup	103	1.2	.3				26.2	17	.4	1	161	70	.03	.03	.2	4
Cherries, maraschino	1 lb	526	.9	.9				133.4	—	—	—	—	—	—	—	—	—
	1	7	tr.	tr.													
Crabapples	1 lb	284	1.7	1.3				74.3	25	1.3	4	459	150	.12	.08	.3	33

*Linoleic acid is unsaturated fat.

4. FRUIT AND FRUIT PRODUCTS (cont.)

Food	Measure	Calories	Protein Gm	Total Fat Gm	Saturated Fat Gm	Lino-leic* Acid Gm	Cholesterol Mg	Carbohydrate Gm	Calcium Mg	Iron Mg	Sodium Mg	Potassium Mg	A IU	Thiamine Mg	Riboflavin Mg	Niacin Mg	C Mg
Cranberries	1 lb	200	1.7	3.0				47.0	61	2.2	9	357	190	.13	.09	.4	47
Cranberry juice cocktail	1 cup	50	.3	.3				11.7	15	.8	2	89	50	.03	.02	.1	12†
Cranberry sauce, canned	1 lb	162	.5	.9				41.2	13	.8	3	25	tr.	.02	.02	.2	100†
Currants, red or white	½ cup	202	.2	.3				170.1	27	.3	5	136	70	.05	.05	.2	8
	1 lb	220	6.2	.9				51.8	141	4.4	2	41	20	.02	.22	.6	182
	½ cup	34	1.0	.1				53.2	22	.7	1	177	530	.18	.03	.1	28
Dates, dry, with pits	1 lb	1,081	8.7	2.0				287.7	233	11.8	4	2,557	80	.35	.38	8.6	0
Dates, dry, pitted	1 lb	1,243	10.0	2.3				330.7	268	13.6	5	2,939	200	.40	.44	9.9	0
	½ cup	244	2.0	.5				64.8	52	2.7	1	576	230	.08	.09	1.9	0
Figs	1 lb	363	5.4	1.4				92.1	159	2.7	6	880	360	.29	.24	1.9	7
	1 1½" diam.	30	.4	.1				7.5	13	.2	1	72	30	.02	.02	.2	1
Figs, canned, water pack	1 lb	218	2.3	.9				56.2	64	1.8	9	703	150	.15	.15	1.1	3
	½ cup	58	.6	.2				14.8	17	.5	2	186	40	.04	.04	.3	1
Figs, canned, heavy syrup	1 lb	381	2.3	.6				98.9	59	1.8	9	676	150	.15	.15	1.1	2
	½ cup	101	.6	.2				26.1	16	.5	2	179	40	.04	.04	.3	tr.
Figs, dried	1 lb	1,243	19.5	5.9				313.4	572	13.6	154	2,903	360	.47	.47	3.2	0
	1 lge (2"x1")	57	.9	.3				14.5	26	.6	7	134	20	.02	.02	.1	0
	½ cup	233	3.7	1.1				58.8	107	2.5	29	544	70	.09	.09	.6	0
Fruit cocktail, canned, water pack	1 lb	168	1.8	.5				44.0	41	1.8	23	762	670	.07	.05	2.1	10
	½ cup	44	.5	.1				11.6	11	.5	6	201	180	.02	.01	.6	3
Fruit cocktail, canned, heavy syrup	1 lb	345	1.8	.5				89.4	41	1.8	23	730	640	.07	.05	2.0	9
	½ cup	97	.5	.1				25.2	11	.5	6	206	180	.02	.01	.6	3
Gooseberries, canned, water pack	1 lb	118	2.3	.5				29.9	54	1.4	5	476	900	—	—	—	50

*Linoleic acid is unsaturated fat.
†Ascorbic acid added.

4. FRUIT AND FRUIT PRODUCTS (cont.)

Food	Measure	Calories	Protein Gm	Total Fat Gm	Saturated Fat Gm	Lino-leic Acid* Gm	Cholesterol Mg	Carbohydrate Gm	Calcium Mg	Iron Mg	Sodium Mg	Potassium Mg	A IU	Thiamine Mg	Riboflavin Mg	Niacin Mg	C Mg
Gooseberries, canned, heavy syrup	1 lb	408	2.3	.5				104.3	50	1.4	5	445	840	—	—	—	47
Grapefruit	1 lb	91	1.1	.2				23.6	36	.9	2	300	180	.08	.04	.4	84
	½ med (3¾")	48	.6	.1				12.5	19	.5	1	159	100	.04	.02	.2	45
Grapefruit segments, canned, water pack	1 lb	136	2.7	.5				34.5	59	1.4	18	653	50	.13	.08	.9	137
	½ cup	37	.7	.1				9.3	16	.4	5	175	10	.03	.02	.2	37
Grapefruit segments, canned, syrup pack	1 lb	318	2.7	.5				80.7	59	1.4	5	612	50	.13	.08	.9	137
	½ cup	89	.8	.1				22.6	16	.4	1	171	10	.04	.02	.2	38
Grapefruit juice, fresh	1 cup	96	1.2	.3				22.6	22	.5	2	398	30†	.09	.04	.4	93
Grapefruit juice, canned, unsweetened	1 cup	101	1.2	.3				24.2	20	1.0	3	400	30	.07	.04	.4	84
Grapefruit juice, canned, sweetened	1 cup	132	1.3	.3				32.0	20	1.0	3	404	30	.07	.04	.4	78
Grapefruit juice, frozen concentrate, unsweetened	1 can (6 oz)	300	3.9	.8				71.5	70	.8	8	1,248	60	.29	.12	1.4	285
diluted with 3 parts water	1 cup	101	1.2	.2				24.2	24	.2	2	420	20	.10	.05	.5	96
Grapefruit juice, frozen concentrate, sweetened	1 can (6 oz)	349	3.4	.7				85.0	59	.7	7	1,075	50	.25	.11	1.2	245
diluted with 3 parts water	1 cup	116	1.0	.2				28.2	20	.2	2	356	20	.07	.02	.5	82
Grapefruit and orange juice, canned, unsweetened	1 cup	106	1.5	.5				24.9	24	.8	3	454	240	.13	.04	.5	84
Grapes, American‡	1 lb	197	3.7	2.9				44.9	46	1.1	9	452	290	.15	.08	.7	10
	¼ cup	33	.6	.5				7.6	8	.2	2	76	50	.03	.01	.1	2
Grapes, European§	1 lb	270	2.4	1.2				69.8	48	1.6	12	698	400	.21	.11	1.0	18
	½ cup	48	.4	.2				12.3	8	.3	2	123	70	.04	.02	.2	3

*Linoleic acid is unsaturated fat.
†For white-fleshed varieties; juice from red-fleshed grapefruit contains 1,080 IU per cup.
‡As Concord, Delaware, Niagara, and Catawba.
§As Malaga, Muscat, Thompson Seedless, Emperor, and Tokay.

4. FRUIT AND FRUIT PRODUCTS (cont.)

Food	Measure	Calories	Protein Gm	Total Fat Gm	Saturated Fat Gm	Oleic Acid Gm	Linoleic* Acid Gm	Cholesterol Mg	Carbohydrate Gm	Calcium Mg	Iron Mg	Sodium Mg	Potassium Mg	A IU	Thiamine Mg	Riboflavin Mg	Niacin Mg	C Mg
Grape juice, canned or bottled	1 cup	166	.5	tr.					41.9	28	.8	5	293	—	.10	.06	.6	tr.
Grape juice, frozen concentrate, sweetened	1 can (6 oz)	395	1.3	tr.					99.8	21	.9	7	254	40	.14	.20	1.5	32
diluted with 3 parts water	1 cup	135	.5	tr.					33.3	8	.3	3	85	10	.05	.08	.5	10
Grape juice drink	1 cup	135	.5	tr.					34.4	8	.3	3	87	tr.	.03	.03	.3	40†
Guava	1 lb	273	3.5	2.6					66.0	101	4.0	18	1,272	1,230	.23	.21	5.1	1,065
Guava	1 med	48	.6	.5					11.6	18	.7	3	223	220	.04	.04	.9	186
Lemon	1 lb	90	3.3	.9					24.9	79	1.8	6	419	50	.13	.06	.4	161
Lemon	1 2⅜" diam.	22	.8	.2					6.0	19	.4	1	101	10	.03	.01	.2	39
Lemon juice, fresh	1 cup	61	1.2	.5					19.5	17	.5	2	344	50	.07	.03	.2	112
Lemon juice, bottled	1 cup	56	1.0	.3					18.5	17	.5	3	344	40	.08	.03	.2	102
	1 T	3	tr.	tr.					1.1	1	tr.	tr.	20	tr.	tr.	tr.	tr.	6
Lemonade, frozen concentrate	1 can (6 oz)	427	.4	.2					111.7	9	.4	4	153	40	.05	.06	.7	66
diluted with 4⅓ parts water	1 cup	109	.2	tr.					28.3	tr.	tr.	tr.	40	tr.	tr.	.02	.2	17
Lime	1 lb	107	2.7	.8					36.2	126	2.3	8	389	50	.10	.08	.7	141
Lime	2" diam.	16	.4	.1					5.4	19	.3	1	58	10	.02	.01	.1	21
Lime juice, fresh	1 cup	64	.7	.2					22.1	22	.5	2	256	20	.05	.02	.2	79
Lime juice, bottled	1 cup	64	.7	.2					22.1	22	.5	2	256	20	.05	.02	.2	52
	1 T	4	tr.	tr.					1.4	1	tr.	tr.	16	tr.	tr.	tr.	tr.	3
Limeade, frozen concentrate	1 can (6 oz)	409	.4	.2					108.2	11	.2	tr.	129	tr.	.02	.02	.2	26
diluted with 4⅓ parts water	1 cup	101	tr.	tr.					27.2	2	tr.	tr.	32	tr.	tr.	tr.	tr.	5
Lychees	1 lb	174	2.4	.8					44.6	22	1.1	8	463	—	tr.	.13	tr.	113
Lychees, dried	1 lb	578	7.9	2.5					147.6	69	3.5	6	2,296	—	—	—	—	—

*Linoleic acid is unsaturated fat.
†Ascorbic acid added.

4. FRUIT AND FRUIT PRODUCTS (cont.)

Food	Measure	Calories	Protein Gm	Total Fat Gm	Saturated Fat Gm	Oleic Acid Gm	Lino-leic* Acid Gm	Choles-terol Mg	Carbo-hydrate Gm	Calcium Mg	Iron Mg	Sodium Mg	Potassium Mg	A IU	Thiamine Mg	Ribo-flavin Mg	Niacin Mg	C Mg
Mangoes	1 lb	201	2.1	1.2					51.1	30	1.2	21	574	14,590	.16	.16	3.2	106
	½ cup diced	36	.4	.2					9.3	5	.2	4	104	2,650	.03	.03	.6	19
Melons																		
Cantaloupe	1 lb	68	1.6	.2					17.0	32	.9	27	569	7,710	.10	.07	1.4	74
	½ 5" melon	57	1.3	.2					14.2	27	.8	23	474	6,430	.08	.06	1.2	62
Casaba	1 lb	61	2.7	tr.					14.7	32	.9	27	569	70	.10	.07	1.4	29
	¾ 7" melon	52	2.3	tr.					12.6	27	.8	23	488	60	.09	.06	1.2	25
Honeydew	1 lb	94	2.3	.9					22.0	40	1.1	34	717	120	.13	.09	1.8	65
	⅙ 6" melon	58	1.4	.6					13.6	25	.7	21	442	70	.08	.06	1.1	40
Melon balls, frozen in syrup	1 lb	281	2.7	.5					71.2	45	1.4	41	853	6,990	.14	.09	2.3	73
	¾ cup	69	.7	.1					17.6	11	.3	10	210	1,720	.03	.02	.6	18
Nectarines	1 lb	267	2.5	tr.					71.4	17	2.1	25	1,227	6,890				54
	2" diam.	73	.7	tr.					19.6	5	.6	7	338	1,900				15
Oranges	1 lb	162	3.3	.7					40.4	136	1.3	3	662	660	.33	.13	1.3	166
	2⅝""	64	1.3	.2					16.0	54	.5	1	262	260	.13	.05	.5	66
Orange juice, fresh	1 cup	111	1.7	.5					25.8	27	.5	3	495	500	.22	.06	.9	124
Orange juice, canned, unsweetened	1 cup	119	2.0	.5					27.8	25	1.0	3	495	500	.18	.05	.7	99
Orange juice, frozen concentrate, unsweetened (6 oz)	1 can	337	4.9	.4					80.9	70	.9	4	1,399	1,510	.64	.11	2.6	337
diluted with 3 parts water	1 cup	112	1.7	.2					26.6	22	.2	2	463	500	.22	.02	.7	112
Orange juice, dehydrated crystals	1 lb (yields 1 gal. juice)	1,724	22.7	7.7					403.3	381	7.7	36	7,838	7,620	3.04	.95	13.3	1,628
	1 oz (yields 1 cup juice)	108	1.4	.5					25.2	24	.5	2	490	480	.19	.06	.8	102
Orange and apricot juice drink	1 cup	124	.8	.3					31.6	13	.3	tr.	233	1,440	.06	.03	.4	40†
	1 lb	119	1.8	.3					30.4	61	.9	9	711	5,320	.12	.13	.9	170
Papayas	1 cup diced	70	1.0	tr.					18.0	36	.5	—		3,190	.07	.08	.5	102

*Linoleic acid is unsaturated fat. †Ascorbic acid added.

4. FRUIT AND FRUIT PRODUCTS (cont.)

Food	Measure	Calories	Protein Gm	Total Fat Gm	Saturated Fat Gm	Lino-leic* Acid Gm	Cholesterol Mg	Carbohydrate Gm	Calcium Mg	Iron Mg	Sodium Mg	Potassium Mg	A IU	Thiamine Mg	Riboflavin Mg	Niacin Mg	C Mg
Peaches	1 lb	150	2.4	.4				38.3	36	2.0	4	797	5,250†	.07	.19	3.8	29
	1 2" diam.	38	.6	.1				9.6	9	.5	1	200	1,320†	.02	.05	1.0	7
Peaches, canned, water pack	1 lb	141	1.8	.5				36.7	18	1.4	9	621	2,040	.04	.11	2.6	14
	½ cup	38	.5	.1				9.9	5	.4	2	167	550	.01	.03	.7	4
Peaches, canned, heavy syrup	1 lb	354	1.8	.5				91.2	18	1.4	9	590	1,950	.04	.11	2.5	13
	¾ cup	100	.5	.1				25.8	5	.4	3	167	550	.01	.03	.7	4
Peaches, dried	1 lb	1,188	14.1	3.2				309.8	218	27.2	73	4,309	17,690	.05	.88	24.2	81
	½ cup	209	2.5	.6				54.6	38	4.8	13	759	3,120	.01	.16	4.3	14
Peaches, frozen, sliced, sweetened	1 piece (½ peach)	33	.4	.1				8.6	6	.8	2	120	490	tr.	.02	.7	2
Peach nectar	1 lb	399	1.8	.5				102.5	18	2.3	9	562	2,950	.05	.18	3.2	181‡
	½ cup	110	.5	.1				28.2	5	.6	2	155	810	.01	.05	.9	50‡
Pears	1 cup	120	.5	.1				30.9	10	.5	3	195	1,070	.03	.05	1.0	18
	1 lb	252	2.9	1.7				63.2	33	1.2	8	537	70	.09	.17	.6	7
	1 3"x2½"	101	1.2	.7				25.3	13	.5	5	215	30	.04	.07	.2	2
Pears, canned, water pack	1 lb	145	.2	.9				37.6	23	.9	5	399	tr.	.07	.09	.6	7
	½ cup	39	.2	.2				10.1	6	.2	1	108	tr.	.02	.02	.2	2
Pears, canned, heavy syrup	1 lb	345	.9	.9				88.9	23	.6	5	381	tr.	.01	.09	.6	6
	¾ cup	97	.3	.3				24.9	6	.3	1	107	tr.	.01	.03	.2	2
Pears, dried	1 lb	1,216	14.1	8.2				305.3	159	5.9	32	2,599	320	.05	.84	2.8	32
	1 piece (½ pear)	40	.5	tr.				10.2	5	.2	1	87	10	tr.	.03	.1	1
Pear nectar	1 cup	125	.7	.5				31.8	7	.3	3	94	tr.	tr.	.05	tr.	tr.
Persimmons, Japanese	1 lb	286	2.6	1.5				73.3	22	1.1	22	647	10,080	.11	.08	.4	41
	1 2½" diam.	79	.7	.4				20.2	6	.3	6	178	2,770	.03	.02	.1	11

*Linoleic acid is unsaturated fat.
†Based on yellow-fleshed varieties; for white-fleshed peaches value is 200 IU's per pound, or 50 per peach.
‡Ascorbic acid added.

4. FRUIT AND FRUIT PRODUCTS (cont.)

Food	Measure	Calories	Protein Gm	Total Fat Gm	Satu-rated Fat Gm	Lino-leic* Acid Gm	Choles-terol Mg	Car-bohy-drate Gm	Cal-cium Mg	Iron Mg	Sodium Mg	Potas-sium Mg	A IU	Thi-amine Mg	Ribo-flavin Mg	Nia-cin Mg	C Mg
Persimmons, native	1 lb	472	3.0	1.5				124.6	100	9.3	4	1,153	170	.21	.06	.6	246
Pineapple, with peel	1 lb	123	.9	.5				32.3	40	1.2	2	344	100	.12	.04	.3	40
peeled	1 cup diced	75	1.0	tr.				19.0	24	.7	—	—					24
Pineapple, canned, water pack	1 lb	177	1.4	.5				46.3	54	1.4	5	449	210	.36	.10	1.0	31
	½ cup	49	.4	.1				12.7	15	.4	1	123	60	.10	.03	.3	9
Pineapple, canned, juice pack	1 lb	263	1.8	.5				68.5	73	1.8	5	667	290	.44	.13	1.2	46
	½ cup	81	.6	.2				20.1	22	.6	2	204	90	.13	.04	.4	14
Pineapple, canned, heavy syrup	1 lb	336	1.4	.5				88.0	50	1.4	5	435	200	.35	.10	1.0	30
	½ cup crushed 2 sm or 1 lge slice with juice	96	.4	.1				25.2	14	.4	1	124	60	.10	.03	.3	9
Pineapple juice, canned, unsweetened	1 cup	136	1.0	.3				33.5	37	.8	3	370	130	.13	.04	.5	22
Pineapple juice, frozen concentrate, unsweetened (6 oz.)	1 can	387	2.8	.2				95.9	85	2.0	7	1,023	110	.50	.12	1.9	91
diluted with 3 parts water	1 cup	129	1.0	tr.				31.9	27	.7	2	339	20	.17	.05	.5	30
Pineapple and grapefruit juice drink	1 cup	135	.5	tr.				33.9	13	.5	tr.	155	30	.04	.02	.2	40
Pineapple and orange juice drink	1 cup	135	.5	.3				33.7	13	.5	tr.	175	130	.06	.02	.2	40
Plums, damson	1 lb	272	2.1	tr.				73.5	74	2.1	8	1,234	1,240	.33	.13	2.2	—
	1" diam.	34	.3	tr.				9.0	9	.3	1	152	150	.04	.02	.3	—
Plums, prune-type	1 lb	320	3.4	.9				84.0	51	2.1	4	725	1,280	.14	.14	2.3	17
	1 avg	20	.2	tr.				5.3	3	.1	tr.	45	1,280	.01	.01	.1	1
Plums, canned, greengage, water pack	1 lb	144	1.7	.4				37.5	39	.9	4	357	720	.06	.08	1.3	9

*Linoleic acid is unsaturated fat.

4. FRUIT AND FRUIT PRODUCTS (cont.)

Food	Measure	Calories	Protein Gm	Total Fat Gm	Saturated Fat Gm	Linoleic* Acid Gm	Cholesterol Mg	Carbohydrate Gm	Calcium Mg	Iron Mg	Sodium Mg	Potassium Mg	A IU	Thiamine Mg	Riboflavin Mg	Niacin Mg	C Mg
Plums, canned, purple, water pack	1 lb	200	1.7	.9				51.8	39	4.4	9	645	5,460	.10	.09	1.7	7
	½ cup	55	.5	.2				14.2	11	1.2	2	177	1,500	.03	.02	.5	2
Plums, canned, purple, heavy syrup	1 lb	361	1.7	.4				94.1	39	3.9	4	618	5,250	.10	.09	1.7	7
	½ cup	102	.5	.1				26.5	11	1.1	1	174	1,480	.03	.03	.5	2
Pomegranate	1 lb	160	1.3	.8				41.7	8	.8	8	658	tr.	.07	.07	.7	10
	4 oz pulp	72	.6	.3				18.6	3	.3	3	294	tr.	.03	.03	.3	5
Prunes, dried, large	1 lb	1,018	8.4	2.4				269.1	204	15.6	32	2,770	6,390	.35	.66	6.3	12
	1 large	20	.2	tr.				5.3	4	.3	1	55	130	.01	.01	.1	tr.
Prunes, dried, medium	1 lb	983	8.1	2.3				259.9	197	15.0	31	2,676	6,170	.34	.64	6.1	12
	1 medium	15	.1	tr.				4.0	3	.3	tr.	41	130	.01	.01	.1	tr.
Prunes, dried, small	1 lb	948	7.8	2.2				250.7	190	14.5	30	2,582	6,100	.33	.61	5.8	12
	1 small	10	.1	tr.				2.8	2	.2	tr.	28	70	tr.	.01	.1	tr.
Prune juice	1 cup	197	1.0	.3				48.6	36	10.5	5	601		.02	.03	1.1	4
Quince	1 lb	158	1.1	.3				42.3	30	1.9	11	545	110	.06	.04	1.1	40
	1 3"x2½"	83	.6	.2				22.3	16	1.0	6	288	60	.03	.04	.3	21
Raisins	1 lb	1,311	11.3	.9				351.1	281	15.9	122	3,461	100	.51	.37	2.4	5
	½ cup	238	2.1	.2				63.8	51	2.9	22	629	20	.09	.07	.4	1
	1½ T (½ oz)	40	.3	tr.				10.8	9	.5	4	107	tr.	.02	.01	.1	tr.
Raspberries, black	1 lb	321	6.6	6.2				69.1	132	4.0	4	876	tr.	.13	.40	4.0	81
	½ cup	49	1.1	1.0				11.3	22	.7	1	144	tr.	.02	.07	.7	13
Raspberries, red	1 lb	251	5.3	2.2				59.8	97	4.0	4	739	590	.13	.40	4.0	111
	½ cup	34	.7	.3				8.1	13	.5	1	100	80	.02	.05	.5	15
Raspberries, black, canned, water pack	1 lb	231	5.0	5.0				48.5	91	2.7	5	612	tr.	.06	.20	2.4	28
	½ cup	62	1.3	1.3				13.0	24	.7	1	164	tr.	.02	.05	.6	8
Raspberries, red, canned, water pack	1 lb	159	3.2	.5				39.9	68	2.7	5	517	410	.06	.20	2.4	39
	½ cup	43	.9	.1				10.7	18	.7	1	139	110	.02	.06	.6	10

*Linoleic acid is unsaturated fat.

4. FRUIT AND FRUIT PRODUCTS (cont.)

Food	Measure	Calories	Protein Gm	Total Fat Gm	Satu-rated Fat Gm	Lino-leic* Acid Gm	Choles-terol Mg	Carbo-hydrate Gm	Cal-cium Mg	Iron Mg	Sodium Mg	Potas-sium Mg	A IU	Thi-amine Mg	Ribo-flavin Mg	Nia-cin Mg	C Mg
Raspberries, red, frozen, sweetened	1 lb	445	3.2	.9				111.6	59	2.7	5	454	320	.09	.27	2.8	94
	½ cup	121	.9	.2				30.5	16	.7	1	124	90	.02	.07	.8	26
Rhubarb	1 lb	62	2.3	.4				14.4	374	3.1	8	979	390	.12	.26	1.2	34
	½ cup diced	9	.3	.1				2.0	51	.4	1	135	50	.02	.04	.2	5
Rhubarb, frozen, sweetened	1 lb	340	2.7	.9				83.9	422	3.6	18	957	380	.09	.23	1.0	34
	½ cup	83	.7	.2				20.5	103	.9	4	233	90	.02	.06	.2	8
Strawberries	1 lb	161	3.0	2.2				36.6	91	4.4	4	714	260	.12	.29	2.6	257
	½ cup	26	.5	.4				6.0	15	.7	1	117	40	.05	.05	.4	42
Strawberries, frozen, sweetened, sliced	1 lb	494	2.3	.9				126.1	64	3.2	5	508	150	.09	.27	2.4	240
	½ cup	136	.6	.2				34.7	18	.9	1	140	40	.02	.07	.7	66
Strawberries, frozen, sweetened, whole	1 lb	417	1.8	.9				106.6	59	2.7	5	472	150	.09	.27	2.3	249
	½ cup	110	.5	.2				28.2	16	.7	1	125	40	.02	.07	.6	66
Tamarinds	1 lb	520	6.1	1.3				136.1	161	6.1	111	1,700	70	.73	.05	2.7	3
Tangerines	1 lb	154	2.7	.7				38.9	134	1.3	7	423	1,410	.20	.07	.4	105
	1 2¾" diam.	39	.7	.2				9.9	34	.3	2	108	360	.05	.01	.1	27
Tangerine juice, fresh	1 cup	107	1.3	.5				25.1	45	.5	3	442	1,050	.15	.04	.3	78
Tangerine juice, frozen concentrate, unsweetened (6 oz)	1 can	341	3.6	1.5				80.6	130	1.5	4	1,291	3,070	.43	.12	.1	202
Tangerine juice, frozen diluted with 3 parts water	1 cup	115	1.2	.5				26.9	45	.5	2	433	1,020	.15	.15	.2	67
Watermelon	1 lb	54	1.0	.4				13.4	15	1.0	2	209	1,230	.06	.06	.3	15
	4"x8" wedge	110	2.0	.8				27.3	31	2.0	4	425	2,500	.12	.12	.6	31

*Linoleic acid is unsaturated fat.

5. VEGETABLES AND VEGETABLE PRODUCTS

We depend on vegetables for a wide assortment of vitamins and minerals. While each particular vegetable has its characteristic nutrient make-up, certain broad generalizations can be made.

Although calcium is most expediently drawn from milk and dairy products, considerable amounts of this mineral are found in dark leafy greens. Unfortunately not all of this calcium is available to our bodies since the presence of oxalic acid in these vegetables inhibits total calcium absorption. Other minerals plentiful in the dark leafy greens include magnesium (not on the table) and iron.

Potassium content of vegetables in general is high, while sodium levels are low; that is, until you consider the salt that is added to some frozen and almost all canned vegetables.

Another vegetable, seaweed (including kelp), is one of the rare food sources of iodine (not included in the table).

When it comes to vitamin contributions, dark leafy greens are again outstanding as a source of B vitamins (particularly the less popularized B_6 and folacin, plus riboflavin) and vitamin A. Orange root vegetables like carrots and sweet potatoes also contain appreciable amounts of vitamin A.

Seed vegetables like fresh beans and peas are similar to cereals in vitamin content, with exceptional thiamine and niacin values. Some amount of vitamin C is found in all vegetables; tomatoes, peppers, and the cabbage family are the most prominent examples.

Cauliflower, broccoli, and mushrooms deserve special mention as a source of the B vitamin complex.

While certain vegetables have been singled out here, in truth, all members of this food group play a significant role in fulfilling our requirement for vitamins, minerals, and trace minerals in particular.

As a further recommendation, vegetables are low on the relative scale of calories. Fruits, flowers, leaves, and stem vegetables provide very little fuel. Bulbs and tubers (which contain food storage for the entire plant) are somewhat higher in carbohydrates and energy value, but when compared to meats, grains, and legumes on a pound for pound basis these root vegetables are still sparing with calories. With the exception of avocados, vegetables contain almost no fat, and in the amounts they are generally eaten offer no real protein nourishment. Vegetables are largely water and fibre, both essential for proper elimination.

To obtain the most food value from vegetables they must be consumed raw, as close to harvest time as possible. The longer they are stored, the greater their vitamin loss.

The process of cooking vegetables produces the largest percentage of vitamin waste in our food supply. Only a few vegetables require heat to be edible, and mushrooms, cauliflower, broccoli, asparagus, zucchini, and spinach are all worth experiencing in their fresh, uncooked form. Thiamine and vitamin C are largely destroyed by heat, and other B vitamins and minerals dissolve in the cooking medium. For this reason any cooking fat or liquid should be served along with the meal or saved for soups or sauces. By using only enough liquid to prevent scorching, or by steaming vegetables and cooking them until barely tender this loss can be minimized. To conserve the vitamins left after the heat of canning be sure to use the liquid portion of the product. Freezing is a much more nutritious form of food processing, although some vitamin destruction comes from the blanching which precedes the cold storage. Once vegetables begin to defrost vitamins diminish rapidly. Never allow frozen vegetables to thaw during storage (purchase only solidly frozen packages) and cook them right from the freezer for maximum nutrition. The native enzymes in vegetables are all heat-sensitive and there is no way to preserve them during processing or cooking.

Aside from being sensitive to heat, vegetables are also affected by the way they are handled during preparation. Since vitamin C is destroyed by exposure to air it is best to prepare vegetables just before they are needed. Tearing greens with your hands rather than shredding them with a knife conserves vitamins, and even beans and asparagus fare better when trimmed by snapping instead of cutting. When you discard the peel or outer layer of a vegetable you throw away nutrients. Unless the skin is inedible or heavily waxed for appearance, peeling is an unnecessary chore. Corn should not be husked until cooking time. Baking soda, which keeps greens greener during cooking, destroys B vitamins. Only carrots truly benefit from rough handling; shredding of this vegetable breaks down the coarse fibers allowing vitamin A to be more readily absorbed.

How to Use the Table

• As with fruit, the most accurate way to determine the weight, and subsequently the nutritional make-up of a vegetable, is to use a scale. When you purchase a known weight of vegetables, dividing by the number of individual units will also give you a fairly good idea of the weight of each portion.

• When weight is unknown use the values for average size or measure per unit that is expressed beneath the pound breakdown in the table.

• All values for fresh vegetables refer to the raw food, including skin and stem ends commonly included in your purchase. In some places where it is important for your calculations the volume of cooked vegetable you obtain from the raw measure is given.

• For canned and frozen vegetables you can divide the number of servings you get into the weight that you find on the package label, or use the cup measures on the table. Unless otherwise mentioned, canned vegetables include an average amount of liquid along with the vegetable.

• If the label on a can of vegetables specifically says "no salt added" subtract 1,070 milligrams of sodium per pound.

• Vegetable juices are evaluated by the cup (8 fluid ounces).

5. VEGETABLES AND VEGETABLE PRODUCTS

Food	Measure	Calories	Protein Gm	Total Fat Gm	Saturated Fat Gm	Linoleic* Acid Gm	Cholesterol Mg	Carbohydrate Gm	Calcium Mg	Iron Mg	Sodium Mg	Potassium Mg	A IU	Thiamine Mg	Riboflavin Mg	Niacin Mg	C Mg
Artichoke, globe	1 lb	16-85†	5.3	.4				19.2	43	2.4	78	780	290	.14	.09	1.7	22
	1 lge (7 oz)	7-37	2.3	.2				8.5	19	1.1	34	341	130	.06	.04	.7	10
Asparagus	1 lb	66	6.4	.5				12.7	56	2.5	5	706	2,290	.46	.51	3.9	84
	4 spears	8	.7	tr.				1.5	6	.3	1	81	260	.05	.06	.4	10
Asparagus, canned spears, green	1 lb	82	8.6	1.4				13.2	82	7.7	1,070	753	2,310	.29	.42	3.7	68
	4 spears	11	1.1	.2				1.7	11	1.0	141	99	300	.04	.06	.5	9
Asparagus, canned spears, white	1 lb	82	7.3	1.4				15.0	68	4.1	1,070	635	230	.23	.26	3.2	68
	4 spears	11	1.0	.2				2.0	9	.5	141	84	30	.03	.03	.4	9
Asparagus, frozen spears	1 lb	109	15.0	.9				17.7	104	5.4	9	1,175	3,540	.82	.68	5.7	132
	4 spears	12	1.7	.1				2.0	12	.6	1	134	400	.09	.08	.7	15
Asparagus, frozen cuts and tips	1 lb	104	15.0	.9				16.3	104	5.9	9	1,084	3,860	.73	.64	5.3	114
	½ cup	21	3.1	.2				3.4	21	1.2	2	224	796	.15	.13	1.1	24
Avocado, California	1 lb	589	7.6	58.6	12	8		20.7	34	2.1	14	2,082	1,000	.37	.68	5.5	49
	1 med, 3⅛" diam.	368	4.8	36.6	8	5		12.9	21	1.3	9	1,301	630	.23	.43	3.4	31
Avocado, Florida	1 med, 3⅜" diam.	389	4.0	33.4	7	4		26.7	30	1.8	12	1,836	880	.33	.60	4.9	43
Bamboo shoots	1 lb	36	3.4	.4				6.8	20	.7	—	701	30	.19	.09	.8	5
Beans, lima, in shell	1 lb	223	15.2	.9				40.1	94	5.1	4	1,179	530	.43	.22	2.5	52
Beans, lima, shelled	1 cup	184	12.6	.8				33.1	78	4.2	3	973	440	.36	.18	2.1	43
Beans, lima, canned	1 lb	322	18.6	1.4				60.8	118	10.9	1,070	1,007	590	.16	.22	2.4	32
	½ cup	92	5.3	.4				17.4	34	3.1	306	288	170	.05	.06	.7	9
Beans, lima, frozen, Fordhook	1 lb	463	28.1	.5				88.5	104	8.6	585	2,223	1,040	.45	.27	5.4	101
	½ cup	87	5.3	.1				16.6	20	1.6	110	417	195	.08	.05	1.0	19

*Linoleic acid is unsaturated fat.
†Caloric values increase with storage.

5. VEGETABLES AND VEGETABLE PRODUCTS (cont.)

Food	Measure	Calories	Protein Gm	Total Fat Gm	Saturated Fat Gm	Lino-leic Acid Gm	Choles-terol Mg	Carbo-hydrate Gm	Minerals Calcium Mg	Iron Mg	Sodium Mg	Potas-sium Mg	Vitamins A IU	Thiamine Mg	Ribo-flavin Mg	Niacin Mg	C Mg
Beans, lima, frozen baby	1 lb	553	34.5	.9				104.3	172	12.7	667	1,987	1,000	.45	.27	5.6	85
	½ cup	104	6.5	.2				19.6	32	2.4	125	373	190	.08	.05	1.1	16
Beans, snap, green	1 lb	128	7.6	.8				28.3	224	3.2	28	970	2,400	.33	.42	2.0	76
	1 cup	32	1.9	.2				7.1	56	.8	7	243	600	.08	.11	.5	19
Beans, snap, green, canned	1 lb	82	4.5	.1				19.1	154	5.4	1,070	431	1,320	.15	.19	1.4	18
	½ cup	22	1.2					5.0	41	1.4	281	113	350	.04	.05	.4	5
Beans, snap, green, frozen, cut	1 lb	118	7.7	.5				27.2	191	3.6	5	758	2,630	.32	.45	2.0	43
	½ cup	21	1.4	.1				4.8	34	.6	1	133	463	.06	.08	.4	8
Beans, snap, frozen, French-style	1 lb	122	7.7	.5				27.7	181	4.1		694	2,400	.32	.41	1.9	45
	½ cup	23	1.4	.1				5.2	34	.8		130	450	.06	.08	.4	8
Beans, snap, yellow or wax	1 lb	108	6.8	.8				24.0	224	3.2	28	970	1,000	.33	.42	2.0	80
	1 cup	27	1.7	.2				6.0	56	.8	7	243	250	.08	.11	.5	20
Beans, snap, yellow, canned	1 lb	86	4.5	.9				19.1	154	5.4	1,070	431	270	.15	.19	1.4	23
	½ cup	23	1.2	.2				5.0	41	1.4	281	113	70	.04	.05	.4	6
Beans, snap, yellow, frozen, cut	1 lb	127	8.2	.5				29.5	163	3.6	5	816	450	.36	.41	2.1	54
	½ cup	22	1.4	.1				5.2	29	.6	1	144	79	.06	.07	.4	10
Bean sprouts—see Legumes and Nuts																	
Beets	1 lb	137	5.1	.3				31.4	51	2.2	190	1,060	80	.10	.15	1.2	32
	1 2″ diam.	22	.8	tr.				5.0	8	.4	30	168	10	.02	.03	.2	5
Beets, canned	1 lb	154	4.1	.5				35.8	64	2.7	1,070	758	50	.04	.11	.5	14
	½ cup	41	1.1	.1				9.7	17	.7	290	205	14	.01	.03	.2	4
Beet greens	1 lb (yields 1⅞ cups cooked)	61	5.6	.8				11.7	302	8.4	330	1,448	15,490	.24	.55	1.0	76

*Linoleic acid is unsaturated fat.

5. VEGETABLES AND VEGETABLE PRODUCTS (cont.)

Food	Measure	Calories	Protein Gm	Total Fat Gm	Saturated Fat Gm	Lino.-* leic Acid Gm	Cholesterol Mg	Carbohydrate Gm	Calcium Mg	Iron Mg	Sodium Mg	Potassium Mg	A IU	Thiamine Mg	Riboflavin Mg	Niacin Mg	C Mg
Broccoli	1 lb	113	12.7	1.1				20.9	364	3.9	53	1,352	8,840	.35	.81	3.2	400
	1 med stalk (about 2.5 oz)	18	2.0	.2				3.3	57	.6	8	211	1,380	.05	.13	.5	63
	½ cup diced	38	4.2	.4				7.0	121	1.3	18	451	2,950	.12	.27	1.1	133
Broccoli, frozen, chopped	1 lb	132	14.5	1.4				23.6	263	3.2	77	1,093	11,790	.32	.59	2.5	318
	½ cup	26	2.9	.3				4.7	53	.6	15	219	2,360	.06	.12	.5	64
Broccoli, frozen, spears	1 lb	177	15.0	.9				23.1	195	3.2	59	1,107	8,620	.32	.59	2.5	359
	⅓ 10-oz pkg	26	3.1	.2				4.8	41	.7	12	231	1,800	.07	.12	.5	75
Brussel sprouts	1 lb (yields 2¼ cups cooked)	188	20.4	1.7				36.4	150	6.3	58	1,627	2,300	.41	.68	3.9	426
	1 lb	163	15.0	.9				33.1	100	4.1	73	1,488	2,590	.45	.50	2.7	395
Brussel sprouts, frozen	¾ cup	34	3.1	.2				6.9	21	.9	15	310	539	.09	.10	.6	82
Cabbage, green	1 lb	98	5.3	.8				22.0	200	1.6	82	951	530	.22	.20	1.3	192
	1 cup coarsely shredded	15	.8	.1				3.4	31	.2	13	147	80	.03	.03	.2	30
Cabbage, red	1 lb	127	8.2	.8				28.2	171	3.3	106	1,094	180	.38	.23	1.7	249
	1 cup coarsely shredded	20	1.3	.1				4.3	26	.5	16	169	30	.06	.04	.3	38
Cabbage, savoy	1 lb	98	9.8	.8				18.8	273	3.7	90	1,098	820	.22	.34	1.2	225
	1 cup coarsely shredded	15	1.5	.1				2.9	42	.6	14	169	126	.03	.05	.2	35
Cabbage, Chinese	1 lb	62	5.3	.4				13.2	189	2.6	101	1,113	660	.20	.18	2.5	110
	1 cup shredded	10	.9	tr.				2.2	31	.4	17	184	109	.03	.03	.4	18

*Linoleic acid is unsaturated fat.

5. VEGETABLES AND VEGETABLE PRODUCTS (cont.)

Food	Measure	Calories	Protein Gm	Total Fat Gm	Saturated Fat Gm	Lino-leic* Acid Gm	Choles-terol Mg	Carbo-hydrate Gm	Calcium Mg	Iron Mg	Sodium Mg	Potas-sium Mg	A IU	Thiamine Mg	Ribo-flavin Mg	Niacin Mg	C Mg
Carrots	1 lb	156	4.1	.7				36.1	138	2.6	175	1,269	40,920	.22	.20	2.2	29
	1 med 5½"x1"	17	.5	.1				4.0	15	.3	19	140	4,500	.02	.02	.2	3
	1 cup grated	38	1.0	.2				8.7	33	.6	42	307	9,910	.05	.05	.5	7
Carrots, canned	1 lb	127	2.7	.9				29.5	113	3.2	1,070	544	45,360	.11	.11	1.6	9
	½ cup	35	.7	.2				8.1	31	.9	294	150	12,480	.03	.03	.2	2
Cauliflower	1 lb	122	12.2	.9				23.6	113	5.0	59	1,338	270	.50	.44	3.0	354
	1 cup diced	61	6.1	.5				11.8	57	2.5	30	669	140	.25	.22	1.5	177
Cauliflower, frozen	1 lb	100	9.1	.9				19.5	86	2.7	50	1,021	140	.27	.27	2.5	254
	½ cup	21	1.9	.2				4.0	18	1.0		211	30	.06	.06	1.2	52
Celery	1 lb	58	3.1	.3				13.3	133	1.0	429	1,160	820	.09	.11	1.1	30
	1 outer stalk	5	.3	tr.				1.2	12	.1	38	102	100	.01	.01	.3	3
	1 cup diced	17	.9	.1				3.9	39	.3	126	341	240	.03	.03	.3	9
Chard, Swiss	1 lb (yields 1¼ cups cooked)	104	10.0	1.3				19.2	367	13.4	613	2,295	27,120	.25	.72	2.2	132
Chicory	1 lb	74	6.7	1.1				14.1	320	3.3	—	1,562	14,880	.22	.37	1.9	82
	1 cup	17	1.6	.3				3.3	75	.8	—	368	3,500	.05	.09	.4	19
Chives	1 T	3	.2	tr.				.6	7	.2	—	25	580	tr.	.01	tr.	6
Chop suey, canned with meat	1 lb	281	20.0	14.5	5		1	19.1	159	8.6	2,499	626	140	.23	.24	3.4	11
	1 cup	155	11.0	8.0	3			10.5	87	4.7	1,374	344	77	.13	.13	1.9	6
Chow mein, chicken, canned	1 lb	172	11.8	.5				32.2	82	2.3	1,315	758	270	.09	.18	1.1	20
	1 cup	98	6.7	.3				18.4	47	1.3	751	433	150	.05	.10	.6	11
Collards	1 lb (yields 2⅓ cups cooked)	139	14.8	2.5				23.1	771	4.6	—	1,388	28,680	.48	.97	5.1	469
Collards, frozen	1 lb	145	14.1	1.8				26.3	866	5.0	82	1,175	30,840	.32	.73	3.1	308
	½ cup	30	2.9	.4				5.4	179	1.0	17	242	6,360	.07	.15	.6	64

*Linoleic acid is unsaturated fat.

5. VEGETABLES AND VEGETABLE PRODUCTS (cont.)

Food	Measure	Calories	Pro-tein Gm	Total Fat Gm	Satu-rated Fat Gm	Lino-leic* Acid Gm	Choles-terol Mg	Car-bohy-drate Gm	Cal-cium Mg	Iron Mg	Sodium Mg	Potas-sium Mg	A IU	Thi-amine Mg	Ribo-flavin Mg	Nia-cin Mg	C Mg
Corn, with husk	1 lb	157	5.7	1.6				36.1	5	1.1	tr.	457	650	.24	.19	2.8	20
Corn, without husk	1 lb	240	8.7	2.5				55.1	7	1.7	tr.	699	1,000	.37	.29	4.2	31
	1 ear, 5"	74	2.5	.8				17.0	2	.5	tr.	215	310	.13	.09	1.3	10
Corn, canned, cream style	1 lb	372	9.5	2.7				90.7	14	2.7	1,070	440	1,520	.13	.23	4.5	23
	½ cup	106	2.7	.8				25.9	4	.7	306	126	430	.04	.07	1.3	7
Corn, canned, vacuum pack	1 lb	376	11.3	2.3				93.0	14	2.3	1,070	440	1,570	.15	.29	4.9	23
	½ cup	79	2.4	.5				19.7	3	.5	226	93	330	.03	.06	1.0	5
Corn, canned, wet pack	1 lb	299	8.6	2.7				71.2	18	1.8	1,070	440	1,220	.12	.22	4.1	23
	½ cup	84	2.4	.8				20.1	5	1.5	301	124	340	.03	.06	1.2	6
Corn, frozen, on cob	1 lb	244	9.0	2.5				56.4	7	2.0	1	634	870	.22	.22	4.7	25
	1 ear	98	3.6	1.0				22.6	3	.8	1	254	350	.17	.09	1.9	10
Corn, frozen, kernels	1 lb	372	14.1	2.3				89.4	14	3.6	1	916	1,590	.50	.32	7.3	38
	½ cup	77	2.9	.5				18.6	3	.7	5	191	330	.10	.07	1.5	8
Cowpeas (including blackeye peas), shelled	1 lb	576	40.8	3.6				98.9	122	10.4	9	2,454	1,680	1.97	.59	7.3	130
	1 cup	180	12.8	1.1				30.9	38	3.3	3	767	530	.62	.18	2.3	41
Cowpeas, canned	1 cup	318	22.7	1.4				56.2	82	6.8	1,070	1,597	270	.42	.21	1.0	14
Cowpeas, frozen	1 cup	140	10.0	.6				24.7	36	3.0	471	703	180	.18	.09	.6	6
	1 lb	594	40.8	1.8				107.0	127	14.1	227	1,755	770	2.04	.54	6.3	58
	1 cup	212	14.5	.6				38.1	45	5.0	81	625	270	.73	.19	2.2	21
Cucumber, with skin	1 lb	65	3.9	.4				14.7	108	4.7	26	689	1,080	.15	.19	.9	48
	7½"x2"	41	2.4	.3				9.2	68	2.9	16	431	680	.09	.12	.6	30
Cucumber, peeled	7½"x2"	21	.9	.1				4.8	26	.5	9	241	tr.	.05	.06	.3	17
	6 slices	5	.2	tr.				1.2	6	.1	2	58	tr.	.01	.02	.1	4
Dandelion greens	1 lb (yields 2¼ cups cooked)	204	12.2	3.2				41.7	848	14.1	345	1,801	63,500	.85	1.17	—	161
Eggplant	1 lb	92	4.4	.7				20.6	44	2.6	7	786	30	.20	.17	2.3	19
	1 med (1¼ lbs; yields 2 cups cooked)	115	5.5	.9				25.8	55	3.3	9	983	40	.25	.21	2.9	24

*Linoleic acid is unsaturated fat.

5. VEGETABLES AND VEGETABLE PRODUCTS (cont.)

Food	Measure	Calories	Protein Gm	Total Fat Gm	Saturated Fat Gm	Linoleic* Acid Gm	Cholesterol Mg	Carbohydrate Gm	Calcium Mg	Iron Mg	Sodium Mg	Potassium Mg	A IU	Thiamine Mg	Riboflavin Mg	Niacin Mg	C Mg
Endive, Belgian	1 lb	61	4.0	.4				12.9	73	2.0	28	735	tr.				—
Endive, curly and escarole	1 cup	7	.5	tr.				2.5	8	.8	3	181					—
	1 lb	80	6.8	.4				16.4	323	6.8	56	1,174	13,170	.27	.56	2.0	42
Fennel	1 cup	12	1.0	.1				2.5	50	1.0	9		2,030				6
	1 lb	118	11.8	1.7				21.5	422	11.4		1,675	14,760	.04	.09	.3	129
Garlic	1 lb	547	24.8	.8				123.0	116	6.0	76	2,112	tr.	1.01	.31	1.9	59
	1 oz	34	1.6	.2				7.7	7	.4	5	132	tr.	.06	.02	.2	4
Ginger root	1 lb	207	5.9	4.2				40.1	97	8.9	25	1,114	40	.10	.17	2.8	17
	1 oz	13	.7	.3				2.5	6	.6	2	70	tr.	.01	.01	.2	—
Horseradish, raw	1 lb	288	10.6	1.0				65.2	464	4.6	26	1,867		.23	.17	.2	268
	1 oz	18	.7	tr.				4.1	29	.3	2	117		.01	.01	.2	17
Horseradish, prepared	1 lb	172	5.9	.9				43.5	277	4.1	435	1,315					—
	1 T	5	.2	tr.				1.4	9	.1	14	41					—
Jerusalem artichoke	1 lb	22–235†	7.2	.3				52.3	44	10.6			50	.64	.17	4.1	12
	1 sm	1–13†	.4	tr.				2.9	2	.6			tr.	.04	.01	.2	1
Kale	1 lb (yields 2¾ cups cooked)	154	17.4	2.3				26.1	723	7.8	218	1,097	29,030	.47	.76	6.0	540
Kale, frozen	1 lb	145	14.5	2.3				24.9	608	5.0	118	1,093	37,200	.36	.82	3.5	290
	½ cup	40	4.0	.6				6.8	167	1.4	32	301	10,230	.10	.23	1.1	80
Kohlrabi	1 lb	96	6.6	.3				21.9	136	1.7	26	1,232	70	.22	.12	1.1	219
Lambsquarter	1 lb	195	19.1	3.6				33.1	1,402	5.4			52,620	.70	2.00	5.5	363
Leeks	1 lb (yields 2¼ cups cooked)	123	5.2	.7				26.4	123	2.6	12	819	90	.26	.13	1.2	40
Lettuce Butterhead, as Boston, Bibb	1 lb	47	4.0	.7				8.4	117	6.7	30	886	3,260	.21	.20	.9	28
	4" head	23	1.9	.3				4.1	57	3.2	15	429	1,580	.10	.10	.4	14
Cos or Romaine	1 lb	52	3.8	.9				10.2	197	4.1	26	766	5,520	.15	.24	1.1	54
	2 leaves	5	.4	.1				1.0	20	.4	3	76	550	.01	.02	.1	5

*Linoleic acid is unsaturated fat.
†Caloric values increase with storage.

5. VEGETABLES AND VEGETABLE PRODUCTS (cont.)

Food	Measure	Calories	Protein Gm	Total Fat Gm	Saturated Fat Gm	Oleic Acid Gm	Lino-*leic Acid Gm	Cholesterol Mg	Carbohydrate Gm	Minerals — Calcium Mg	Iron Mg	Sodium Mg	Potassium Mg	Vitamins — A IU	Thiamine Mg	Riboflavin Mg	Niacin Mg	C Mg
Crispshead, as Iceberg	1 lb, or 1 head 4¾"	56	3.9	.4					12.5	86	2.2	39	754	1,420	.27	.25	1.2	28
Looseleaf	1 lb	52	3.8	.9					10.2	197	4.1	26	766	5,520	.15	.24	1.1	54
	2 leaves	6	.4	.1					1.1	22	.5	3	84	610	.02	.03	.03	6
Mushrooms	1 lb	123	11.9	1.3					19.4	26	3.5	66	1,822	tr.	.40	2.02	18.6	14
	1 cup or 9 sm	25	2.4	.3					3.9	5	.7	13	364	tr.	.08	.40	3.7	3
Mushrooms, canned	1 lb	77	8.6	.5					10.9	27	2.3	1,814	894	tr.	.07	1.12	8.9	8
	½ cup	21	2.3	.1					2.9	7	.6	487	240	tr.	.02	.30	2.4	2
Mustard greens	1 lb (yields 1¼ cups cooked)	98	9.5	1.6					17.8	581	9.5	102	1,197	22,220	.34	.70	2.7	308
Okra	1 lb (yields 2¾ cups cooked)	140	9.4	1.2					29.6	359	2.3	12	971	2,030	.66	.80	4.0	122
Okra, frozen	1 lb	177	10.4	.5					40.8	426	2.7	9	993	2,180	.77	.95	4.7	72
	⅔ cup	44	2.6	.1					10.2	107	.7	2	248	545	.19	.24	1.2	18
Olives, green, canned	1 lb	275	2.3	29.4					5.5	179	3.4	1,733	72	140	tr.	tr.	tr.	
	4 med or 2 giant	10	tr.	1.0					.2	6	.1	61	3	tr.				
Olives, black, mission, canned	1 lb	392	2.6	42.9	5	3			6.8	226	3.6	1,733	72	140	tr.	tr.	tr.	
	2 lge	9	tr.	.9					.1	5	.1	38	2	tr.				
Olives, black, Sevillano, canned	1 lb	198	2.3	20.3	2	1			5.8	158	3.4	1,765	94	130	tr.	tr.	tr.	
	2 lge	3	tr.	.4					.1	3	tr.	31	2	tr.				
Olives, Greek-style, oil cured	1 lb	1,227	8.0	129.9	11	7			31.6	—	—	11,932	263	—				
	2	27	.2	2.9														
Onions	1 lb	157	6.2	.4					35.9	111	2.1	41	648	160	.14	.15	.8	42
	2½" diam.	38	1.5	.1					8.7	27	.5	10	157	40	.03	.04	.2	10
Parsley	1 T	2	.1	tr.					.3	8	.2	2	29	340	.01	.01	tr.	7

*Linoleic acid is unsaturated fat.

5. VEGETABLES AND VEGETABLE PRODUCTS (cont.)

Food	Measure	Calories	Protein Gm	Total Fat Gm	Saturated Fat Gm	Lino-leic Acid Gm	Cholesterol Mg	Carbohydrate Gm	Calcium Mg	Iron Mg	Sodium Mg	Potassium Mg	A IU	Thiamine Mg	Riboflavin Mg	Niacin Mg	C Mg
Parsnips	1 lb	293	6.6	1.9				67.5	193	2.7	46	2,086	120	.30	.35	.7	62
	1 med (3/lb)	98	2.2	.6				22.5	64	.9	15	695	40	.10	.12	.2	21
Peas, edible pod	1 lb	228	14.7	.9				51.7	267	3.0	—	733	2,930	1.21	.52	—	90
	10 pods	10	.6	tr.				2.3	12	.1	—	32	130	.05	.02	—	4
Peas, green, in pod	1 lb	145	10.9	.7				24.8	45	3.3	3	545	1,100	.60	.23	4.9	47
Peas, green, shelled	1 lb	381	28.6	1.8				65.3	118	8.6	9	1,433	2,900	1.58	.62	13.0	124
	1 cup	113	8.5	.5				19.4	35	2.6	3	426	860	.47	.18	3.9	37
Peas, green, canned Alaska, Early, or June	1 lb	299	15.9	1.4				56.7	91	7.7	1,070	435	2,040	.43	.24	3.9	40
	½ cup	82	4.4	.4				15.5	25	2.1	293	119	560	.07	.07	1.1	10
Peas, green, canned, sweet	1 lb	259	15.4	1.4				47.2	86	6.8	1,070	435	2,040	.52	.26	4.5	40
	½ cup	68	4.0	.4				12.4	23	1.8	280	114	530	.14	.07	1.2	10
Peas, green, frozen	1 lb	331	24.5	1.4				58.1	91	9.1	585	680	3,080	1.45	.45	9.3	85
	½ cup	68	5.1	.3				12.0	19	1.9	121	140	640	.30	.09	1.9	18
Peas and carrots, frozen	1 lb	249	15.0	1.4				47.2	118	5.4	417	776	42,180	.91	.32	6.1	45
	½ cup	51	3.1	.3				9.7	24	1.1	86	160	8,700	.09	.07	1.3	9
Peppers, hot chili, green	1 lb	123	5.9	.3				30.1	33	2.3	—	—	2,550	.20	.20	5.6	778
	1 avg	4	.1	tr.				.9	1	.1	—	—	80	.01	tr.	.2	24
Peppers, hot chili, green, canned	1 lb	113	4.1	.5				27.7	32	2.3	—	—	2,770	.08	.22	3.7	308
	4" long	7	.3	tr.				1.7	2	.2	—	—	170	.01	.02	.2	19
Green chili sauce, canned	1 lb	91	3.2	.5				22.7	23	1.8	—	—	2,770	.14	.14	3.2	308
	1 T	4	.2	tr.				1.0	8	.1	—	—	120	tr.	tr.	.2	14
Peppers, hot chili, red	1 lb	405	16.1	10.0				78.8	126	5.2	—	—	94,070	.96	1.57	19.2	1,607
	1 avg	25	1.0	.6				4.9	8	.3	—	—	5,880	.06	.10	1.2	100
Red chili sauce, canned	1 lb	95	4.1	2.7				17.7	41	2.3	—	—	43,500	tr.	.05	2.7	136
	1 T	6	.2	.7				1.8	2	.1	—	—	1,910	tr.	.02	.1	6
Peppers, sweet, green	1 lb	82	4.5	.7				17.9	33	2.6	48	792	1,540	.28	.30	2.0	476
	1 med (5/lb)	16	.9	.1				3.6	7	.5	10	158	310	.06	.06	.4	95

*Linoleic acid is unsaturated fat.

5. VEGETABLES AND VEGETABLE PRODUCTS (cont.)

Food	Measure	Calories	Protein Gm	Total Fat Gm	Saturated Fat Gm	Oleic Acid Gm	Lino-leic* Gm	Choles-terol Mg	Carbo-hydrate Gm	Calcium Mg	Iron Mg	Sodium Mg	Potassium Mg	A IU	Thiamine Mg	Ribo-flavin Mg	Niacin Mg	C Mg
Peppers, sweet, red	1 lb	112	5.1	1.1					25.8	47	2.2	—	—	16,150	.28	.29	1.9	740
Pickles, dill	1 med (5/lb)	22	1.0	.2					5.2	9		6,477	907	3,320	.06	.06	.4	148
Pickles, sour	1 lb	50	3.2	.2					10.0	118	4.5	1,924	269	450	tr.	.09	tr.	28
	1¼"x1¾"	15	1.0	.3					3.0	35	1.3	6,137		130	tr.	.03	tr.	8
Pickles, sweet	1 lb	45	2.3	.3					9.1	77	14.5	1,823		450	tr.	.09	tr.	30
	1¼"x1¾"	13	.7	.3					2.7	23	4.3			130	tr.	.03	tr.	9
Pickles, sweet	1 lb	662	3.2	1.8					165.6	54	5.4			410	tr.	.09	.1	26
	2 slices or 2½" gherkin	22	.1	tr.					5.5	2	.2				tr.	tr.	tr.	1
Chow Chow, sour	1 lb	132	6.4	5.9					18.6	145	11.8	6,069		10				
	1 T	7	.3	.3					1.0	8	.6	334						
Chow Chow, sweet	1 lb	526	6.8	4.1					122.5	104	6.8	2,390						
	1 T	29	.3	.2					6.7	6	.4	131						
Pickle relish, sour	1 lb	86	3.2	4.1					12.2	132	5.0	3,230						
	1 T	3	.1	.1					.4	4	.2	107						
Pickle relish, sweet	1 lb	626	2.7	2.7					154.2	91	3.6							
	1 T	21	tr.	tr.					5.1	3	.1							
Pimiento, canned	1 lb	122	4.1	2.3					26.3	32	6.8	11		10,430	.11	.29	1.7	430
	4 oz	31	1.0	1.6					6.6	8	1.7	16		2,610	.03	.07	.4	108
Plantain	1 lb	389	3.6	1.3					101.9	23	2.3	11	1,257	†	.20	.13	2.0	46
Potatoes	1 lb	279	7.7	.4					62.8	26	2.2	16	1,495	tr.	.39	.14	2.4	73
Potatoes, canned	1 med (3/lb)	93	2.6	.9					20.9	9	.7	4	498	tr.	.13	.05	1.8	24
	1 lb	200	5.0	.5					44.5	18	1.4	1,070	1,134	tr.	.17	.10	2.9	58
	1 cup	110	2.8						24.5	10	.8	589	624	tr.	.09	.06	1.6	32
Potatoes, dehydrated, mashed, flakes	1 lb	1,651	32.7	2.7					381.0	159	7.7	404	7,258	tr.	1.05	.27	24.4	—
	⅓ cup (yields ½ cup potatoes)	69	1.4	.1					15.9	7	.3	17	303	tr.	.04	.01	1.0	—

*Linoleic acid is unsaturated fat.
†Values range from 30 IU's for white-fleshed varieties to 3,900 IU's for those with deep yellow flesh.

5. VEGETABLES AND VEGETABLE PRODUCTS (cont.)

Food	Measure	Calories	Pro-tein Gm	Total Fat Gm	Satu-rated Fat Gm	Lino-* leic Acid Gm	Choles-terol Mg	Car-bohy-drate Gm	Cal-cium Mg	Iron Mg	Sodium Mg	Potas-sium Mg	A IU	Thi-amine Mg	Ribo-flavin Mg	Nia-cin Mg	C Mg
Potatoes, frozen, diced	1 lb	331	5.4	tr.				78.9	45	3.2	36	771	tr.	.32	.05	2.9	41
	1 cup	138	2.2	tr.				33.0	19	1.3	15	322	tr.	.13	.02	1.2	17
Potatoes, frozen, French fried	1 lb	771	12.7	29.5	7	1	15	118.4	32	6.4	1,070	2,295	tr.	.64	.09	9.7	91
	10 pieces	97	1.6	3.7	1		2	14.8	4	.8	134	288	tr.	.08	.01	1.2	11
Potatoes, frozen, mashed	1 lb	340	7.7	.5				77.6	73	3.2	358	1,039	140	.32	.14	3.7	29
	½ cup	73	1.7	.1				16.7	16	.7	77	223	30	.07	.03	.8	6
Potato chips	1 lb	2,576	24.0	180.5	45		90	226.8	181	8.2	up to 4,500	5,126	tr.	.93	.31	21.7	73
	3 oz	483	4.5	33.8	8		17	42.5	34	1.5	up to 840	961	tr.	.17	.06	4.1	14
Potato sticks	10	113	1.1	7.9	2		4	1.0	8	.4	up to 200	226	tr.	.04	.01	1.0	3
	1 lb	2,468	29.0	165.1	41		83	230.4	200	8.2	up to 4,500	5,126	tr.	.93	.31	21.7	181
	1½ oz	231	2.7	15.5	4		8	21.6	19	.8	up to 425	481	tr.	.09	.03	2.0	17
Pumpkin	1 lb	83	3.2	.4				20.6	67	2.5	2	1,080	5,080	.14	.35	2.8	30
Pumpkin, canned	1 lb	150	4.5	1.4				35.8	113	1.8	9	1,089	29,030	.15	.24	2.5	24
	¼ cup	38	1.1	.4				9.0	28	.2	2	273	7,280	.04	.06	.6	6
Radish, common	1 lb	69	4.1	tr.				14.7	122	4.1	73	1,314	40	.13	.12	1.3	106
	4 sm	7	.4	tr.				1.5	12	.4	7	130	tr.	.01	.01	.1	10
Radish, Oriental	1 lb	67	3.2	.4				14.9	124	2.1	—	637	40	.11	.07	1.3	113
	2 oz	8	.4	tr.				1.9	16	.3	—	80	tr.	.01	.01	.2	10
Rutabaga	1 lb	177	4.2	.9				42.4	254	2.3	19	922	2,240	.07	.26	4.3	166
	½ cup diced	29	.7	tr.				6.9	41	.4	3	150	360	.04	.04	.7	27
Sauerkraut, canned	1 lb	82	4.5	1.2				18.1	163	2.3	3,388	635	240	.14	.17	.8	64
	½ cup	21	1.2	.2				4.7	42	.6	876	164	60	.04	.04	.2	17
Sauerkraut juice	1 cup	25	1.8	tr.				5.8	93	2.8	1,968	—	tr.	.08	.10	.5	45
Scallions	1 lb	76	1.8	.3				17.6	67	1.0		388	tr.	.08	.07	.7	42
	6	23	.6	.1				5.2	20	.3		115	tr.	.02	.02	.2	12

*Linoleic acid is unsaturated fat.

5. VEGETABLES AND VEGETABLE PRODUCTS (cont.)

Food	Measure	Calories	Protein Gm	Total Fat Gm	Saturated Fat Gm	Linoleic Acid Gm	Cholesterol Mg	Carbohydrate Gm	Calcium Mg	Iron Mg	Sodium Mg	Potassium Mg	A IU	Thiamine Mg	Riboflavin Mg	Niacin Mg	C Mg
Seaweed, agar	1 lb	—	—	1.4				—	2,572	28.6							—
Seaweed, dulse	1 oz	—	—	tr.				—	161	1.8							—
Seaweed, Irish moss	1 lb	—	—	14.5				—	1,343		9,458	36,560					—
Seaweed, kelp	1 T	—	—	.3				—	29	40.4	207	800					—
	1 lb	—	—	.2				—	4,014	.9	13,118	12,900					—
	1 T	—	—	5.0				—	88		289	284					—
	1 lb	—	—	.1				—	4,958		13,640	23,918					—
Shallot	1/4"	907	78.8	63.5				0	109		300	526					—
Soybeans, in pod	1 lb	322	26.2	14.5				31.7	161	6.7			1,660	1.06	.38	3.3	69
Soybeans, shelled	1 lb	608	49.4	23.1				59.9	304	12.7			3,130	2.00	.72	6.2	130
Soybeans, canned	1 lb	100	8.2	3.8				9.9	50	2.1	1,070		517	.33	.12	1.0	21
Spinach, in bulk	½ cup	340	29.5	14.5				28.6	249	13.2	159			.40	.40		39
	2/3 cup (1 lb yields 2 cups cooked)	50	4.4	2.2				4.2	37	2.0				.06	.06		6
Spinach, packaged (trimmed)	1 lb	85	10.5	1.0				14.0	304	10.1	232	1,535	26,450	.32	.65	2.0	167
	1 lb	118	14.5	1.4				19.5	422	14.1	322	2,132	36,740	.44	.91	2.8	231
Spinach, canned	1 cup	15	1.8	.2				2.4	53	1.8	40	267	4,590	.06	.11	.4	29
	1 lb	86	9.1	1.8				13.6	386	9.5	273	1,134	24,950	.09	.45	1.5	62
Spinach, frozen, chopped	½ cup	22	2.3	.5				3.5	99	2.4		290	6,370	.02	.11	.4	16
	½ cup	109	14.1	.4				17.2	513	9.5	259	1,606	35,830	.41	.73	2.2	133
Spinach, frozen, leaf	1 lb	27	3.5	.4				4.3	128	2.4	65	402	8,960	.10	.18	.6	33
	½ cup	113	13.6	1.4				19.1	476	11.3	240	1,746	36,740	.45	.73	2.3	159
Squash, yellow, summer	2/3 cup	23	2.8	.3				3.9	98	1.8	50	360	7,580	.09	.15	.5	33
	1 lb	89	2.4	.9				19.1	124	1.8	4	898	2,040	.24	.38	4.6	111
Squash, zucchini	1 med, 5"	40	2.4	.4				8.6	56	.8	2	404	920	.11	.17	2.1	50
	1 lb	73	5.2	.4				15.5	121	1.7	4	870	1,380†	.23	.37	4.4	82
	1 med, 6"	26	1.8	.1				5.4	42	.6	1	305	480	.08	.13	1.5	29

*Linoleic acid is unsaturated fat.
†Primarily in skin.

5. VEGETABLES AND VEGETABLE PRODUCTS (cont.)

Food	Measure	Calories	Protein Gm	Total Fat Gm	Saturated Fat Gm	Lino-leic* Acid Gm	Choles-terol Mg	Car-bohy-drate Gm	Cal-cium Mg	Iron Mg	Sodium Mg	Potas-sium Mg	A IU	Thi-amine Mg	Ribo-flavin Mg	Nia-cin Mg	C Mg
Squash, winter, acorn	1 lb	152	5.2	.3				38.6	107	3.1	3	1,324	4,140	.16	.38	2.0	49
Squash, winter, butternut	1 lb	171	4.4	.3				44.4	102	2.5	3	1,546	18,100	.14	.35	1.8	29
Squash, winter, Hubbard	1 lb (yields 1 cup mashed)	117	4.2	.9				28.1	57	1.8	3	650	12,870	.13	.33	1.7	32
Squash, frozen, summer	1 lb	95	6.4	.9				21.3	64	3.2	14	758	680	.32	.18	2.0	44
	½ cup	21	1.4	.1				4.8	14	.7	3	171	150	.07	.04	.5	10
Squash, frozen, winter	1 lb	172	5.4	1.4				41.7	113	4.5	5	939	17,690	.14	.32	2.2	44
	½ cup	52	1.6	.4				12.5	34	1.4	5	282	5,300	.04	.10	.7	13
Succotash, frozen	1 lb	440	19.5	1.8				97.5	64	5.0	204	1,238	1,360	.50	.27	6.7	42
	½ cup	91	4.0	.4				20.1	13	1.0	42	255	280	.10	.06	1.4	9
Sweet potatoes	1 lb	419	6.2	1.5				96.6	118	2.6	37	1,235	32,330	.36	.22	2.2	77
	1 5"x2"	157	2.3	.6				36.2	44	1.0	14	893	12,120	.14	.08	.8	29
Sweet potatoes, canned in syrup	1 lb	517	4.5	.9				124.7	59	3.2	218	544	22,680	.15	.14	2.5	36
	1 potato	199	1.7	.3				48.0	23	1.2	84	209	8,730	.06	.05	1.0	14
	½ cup	136	1.2	.2				32.7	15	.8	57	143	5,950	.04	.04	.7	9
Sweet potatoes, canned, vacuum or solid pack	1 lb	490	9.1	.9				112.9	113	3.6	218	907	35,380	.21	.20	2.9	62
	½ cup	118	2.2	.2				27.1	27	.9	52	218	8,490	.05	.05	.7	15
Tomatoes	1 lb	100	5.0	.9				21.3	59	2.3	14	1,107	4,080	.29	.18	3.0	102
	1 3" diam.	44	2.2	.4				9.4	26	1.0	6	487	1,800	.13	.08	1.3	45
Tomatoes, canned	1 lb	95	4.5	.5				19.5	27	2.3	590	984	4,080	.24	.13	3.1	76
	1 cup	50	2.4	tr.				10.3	14	1.2	313	522	2,160	.13	.07	1.6	40
Tomato chili sauce	1 T	16	.4	tr.				3.7	3	.1	200	55	210	.01	.01	.2	4
Tomato juice	1 cup	46	2.2	.2				10.4	17	2.2	486	552	1,940	.12	.07	1.9	39
Tomato juice cocktail	1 cup	51	1.7	.2				12.2	24	2.2	486	537	1,940	.12	.05	1.5	39
Tomato ketchup	1 T	16	.3	.1				3.8	3	.1	156	55	210	.01	.01	.2	2
Tomato paste	1 lb	372	15.4	1.8				84.4	122	15.9	172†	4,028	14,970	.88	.54	14.2	221
	6 oz	140	5.8	.7				31.7	46	6.0	65	1,511	5,610	.33	.20	5.3	83

*Linoleic acid is unsaturated fat.
†Values apply to unsalted product.

5. VEGETABLES AND VEGETABLE PRODUCTS (cont.)

Food	Measure	Calories	Protein Gm	Total Fat Gm	Saturated Fat Gm	Lino-* Add Gm	Cholesterol Mg	Carbohydrate Gm	Calcium Mg	Iron Mg	Sodium Mg	Potassium Mg	A IU	Thiamine Mg	Riboflavin Mg	Niacin Mg	C Mg
Tomato puree	1 lb	177	7.7	.9				40.4	59	7.7	1,810	1,932	7,260	.39	.24	6.3	148
	1 cup	97	4.2	.5				22.1	32	4.2	992	1,059	3,980	.21	.13	3.5	81
Turnips	1 lb	117	3.9	.8				25.7	152	2.0	191	1,045	tr.	.16	.26	2.2	140
Vegetable juice cocktail	1 cup	43	2.3	.3				9.0	30	1.3	500	555	1,750	.13	.08	2.0	23
Vegetable main dishes, canned—see Miscellaneous																	
Vegetables, mixed, frozen	1 lb	295	15.0	1.4				62.1	118	6.4	268	943	22,680	.59	.32	5.3	42
	½ cup	61	3.1	.3				12.8	24	1.3	55	195	4,680	.12	.07	1.1	9
Waterchestnuts	1 lb	272	4.9	.7				66.4	14	2.1	70	1,746	0	.49	.70	3.5	14
	4	15	.3	tr.				3.7	1	.1	4	96	0	.03	.04	.2	tr.
Watercress	1 lb	79	9.2	1.3				12.5	630	7.1	217	1,177	20,450	.35	.68	3.6	330
	½ cup	3	.3	tr.				.5	24	.3	8	44	770	.01	.03	.1	12
Yams	1 lb	394	8.2	.8				90.5	78	2.3	—	2,341	tr.	.39	.16	2.0	36
	1 med, 5½"	108	2.3	.2				24.9	21	.6	—	644	tr.	.10	.04	.6	10

*Linoleic acid is unsaturated fat.

6. FLOUR, CEREAL GRAINS, AND GRAIN PRODUCTS

A century ago most Americans ate grains in the form of heavy-textured breads, hot gritty cereals, and rich, nutty-flavored soups and casseroles. Today when we think of grains we tend to picture soft white bread and rolls, packaged cold breakfast cereals, or a mound of rice or pasta smothered in gravy. No other food group has undergone as much change as flour, cereals, and grain products since the advent of modern technology. Where grains were formerly milled between slowly rotating stones to crush them into flour they are now whizzed through high-friction steel rollers which rapidly sift out the tough bran and germ coating leaving only the fine-textured endosperm. Cereal grains such as rice and barley can be hulled by machine in a fraction of the time it takes more primitive methods to separate them.

These advances in food production are not without penalty. Where whole grains are rich in iron, B vitamins, and vitamin E, white flour, white rice, pearled barley, and products made from these raw ingredients have much less iron, few B vitamins, and no vitamin E. The reason is that the majority of vitamins and minerals are contained in the bran and germ coatings which are separated in the milling. To compensate for the loss, flour and rice are often enriched. By legal definition the term *enriched* designates the addition of 13.0 to 16.5 milligrams iron, 2.0 to 2.5 milligrams thiamine, 1.2 to 1.5 milligrams riboflavin, and 16 to 20 milligrams niacin per pound of grain. Enriched grains may also have 500 to 625 milligrams calcium and 250 to 1,000 international units vitamin A added per pound. When compared with whole grains, enriched grains are higher in riboflavin, but still lower in iron, thiamine, and niacin. Since calcium enrichment is not usual, they also remain lower in calcium, although with the exception of oats, most grains and cereals cannot be considered a good source of this mineral in the first place. The other B vitamins that are removed during milling are not replaced in grain enrichment so that not only the quantity but the balance of B vitamins differs among whole, enriched, and unenriched cereals and flour.

Whole grains are a good source of potassium and also of phosphorous and magnesium (which do not appear on the table).

On the average, 8 to 12 percent of all grain is protein. Although individual grains differ in their amino-acid assortment, those amino acids in the bran and germ frequently supplement those in the endosperm, making the quality as well as the quantity of protein in whole grains higher than that in their enriched and unenriched counterparts. In any case, no grain supplies adequate amounts of all the essential amino acids in an average-size serving, so they cannot be considered as efficient for growth as the higher-quality protein in egg, meat, and milk. However, small amounts of milk or cheese added to grain dishes greatly increase their protein value. Grains and grain products served along with beans, nuts, or seeds and their related products such as bean flours and nut butters also provide complete protein.

All grains have similar energy-generating potential. A pound of flour, pasta, rice, and hot or cold cereal provides about 1,600 calories, or about 100 calories per 1-ounce serving. The size of an ounce, however, may vary greatly with each grain form, so, for example, 3 tablespoons of whole wheat, 2⅛ cups puffed wheat, or one large shredded wheat biscuit can all weigh one ounce.

While wheat, oats, and rice are the most familiar grains in our culture, other less conventional grains offer important vitamins and minerals as well as supplementary protein. You will find them listed in the table and should consider them not only in relation to their nutritional significance, but in terms of their exciting potential in varying the menu in form and flavor. For the most part, grains offer a wealth of food value on a low budget.

While high in carbohydrate, grains contain little fat, and although whole grains contain a higher percentage of fat (found largely in the germ) than refined grains, this fat is unsaturated and rich in vitamin E. Despite their high food value in some aspects, grains are low in vitamins A, C, D, and riboflavin.

Bread, cookies, cakes, pastries, and other prepared flour products reflect not only the nutritional value of the grain that is their essential foundation, but the other ingredients like milk, egg, fat, and sugar which go into their manufacture. Varying the recipe can greatly alter the food composition so that baked goods made with butter, for example, will contain more saturated fat than those made with a vegetable oil, and those prepared with milk will contain more protein than their counterparts made with water.

Cooking has no appreciable effect on the food value of grain products. For the most part, though, we do not eat these items plain, but serve them in combination with milk, butter, sugar, sauces, or gravy. Don't forget to include these items as well as any fat or nutritionally significant liquid used in cooking when computing food value.

How to Use the Table

• Flour, cereals, and similar grain products like pasta or bread are commonly purchased by the pound. Since they are never consumed in such large quantity they are measured here in both pound units and more common serving sizes. When no information on volume is available, one ounce of cereal is considered to be a standard serving.

• The figures on this table for grains that require cooking refer to dry, uncooked measures, with the approximate volume that results from cooking noted. Whenever possible a cooked measure is evaluated too.

• Crackers, cookies, cakes, pies, and other similar foods are measured by units, as a specified number of cookies, ⅙ of a 9-inch pie, a 3-inch square of gingerbread, etc. The value of an entire cake or pie may also be given, and for baked goods made from a mix, the nutritive contents of the most common size package of mix is expressed.

• While the cookies, pies, cakes, and breads here are based on commercial products and standard home recipes, not every variety can be represented. Foods not listed in the table can be compared to the most similar items. You can also determine the precise make-up of home-baked goods from the recipe as illustrated on page 138.

6. FLOUR, CEREAL GRAINS, AND GRAIN PRODUCTS

Food	Measure	Calories	Protein Gm	Total Fat Gm	Saturated Fat Gm	Linoleic Acid* Gm	Cholesterol Mg	Carbohydrate Gm	Calcium Mg	Iron Mg	Sodium Mg	Potassium Mg	A IU	Thiamine Mg	Riboflavin Mg	Niacin Mg	C Mg
Barley, pearled	1 lb	1,583	37.2	4.5				357.4	73	9.1	14	726	0	.55	.23	14.1	0
	¾ cup (yields 1 cup cooked)	174	4.1	.5				39.3	8	1.0	2	80	0	.06	.03	1.6	0
Biscuits, baking powder, home recipe, enriched flour	1 2" diam.	103	2.1	4.8	1	tr.		12.8	34	.4	175	33	tr.	.06	.06	.5	tr.
Biscuits, baking powder, home recipe, unenriched flour	1 2" diam.	103	2.1	4.8	1	tr.		12.8	34	.1	175	33	tr.	.01	.03	.1	tr.
Biscuit dough, enriched flour, chilled in cans	½ lb	628	16.6	14.5	3	2		105.3	120	3.9	1,969	148	tr.	.60	.39	4.8	0
	1 biscuit	63	1.7	1.5	tr.	tr.		10.5	12	.4	197	15	tr.	.06	.04	.5	0
Biscuits, from mix	1 2" diam.	91	2.0	2.6	1	tr.		14.6	19	.6	272	32	tr.	.08	.07	.6	tr.
Boston brown bread	1 lb	957	24.9	5.9				206.8	408	8.6	1,139	1,325	0	.50	.28	5.3	0
	¾" slice	101	2.6	.6				21.8	43	.9	120	140	0	.05	.03	.6	0
Bran—see Wheat Bran																	
Bran flakes (40% bran)	1 lb	1,374	46.3	8.2				365.6	322	20.0	4,196	—	0	1.84	.77	27.9	0
	1 cup (1.2 oz)	106	3.6	.6				28.2	25	1.5	323	—	0	.14	.06	2.1	0
Bran flakes with raisins	1 lb	1,302	37.6	6.4				359.7	254	18.1	3,629	—	0	1.43	.58	24.0	0
	1 cup (1.8 oz)	143	4.1	.7				39.6	28	2.0	399	—	0	.16	.06	2.6	0
Bread																	
cracked wheat	1 lb	1,193	39.5	10.0				236.3	399	5.0	2,400	608	tr.	.53	.42	5.8	tr.
	1 slice (18/lb)	66	2.2	1.0				13.1	22	.3	133	34	tr.	.03	.02	.3	tr.
French, enriched	1 lb	1,315	41.3	13.6				251.3	195	10.0	2,631	408	tr.	1.26	.98	11.3	tr.
	1 slice (16/lb)	82	2.6	.9				15.7	12	.6	164	26	tr.	.08	.06	.7	tr.
French, unenriched	1 lb	1,315	41.3	13.6				251.3	195	3.2	2,631	408	tr.	.39	.39	3.6	tr.
	1 slice (16/lb)	82	2.6	.9				15.7	12	.2	164	26	tr.	.02	.02	.2	tr.
Italian, enriched	1 lb	1,252	41.3	3.6				255.8	77	10.0	2,654	336	0	1.31	.93	11.7	0
	1 slice (16/lb)	78	2.6	.2				16.0	5	.6	166	21	0	.08	.06	.7	0
Italian, unenriched	1 lb	1,252	41.3	3.6				255.8	77	3.2	2,654	336	0	.39	.27	3.6	0
	1 slice (16/lb)	78	2.6	.2				16.0	5	.2	166	21	0	.02	.02	.2	0

*Linoleic acid is unsaturated fat.

6. FLOUR, CEREAL GRAINS, AND GRAIN PRODUCTS (cont.)

Food	Measure	Calories	Protein Gm	Total Fat Gm	Saturated Fat Gm	Lino-* leic Acid Gm	Cholesterol Mg	Carbohydrate Gm	Calcium Mg	Iron Mg	Sodium Mg	Potassium Mg	A IU	Thiamine Mg	Riboflavin Mg	Niacin Mg	C Mg
Bread (cont.)																	
Raisin	1 lb	1,188	29.9	12.7				243.1	322	5.9	1,656	1,057	tr.	.24	.42	3.0	tr.
	1 slice (18/lb)	66	1.7	.7				13.5	18	.3	92	59	tr.	.01	.02	.2	tr.
Rye, American	1 lb	1,102	41.3	5.0				236.3	340	7.3	2,527	658	0	.81	.33	6.4	0
	1 slice (18/lb)	61	2.3	.3				13.1	19	.4	140	37	0	.05	.02	.4	0
Pumpernickel	1 slice (14/lb)	79	3.0	.4				16.9	24	.5	181	47	0	.06	.02	.5	0
	1 lb	1,116	41.3	5.4				240.9	381	10.9	2,581	2,059	0	1.05	.63	5.4	0
White, enriched	1 slice (14/lb)	80	3.0	4.5				17.2	27	.8	184	147	0	.08	.05	.5	tr.
	1 lb	1,225	39.5	14.5	3	2		229.1	381	11.3	2,300	476	tr.	1.13	.95	10.8	tr.
	1 slice (18/lb)	68	2.2	.8				12.7	21	.6	128	26	tr.	.07	.05	.6	tr.
White, unenriched	1 slice (16/lb)	77	2.5	.9				14.3	24	.2	144	30	tr.	.07	.06	.7	tr.
	1 lb	1,225	39.5	14.5	3	2		229.1	381	3.2	2,300	476	tr.	.31	.39	5.0	tr.
Whole wheat, made with water	1 lb	1,093	41.3	11.8				223.6	381	10.4	2,404	1,161	tr.	1.37	.47	12.7	tr.
	1 slice (16/lb)	68	2.6	.7				14.0	24	.7	150	73	tr.	.09	.03	.8	tr.
Whole wheat, made with nonfat dry milk	1 lb	1,102	47.6	13.6				216.4	449	10.4	2,390	1,238	tr.	1.07	.56	12.9	tr.
	1 slice (18/lb)	61	2.6	.8				12.0	25	.6	133	69	tr.	.06	.03	.8	tr.
Breadcrumbs, dry	1 lb	1,778	57.2	20.9	4	3		332.9	553	16.3	3,338	689	tr.	1.00	1.36	15.9	tr.
	1 cup	392	12.6	4.6				73.4	122	3.6	736	152	tr.	.22	.30	3.5	tr.
Bread stuffing mix prepared with water and fat	1 lb	1,683	58.5	17.2	4	2		328.4	562	14.5	6,037	780	tr.	.99	1.17	14.7	tr.
	1 cup	679	12.3	41.4				67.5	125	3.1	1,699	171	1,230	.16	.23	2.8	tr.
prepared with egg, water and fat	1 cup	425	9.0	26.2				40.3	82	2.0	1,031	119	860	.11	.18	1.7	tr.
Buckwheat (kasha)	1 lb	1,520	53.1	10.9				330.7	517	14.1	—	2,032	0	2.71	—	20.0	0
	½ cup (yields 1 cup cooked)	261	9.1	1.9				56.8	89	2.4	—	349	0	.47	—	3.4	0

*Linoleic acid is unsaturated fat.

6. FLOUR, CEREAL GRAINS, AND GRAIN PRODUCTS (cont.)

Food	Measure	Calories	Protein Gm	Total Fat Gm	Saturated Fat Gm	Linoleic Acid Gm	Cholesterol Mg	Carbohydrate Gm	Calcium Mg	Iron Mg	Sodium Mg	Potassium Mg	A IU	Thiamine Mg	Riboflavin Mg	Niacin Mg	C Mg
Buckwheat flour, dark	1 lb	1,510	53.1	11.3				326.6	150	12.7	—	—	0	2.61	.68	13.2	0
	1 cup, sifted	333	11.7	2.5				72.0	33	2.8	—	—	0	.58	.15	2.0	0
Buckwheat flour, light	1 lb	1,574	29.0	5.4				360.6	50	4.5	—	1,452	0	.35	.19	1.8	0
	1 cup, sifted	340	6.3	1.2				77.8	11	1.0	—	313	0	.08	.04	.4	0
Bulgar	1 lb	1,605	50.8	6.8				343.4	132	16.8	—	1,039	0	1.27	.64	20.5	0
	½ cup (yields 1½ cups cooked)	300	9.5	1.3				64.4	25	3.2	—	195	0	.24	.12	3.8	0
Cakes, home recipe																	
Angel food	8″ cake	1,289	34.0	1.0				288.5	43	1.0	1,356	421	0	.03	.67	.8	0
	1/12 cake	107	2.8	tr.				24.0	4	.1	113	35	0	tr.	.06	.1	tr.
Boston cream pie	8″ cake	1,644	27.6	51.8				274.9	369	2.8	1,025	491	1,150	.18	.61	1.2	tr.
	1/8 cake	206	3.5	6.5				34.4	46	.4	128	61	140	.02	.08	.2	tr.
Fruitcake, dark	1-lb loaf	1,719	21.8	69.4				270.8	327	11.8	717	2,250	540	.61	.64	3.8	tr.
	½″ slice	107	1.4	4.3				16.9	20	.7	45	141	30	.04	.04	.2	tr.
Fruitcake, light	1-lb loaf	1,765	27.2	74.8	16†	9†		260.4	308	7.3	875	1,057	320	.44	.49	3.0	tr.
	½″ slice	110	1.7	4.7	1†	1†		16.3	19	.5	55	66	20	.03	.03	.2	tr.
Plain cake, no icing	9″ square	2,823	34.9	107.9	29†	9†		433.7	496	3.1	2,327	612	1,320	.19	.67	1.5	tr.
	3″x3″ piece	314	3.9	12.0	3†	1†		48.2	55	.3	259	68	150	.02	.07	.2	tr.
Plain cake, boiled white icing	9″ square	3,606	38.8	107.5				632.9	501	3.2	2,682	655	1,330	.18	.75	1.6	tr.
	3″x3″ piece	400	4.3	11.9				70.3	56	.4	298	73	150	.02	.08	.2	tr.
Poundcake, old-fashioned	1-lb loaf	2,146	25.9	133.8	32†	10†		213.2	95	3.6	499	272	1,270	.14	.41	.8	0
	½″ slice	134	1.6	8.4	2†	1†		13.3	6	.2	31	17	80	.01	.03	tr.	tr.
Spongecake	10″ cake	2,342	60.0	45.0	14†	3		426.7	236	9.4	1,318	687	3,550	.37	1.11	1.2	tr.
	1/12 cake	195	5.0	3.8	1	tr.		35.6	20	.8	110	57	300	.03	.09	.1	tr.

*Linoleic acid is unsaturated fat.
†Value for cakes made with vegetable shortening; when made with butter, saturated-fat content is about doubled and linoleic acid (polyunsaturated fat) content is about half.

6. FLOUR, CEREAL GRAINS, AND GRAIN PRODUCTS (cont.)

Food	Measure	Calories	Pro-tein Gm	Total Fat Gm	Satu-rated Fat Gm	Lino-leic Acid* Gm	Choles-terol Mg	Carbo-hydrate Gm	Cal-cium Mg	Iron Mg	Sodium Mg	Potas-sium Mg	A IU	Thi-amine Mg	Ribo-flavin Mg	Nia-cin Mg	C Mg
White cake, 2-layer with white icing	9" cake	4,492	39.6	154.5				753.4	576	1.3	2,802	695	1,320	.11	.77	1.6	tr.
	⅛ cake	562	5.0	19.3				94.2	72	.2	350	87	160	.01	.10	.2	tr.
Yellow cake, 2-layer with chocolate icing	9" cake	4,373	50.4	155.8				723.6	813	7.1	2,490	1,294	1,930	.26	1.00	2.6	tr.
	⅛ cake	547	6.3	19.5				90.5	102	.9	311	162	240	.03	.13	.3	tr.
Cake mixes and cakes prepared from mix																	
Angel food	14.5 oz mix	1,582	34.5	.8				363.8	444	1.6	781	460	0	.04	.72	.8	0
	10" cake	1,642	36.2	1.3				376.5	602	2.0	925	380	0	.03	.70	.7	0
	1/12 cake	137	3.0	.1				31.4	50	.2	77	32	0	tr.	.06	.1	0
Coffeecake	16 oz mix	1,955	26.8	49.9				350.2	163	9.1	2,781	395	tr.	1.36	.64	10.9	tr.
	9" square	1,644	32.2	48.9				267.4	312	8.2	2,199	556	820	.89	.83	7.4	tr.
	3"x3" piece	183	3.6	5.4				29.7	35	.9	244	62	90	.10	.09	.8	tr.
Cupcake																	
plain	18.5 oz mix	2,298	19.4	71.3	16	1	6	397.5	908	2.1	3,125	242	40	.27	.31	1.6	0
plain	1 2½" diam.	87	1.2	3	1	1	1	13.9	40	.1	113	21	40	.01	.03	.1	tr.
chocolate iced	1 2½" diam.	129	1.6	4.5	2	1	1	21.3	47	.3	120	42	60	.01	.04	.1	tr.
Devil's food 2-layer with chocolate icing	18.5 oz mix	2,130	25.2	61.4				403.9	420	6.2	2,397	635	0	.14	.45	2.4	tr.
Gingerbread	9" cake	3,747	48.7	135.9	56	7		644.1	653	8.8	2,894	1,437	1,660	.34	.93	3.4	tr.
	1/12 cake	312	4.1	11.3	5	1		53.7	54	.7	241	120	140	.03	.08	.3	tr.
	14 oz mix	1,687	21.4	41.3				310.4	714	5.6	1,838	1,659	tr.	.14	.54	1.4	tr.
	8" square	1,571	17.7	38.6				290.8	512	9.2	1,730	2,081	tr.	.15	.49	4.9	tr.
	2"x4" piece	196	2.2	4.8				36.4	64	1.2	216	260	tr.	.02	.06	.6	tr.

*Linoleic acid is unsaturated fat.

6. FLOUR, CEREAL GRAINS, AND GRAIN PRODUCTS (cont.)

Food	Measure	Calories	Protein Gm	Total Fat Gm	Saturated Fat Gm	Lino-leic* Acid Gm	Choles-terol Mg	Carbo-hydrate Gm	Cal-cium Mg	Iron Mg	Sodium Mg	Potas-sium Mg	A IU	Thi-amine Mg	Ribo-flavin Mg	Nia-cin Mg	C Mg
White cake 2-layer with chocolate icing	18.5 oz mix	2,277	21.5	62.4				411.2	786	1.0	1,956	461	tr.	.12	.35	1.6	tr.
	9" cake	3,994	44.4	121.7	56	7		714.8	1,126	5.8	2,584	1,320	680	.18	.90	2.5	tr.
	1/12 cake	333	3.7	10.1	5	1		59.6	94	.5	215	110	60	.02	.08	.2	tr.
Yellow cake 2-layer with chocolate icing	18.5 oz mix	2,298	20.9	67.6				407.0	734	1.0	2,135	451	tr.	.12	.36	1.5	tr.
	9" cake	3,724	45.3	125.0	56	7		636.6	1,006	6.6	2,509	1,203	1,560	.24	.95	2.2	tr.
	1/12 cake	310	3.8	10.4	5	1		53.0	84	.6	209	100	130	.02	.08	.2	tr.
Chestnut flour—see Legumes and Nuts																	
Cookies																	
Assorted, packaged	1 cookie	54	.6	2.3				8.1	4	.1	41	8	10	tr.	tr.	.1	tr.
Brownie, with nuts, home recipe, enriched flour	1 brownie	97	1.3	6.2	1	1		10.2	8	.4	50	38	40	.04	.03	.1	tr.
Brownie with nuts, frozen, commercial with chocolate icing	1 brownie	119	1.4	5.8	1	1		17.3	11	.4	57	51	60	.02	.02	.1	tr.
Butter	1 cookie	23	.3	.8				3.5	6	tr.	21	3	30	tr.	tr.	tr.	0
Chocolate wafer	1 wafer	29	.5	1.0				4.6	3	.1	9	8	10	tr.	tr.	tr.	tr.
Chocolate-chip, home recipe, enriched flour	1 cookie	52	.5	3.0	1	1		6.0	3	.2	35	12	10	.01	.01	.1	tr.
Chocolate-chip, commercial	1 cookie (2")	47	.5	2.1	1	tr.		7.0	4	.2	40	13	10	tr.	.01	tr.	tr.
Coconut bars	1 cookie	43	.5	2.1				5.5	6	.1	13	20	10	.01	.01	tr.	0
Fig bars	1 cookie	55	.6	.9				11.5	12	.2	39	30	20	.01	.01	.1	tr.
Gingersnaps	1 cookie	25	.3	.5				4.8	4	.1	34	28	tr.	tr.	tr.	.1	tr.
Macaroons	1 cookie	81	.6	3.9	3	tr.		11.2	5	.1	6	79	0	.01	.03	tr.	0
Marshmallow	1 cookie	65	.6	2.1				11.5	5	.1	33	14	40	tr.	tr.	tr.	tr.
Molasses	1 cookie (2")	48	.7	1.2				8.6	6	.2	44	16	10	.01	.01	.1	0

*Linoleic acid is unsaturated fat.

6. FLOUR, CEREAL GRAINS, AND GRAIN PRODUCTS (cont.)

Food	Measure	Calories	Pro-tein Gm	Total Fat Gm	Satu-rated Fat Gm	Lino-leic* Acid Gm	Choles-terol Mg	Car-bohy-drate Gm	Cal-cium Mg	Iron Mg	Sodium Mg	Potas-sium Mg	A IU	Thi-amine Mg	Ribo-flavin Mg	Nia-cin Mg	C Mg
Oatmeal with raisins	1 cookie (2")	75	1.0	2.6				12.3	4	.5	27	62	10	.02	.01	.1	tr.
Peanut	1 cookie (2")	59	1.2	2.4				8.4	5	.1	22	22	30	.01	.01	.3	tr.
Raisin	1 cookie	54	.6	.8				11.5	10	.3	7	39	30	.01	.01	.1	tr.
Sandwich type	1 cookie	49	.5	2.2				6.9	3	.1	48	4	0	tr.	tr.	tr.	0
Shortbread	1 cookie	37	.5	1.7				4.8	5	tr.	4	5	10	tr.	tr.	tr.	0
Sugar, soft thick, home type with enriched flour	1 cookie (2½")	94	1.3	3.6				14.5	17	.3	68	16	20	.03	.03	.3	tr.
Sugar wafer	1 wafer	41	.4	1.7				6.2	2	tr.	16	5	10	tr.	tr.	tr.	0
Vanilla wafer	1 cookie	18	.2	.6				3.0	2	tr.	10	3	10	tr.	tr.	tr.	0
Corn flakes	1 lb	1,751	35.8	1.8				386.9	77	6.4	4,559	544	0	1.94	.36	9.3	0
	1 cup (.9 oz)	96	2.0	.1				21.3	4	.4	251	30	0	.11	.02	.5	0
Corn flakes, sugar-coated	1 lb	1,751	20.0	.9				414.1	54	4.5	3,515	—	0	1.85	.16	8.6	0
	1 cup (1.4 oz)	154	1.8	.1				36.4	5	.4	309	—	0	.16	.01	.8	0
Corn flour	1 lb	1,669	35.4	11.8	1	5		348.4	27	8.2	5	5	1,540†	.91	.27	6.4	0
	1 cup	407	8.6	2.9	tr.	1		84.9	7	2.0	1	1	380†	.22	.07	1.6	0
Corn grits, degermed, enriched	1 lb	1,642	39.5	3.6				354.3	18	13.0	5	363	2,000†	2.00	1.20	16.0	0
	¾ cup	134	3.2	.3				28.8	1	1.1	tr.	30	160†	.16	.10	1.3	0
	1 cup cooked	125	2.9	.2				27.0	2	.7	502	27	150†	.10	.07	1.0	0
Corn grits, degermed, unenriched	1 lb	1,642	39.5	3.6				354.3	18	4.5	5	363	2,000†	.59	.18	5.4	0
	¾ cup	134	3.2	.3				28.8	1	.4	tr.	30	160†	.05	.01	.4	0
	1 cup cooked	125	2.9	.2				27.0	2	.2	502	27	150†	.05	.02	.5	0
Corn muffins—see Muffins, corn																	
Corn, puffed	1 lb	1,810	36.7	19.1				366.5	91	26.3	4,808	—	0	4.00	.83	12.1	0
	1 cup (1 oz)	113	2.3	1.2				22.9	6	1.6	301	—	0	.25	.05	.8	0

*Linoleic acid is unsaturated fat.
†Based on yellow varieties; white varieties contain only a trace of vitamin A.

6. FLOUR, CEREAL GRAINS, AND GRAIN PRODUCTS (cont.)

Food	Measure	Calories	Protein Gm	Total Fat Gm	Saturated Fat Gm	Lino-* leic Acid Gm	Cholesterol Mg	Carbohydrate Gm	Calcium Mg	Iron Mg	Sodium Mg	Potassium Mg	A IU	Thiamine Mg	Riboflavin Mg	Niacin Mg	C Mg
Corn, puffed, sweetened	1 lb	1,719	18.1	.9				407.3	50	8.2	1,361	—	0	1.92	.77	9.6	0
	1 cup (1 oz)	113	1.2	.1				26.9	3	.5	90	—	0	.12	.05	.6	0
Corn, puffed, sweetened, cocoa-flavored	1 lb	1,769	28.1	10.0				393.3	91	27.2	3,856	—	0	3.60	.83	11.5	0
	1 cup (1 oz)	111	1.8	.6				24.6	6	1.7	241	—	0	.23	.05	.7	0
Corn, puffed, sweetened, fruit-flavored	1 lb	1,792	25.4	12.2				396.4	136	22.7	2,722	—	0	4.50	.76	11.3	0
	1 cup (1 oz)	112	1.6	.8				24.8	9	1.4	170	—	0	.28	.05	.7	0
Corn, rice, and wheat flakes	1 lb	1,765	33.6	3.2				390.5	177	8.2	4,309	—	0	1.77	—	14.5	0
	1 cup (1 oz)	110	2.1	.2				24.4	11	.5	269	—	0	.11	—	.9	0
Cornmeal, whole ground	1 lb	1,610	41.7	17.7		2	8	334.3	91	10.9	5	1,288	2,310†	1.72	.50	9.1	0
	1 cup (yields 4 cups cooked)	432	11.2	4.8				89.8	24	2.9	1	346	620†	.46	.13	2.4	0
Cornmeal, bolted	1 lb	1,642	40.8	15.4	tr.	2	8	337.9	77	8.2	5	1,125	2,180†	1.36	.36	8.6	0
	1 cup (yields 4 cups cooked)	441	11.0	4.1				90.7	21	2.2	1	302	590†	.37	.10	2.3	0
Cornmeal, degermed, enriched	1 lb	1,651	35.8	5.4		2		355.6	27	13.0	5	544	2,000†	2.00	1.20	16.0	0
	1 cup	501	10.9	1.6				108.0	8	3.9	2	165	610†	.61	.36	4.9	0
	1 cup cooked	120	2.6	.5				25.7	2	1.0	264	38	140†	.14	.10	1.2	0
Cornmeal, degermed, unenriched	1 lb	1,651	35.8	5.4				355.6	27	5.0	5	544	2,000†	.64	.23	4.5	0
	1 cup	501	10.9	1.6				108.0	8	1.5	2	165	610†	.19	.07	1.4	0
	1 cup cooked	120	2.6	.5				25.7	2	.5	264	38	140†	.05	.02	.2	0
Cornstarch	1 lb	1,642	1.4	tr.				397.4	0	0	tr.	tr.	0	0	0	0	0
	1 cup	463	tr.	tr.				111.9	0	0	tr.	tr.	0	0	0	0	0
	1 T	29	tr.	tr.				2.0	0	0	tr.	tr.	0	0	0	0	0
Cottonseed flour	1 lb	1,615	218.2	29.9				149.7	1,284	57.2	—	—	270	5.49	3.80	29.3	—
	1 oz	101	13.6	1.9				9.4	80	3.6	—	—	20	.34	.24	1.8	—

*Linoleic acid is unsaturated fat.
†Based on yellow varieties; white varieties contain only a trace of vitamin A.

6. FLOUR, CEREAL GRAINS, AND GRAIN PRODUCTS (cont.)

Food	Measure	Calo-ries	Pro-tein Gm	Total Fat Gm	Satu-rated Fat Gm	Oleic Acid Gm	Lino-leic* Acid Gm	Choles-terol Mg	Carbo-hydrate Gm	Calcium Mg	Iron Mg	Sodium Mg	Potas-sium Mg	A IU	Thi-amine Mg	Ribo-flavin Mg	Nia-cin Mg	C Mg
Crackers																		
Animal	2 oz box	243	3.7	5.3					45.3	29	.3	172	54	70	.02	.06	.2	tr.
Butter	1 cracker	14	.2	.5					2.0	4	tr.	33	3	10	tr.	tr.	tr.	0
Cheese	1 cracker	14	.3	.6					1.8	10	tr.	31	3	10	tr.	tr.	tr.	0
Graham, plain	2 squares	54	1.1	1.3					9.9	6	.2	94	54	10	.01	.03	.2	0
Graham, sugar-honey	2 squares	57	.9	1.6					10.7	12	.2	70	38	—	.01	tr.	.1	0
Graham, chocolate-covered	2 squares	108	1.2	5.3					15.4	42	.6	92	73	0	.02	.06	.3	0
Saltines	4 crackers	48	1.0	1.3					7.8	2	.1	121	13	0	tr.	tr.	.1	0
Sandwich type, peanut-cheese	1 sandwich	35	1.1	1.7					4.0	4	tr.	70	16	tr.	tr.	tr.	.3	0
Soda	2 crackers	50	1.1	1.5					8.0	3	.2	125	14	0	tr.	tr.	.1	0
Whole-wheat	2 crackers	24	.5	.9					4.1	1	tr.	33		0	tr.	tr.	.1	0
Cream puff, custard filling	1	244	6.8	14.6	4		1		21.5	85	.7	87	127	370	.04	.18	.1	tr.
Danish pastry	1 lge ring (12 oz)	1,436	25.2	80.0					155.1	170	3.1	1,245	381	1,060	.23	.50	2.6	tr.
	1 4¾" diam	274	4.8	15.2					30.0	32	.6	237	73	200	.04	.10	.5	tr.
Doughnut, enriched flour	1	125	1.5	5.9	1	4	tr.		16.4	13	.5	160	29	30	.05	.05	.4	0
Eclair	1	262	6.8	15.0	4		1		25.5	88	.8	90	134	0	.05	.18	.1	0
Farina, enriched, regular	1 lb	1,683	51.7	4.1					349.3	113	13.0	1	376	0	2.00	1.20	16.0	0
	¼ cup	167	5.1	.4					35.6	11	1.3	9	37	0	.20	.12	1.6	0
	1 cup cooked	100	3.1	.2					20.8	10	.7	344	21	0	.10	.07	1.0	0
Farina, enriched, quick cooking	1 lb	1,642	51.7	4.1					339.7	2,268	—	1,134	376	0	2.00	1.20	16.0	0
	¼ cup cooked	163	5.1	.4					33.6	225	—	112	37	0	.20	.12	1.6	0
	1 cup cooked	105	3.2	.2					21.8	147	—	466	25	0	.12	.07	1.0	0
Macaroni, enriched	1 lb	1,674	56.7	5.4					341.1	122	13.0	9	894	0	4.00	1.70	27.0	0
	1 cup	442	15.0	1.4					90.1	32	3.4	2	236	0	1.06	.45	7.1	0
	1 cup cooked firm (8-10 min)	192	6.5	.7					39.1	14	1.4	1	103	0	.23	.13	1.8	0
	1 cup cooked tender (14-20 min)	155	4.8	.6					32.2	11	1.3	1	85	0	.20	.11	1.5	0

*Linoleic acid is unsaturated fat.

6. FLOUR, CEREAL GRAINS, AND GRAIN PRODUCTS (cont.)

Food	Measure	Calories	Protein Gm	Total Fat Gm	Saturated Fat Gm	Linoleic* Acid Gm	Cholesterol Mg	Carbohydrate Gm	Calcium Mg	Iron Mg	Sodium Mg	Potassium Mg	A IU	Thiamine Mg	Riboflavin Mg	Niacin Mg	C Mg
Macaroni, unenriched	1 lb	1,674	56.7	5.4				341.1	122	5.9	9	894	0	.42	.29	7.7	0
	1 cup	442	15.0	1.4				90.1	32	1.6	2	236	0	.11	.08	2.0	0
	1 cup cooked firm (8-10 min)	192	6.5	.7				39.1	14	.7	1	103	0	.03	.03	.5	0
	1 cup cooked tender (14-20 min)	155	4.8	.6				32.2	11	.6	1	103	0	.01	.01	.4	0
Macaroni and cheese, canned	1 lb	431	17.7	18.1	8	3		48.5	376	1.8	1,379	263	500	.23	.44	1.9	tr.
	1 cup	228	9.3	9.6	4	2		25.6	199	1.0	728	139	260	.12	.23	1.0	tr.
Millet	1 lb	1,483	44.9	13.2				330.7	91	30.8	—	1,950	0	3.30	1.70	10.6	0
	⅓ cup (yields 1 cup cooked)	196	5.9	1.7				43.7	12	4.1		257	0	.44	.22	1.4	0
Muffins, plain, enriched flour	3″ diam.	117	3.1	4.0	1	tr.		16.9	42	.6	176	50	40	.07	.09	.6	tr.
Muffins, plain, unenriched	3″ diam.	117	3.1	4.0	1	tr.		16.9	42	.2	176	50	40	.02	.06	.2	tr.
Muffins, blueberry†	3″ diam.	112	2.9	3.7	1	tr.		16.7	34	.6	252	46	90	.06	.08	.5	tr.
Muffins, bran†	3″ diam.	104	3.1	3.9	1	tr.		17.2	57	1.5	179	172	90	.06	.10	1.6	tr.
Muffins, corn, made with enriched degermed cornmeal†	3″ diam.	125	2.8	4.0	1	tr.		19.2	42	.7	192	54	120	.08	.09	.7	tr.
Muffins, corn, made with whole-ground cornmeal†	3″ diam.	115	2.9	4.1	1	tr.		20.0	45	.6	198	53	120	.07	.07	.4	tr.
Muffin mix, corn†	1 lb	1,892	28.1	52.2	12	5		325.7	1,361	8.2	2,994	345	680	1.09	.73	9.5	tr.
	1 muffin	129	2.8	4.2	1	1		20.0	96	.6	191	44	100	.07	.08	.6	tr.
Noodles, enriched	1 lb	1,760	58.1	20.9	7	1		326.6	141	13.0	23	617	1,000	4.00	1.70	27.0	0
	1 cup	242	8.0	2.9	1	tr.		45.0	19	1.8	3	65	140	.55	.23	3.7	0
	1 cup cooked	200	6.6	2.4	1	tr.		37.3	16	1.4	3	70	110	.22	.13	1.9	0
Noodles, unenriched	1 lb	1,760	58.1	20.9	7	1		326.6	141	8.6	23	617	1,000	.75	.40	9.7	0
	1 cup	242	8.0	2.9	1	tr.		45.0	19	1.2	3	65	140	.10	.06	1.3	0
	1 cup cooked	200	6.6	2.4	1	tr.		37.3	16	1.0	3	70	110	.05	.03	.6	0

*Linoleic acid is unsaturated fat.
†Made with enriched flour.

6. FLOUR, CEREAL GRAINS, AND GRAIN PRODUCTS (cont.)

Food	Measure	Calories	Protein Gm	Total Fat Gm	Saturated Fat Gm	Linoleic Acid Gm*	Cholesterol Mg	Carbohydrate Gm	Calcium Mg	Iron Mg	Sodium Mg	Potassium Mg	A IU	Thiamine Mg	Riboflavin Mg	Niacin Mg	C Mg
Noodles, chow mein, canned	1 lb	2,218	59.9	106.6				263.1	—	—	—	—	—	—	—	—	—
	1 cup	222	6.0	10.7				26.3	—	—	—	—	—	—	—	—	—
Oat cereals, hot with wheat germ and soy grits	1 lb	1,733	93.0	40.8	7	18		265.8	318	32.2	36	—	0	4.80	.76	6.4	0
	1 oz	108	5.8	2.6	tr.	1		16.6	20	2.0	2	—	0	.30	.05	.4	0
Oat flakes, maple-flavored, instant-cooking	1 lb	1,742	66.2	19.1				328.0	227	15.9	5	—	0	1.59	—	—	0
	½ cup (yields 1 cup cooked)	179	6.8	2.0				33.8	23	1.6	tr.	—	0	.16			0
Oat granules, maple-flavored, quick-cooking	1 lb	1,737	67.1	18.1				328.9	272	17.2	5	—	0	1.81	—	—	0
	½ cup (yields 1 cup cooked)	217	8.4	2.3				41.1	34	2.1	1	—	0	.23			0
Oats and wheat	1 lb	1,651	66.7	22.7	5	9		309.8	240	17.7	1	—	0	2.24	.80	12.0	0
	1 oz	103	4.2	1.4	tr.	1		19.4	15	1.1	1	—	0	.14	.05	.8	0
Oatmeal (rolled oats)	1 lb	1,769	64.4	33.6				309.4	240	20.4	9	1,597	0	2.72	.64	4.5	0
	1 oz (⅔ cup)	111	4.0	2.1				19.3	15	1.3	1	100	0	.17	.04	.3	0
	1 cup cooked	132	4.8	2.4				23.3	22	1.4	523	146	0	.19	.05	.2	0
Oat cereals, cold: Shredded oats	1 lb	1,719	85.3	9.5				326.6	1,202	24.0	2,767	—	0	3.22	1.50	38.6	0
	1 oz	107	5.3	.6				20.4	75	1.5	173	—	0	.20	.09	2.4	0
Puffed oats	1 lb	1,801	54.0	24.9				341.1	803	21.3	5,747	—	0	4.46	.79	8.8	0
	1 oz (1⅛ cup)	113	3.4	1.6				21.3	50	1.3	359	—	0	.28	.05	.6	0
Puffed oats, sugar-coated	1 lb	1,796	30.4	15.4				388.3	327	20.0	2,667	—	0	4.69	.55	7.8	0
	1 oz	112	1.9	1.0				24.3	20	1.3	167	—	0	.29	.03	.5	0
Oat flakes	1 lb	1,801	67.6	25.9				320.7	680	38.6	5,443	—	0	3.22	1.50	38.6	0
	1 oz (⅔ cup)	113	4.2	1.6				20.0	42	2.4	340	—	0	.20	.09	2.4	0

*Linoleic acid is unsaturated fat.

6. FLOUR, CEREAL GRAINS, AND GRAIN PRODUCTS (cont.)

Food	Measure	Calories	Protein Gm	Total Fat Gm	Saturated Fat Gm	Lino-leic* Acid Gm	Choles-terol Mg	Carbo-hydrate Gm	Calcium Mg	Iron Mg	Sodium Mg	Potas-sium Mg	A IU	Thi-amine Mg	Ribo-flavin Mg	Nia-cin Mg	C Mg
Pancakes, home recipe, enriched flour	1 4" pancake	62	1.9	1.9	1	tr.		9.2	27	.4	115	33	30	.05	.06	.4	tr.
Pancakes, home recipe, unenriched flour	1 4" pancake	62	1.9	1.9	1	tr.		9.2	27	.2	115	33	30	.01	.04	.1	tr.
Pancake and waffle mix																	
Plain and buttermilk, enriched flour	1 lb	1,615	39.0	8.2				343.4	2,041	14.1	6,500	735	0	2.00	1.53	13.0	0
	1 cup	485	11.7	2.5				103.0	612	4.2	1,950	221	0	.60	.46	3.9	0
	1 4" pancake	61	1.9	2.0				8.7	58	.3	152	42	70	.04	.06	.2	tr.
Plain and buttermilk, unenriched flour	1 lb	1,615	39.0	8.2				343.4	2,041	6.4	6,500	735	0	.54	.36	5.0	0
	1 cup	485	11.7	2.5				103.0	612	1.9	1,950	221	0	.16	.11	1.5	0
	1 4" pancake	61	1.9	2.0				8.7	58	.2	152	42	70	.02	.05	.1	tr.
Buckwheat	1 lb	1,488	47.6	8.6				318.9	2,114	14.1	6,051	2,154	tr.	1.63	.54	10.0	0
	1 cup	446	14.3	2.6				95.7	634	4.2	1,815	646	tr.	.49	.16	3.0	0
	1 4" pancake	54	1.8	.5				6.4	59	.4	125	66	60	.03	.04	.1	0
Pastina, egg	1 lb	1,737	58.5	18.6	6	1	tr.	325.7	159	13.0	23		1,000	4.00	1.70	27.0	0
	1 oz (2½ T)	109	3.7	1.2				20.4	10	.8	1		60	.25	.11	1.7	0
Pastina, carrot	1 lb	1,683	54.0	7.3				343.4	172	13.0			3,310	4.00	1.70	27.0	0
Pastina, spinach	1 lb	1,669	56.2	7.3				339.4	286	13.0			2,900	4.00	1.70	27.0	0
	1 oz (2½ T)	104	3.5	.5				21.2	18	.8	125		180	.25	.11	1.7	0
Pies, made with vegetable shortening and unenriched flour																	
Apple	⅙ of 9" pie	402	3.5	17.4	4	1		59.9	12	.5	473	126	50	.03	.03	.6	1
Banana custard	⅙ of 9" pie	338	6.9	14.2	4	1		47.0	101	.8	297	311	380	.06	.20	.5	2
Blackberry	⅙ of 9" pie	382	4.1	17.2	4	1		54.1	30	.8	421	157	140	.03	.03	.5	5
Blueberry	⅙ of 9" pie	381	3.8	17.0	4	1		54.9	17	.9	421	102	40	.03	.03	.4	6

*Linoleic acid is unsaturated fat.

6. FLOUR, CEREAL GRAINS, AND GRAIN PRODUCTS (cont.)

Food	Measure	Calories	Protein Gm	Total Fat Gm	Saturated Fat Gm	Lino-leic* Acid Gm	Cholesterol Mg	Carbohydrate Gm	Calcium Mg	Iron Mg	Sodium Mg	Potassium Mg	A IU	Thiamine Mg	Riboflavin Mg	Niacin Mg	C Mg
Pies, made with vegetable shortening and unenriched flour (cont.)																	
Butterscotch	1/6 of 9" pie	404	6.7	16.7				58.0	113	1.4	324	144	390	.04	.16	.3	tr.
Cherry	1/6 of 9" pie	410	4.1	17.8	4	1		60.4	22	.5	478	165	690	.04	.03	.7	tr.
Chocolate chiffon	1/6 of 9" pie	456	9.4	21.3				60.7	33	1.7	350	153	432	.04	.13	.3	0
Coconut custard	1/6 of 9" pie	356	9.1	18.9				37.7	142	1.1	374	247	350	.09	.28	.4	0
Custard	1/6 of 9" pie	330	9.2	16.8				35.4	145	.9	435	207	350	.08	.25	.5	0
Lemon chiffon	1/6 of 9" pie	339	7.6	13.7				47.4	25	1.0	283	88	180	.04	.09	.2	3
Lemon meringue	1/6 of 9" pie	356	5.2	14.3				52.7	20	.7	394	70	240	.05	.12	.3	4
Mince	1/6 of 9" pie	426	3.9	18.1	4	1		64.8	44	1.6	704	280	tr.	.11	.06	.6	1
Peach	1/6 of 9" pie	401	3.9	16.8	4	1		60.1	16	.8	421	234	1,150	.03	.06	1.1	5
Pecan	1/6 of 9" pie	574	7.0	31.5	4	5		70.5	65	3.8	304	169	1,220	.22	.10	.5	tr.
Pineapple chiffon	1/6 of 9" pie	312	7.1	13.1				42.4	26	1.0	277	106	380	.05	.10	.5	1
Pumpkin	1/6 of 9" pie	319	6.0	17.0				37.1	77	.8	324	242	3,740	.05	.15	.8	tr.
Raisin	1/6 of 9" pie	424	4.1	16.8	4	1		67.6	28	1.4	448	302	70	.05	.04	.5	1
Rhubarb	1/6 of 9" pie	398	3.9	16.8	4	1		60.1	101	1.1	425	250	70	.03	.06	.4	5
Strawberry	1/6 of 9" pie	311	3.0	12.4	4	1		48.6	25	1.1	305	189	60	.03	.07	.7	40
Sweet potato	1/6 of 9" pie	322	6.8	17.1				35.9	104	.8	330	247	3,630	.07	.18	.5	6
Piecrust, baked, enriched flour	1 9" shell	900	11.0	60.1	13	4		78.8	25	3.1	1,100	90	0	.36	.25	3.2	0
Piecrust, baked, unenriched flour	1 9" shell	900	11.0	60.1	13	4		78.8	25	.9	1,100	90	0	.05	.05	.9	0
Piecrust mix	10 oz (double crust)	1,480	20.4	92.6	21	8		140.3	131	1.4	1,964	179	0	.12	.11	1.9	0
Pizza	14" pie	1,413	71.8	49.6	20	3		169.5	1,323	5.9	4,204	779	3,780	.36	1.20	5.9	51
	3/6 pie	177	9.0	6.2	tr.	tr.		21.2	165	.7	525	97	470	.04	.15	.7	6
Pizza, frozen	14" pie	1,372	53.3	39.5	15	3		198.2	874	5.4	3,623	640	2,690	.34	1.00	5.5	32
	1/6 pie	172	6.7	4.9	2	tr.		24.8	109	.7	453	80	340	.04	.12	.7	4

*Linoleic acid is unsaturated fat.

6. FLOUR, CEREAL GRAINS, AND GRAIN PRODUCTS (cont.)

Food	Measure	Calories	Protein Gm	Total Fat Gm	Saturated Fat Gm	Linoleic* Acid Gm	Cholesterol Mg	Carbohydrate Gm	Calcium Mg	Iron Mg	Sodium Mg	Potassium Mg	A IU	Thiamine Mg	Riboflavin Mg	Niacin Mg	C Mg
Popcorn, popped plain	1 lb	1,751	57.6	22.7	2	12		347.9	50	12.2	14	—	—	—	.54	10.0	0
	1 cup	23	.8	.3	tr.	tr.		4.6	1	.2	tr.	—	—	—	.01	.1	0
with oil and salt	1 lb	2,068	44.5	98.9	72	9		268.1	36	9.5	8,800	—	—	—	.42	7.7	0
	1 cup	41	.9	2.0	1	tr.		5.3	1	.2	174	—	—	—	.01	.2	0
sugar-coated	1 lb	1,737	27.7	15.9	5	6		387.4	23	5.9	5	—	—	—	.26	4.8	0
	1 cup	134	2.1	1.2	tr.	tr.		29.8	2	.5	tr.	—	—	—	.02	.4	0
Potato flour	1 lb	1,592	36.3	3.6				362.4	150	78.0	154	7,203	tr.	1.91	.61	15.2	86
	1 cup	525	12.0	1.2				119.6	50	25.7	51	2,378	tr.	.63	.20	5.0	28
	1 T	33	.7	.1				7.5	3	1.6	3	148	tr.	.04	.01	.3	2
Pretzels Dutch twisted	1	62	1.6	.7				12.1	4	.2	268	21	0	tr.	.1	.1	0
thin twisted	1	23	.6	.3				4.5	1	.1	200	8	0	tr.	tr.	tr.	0
stick, thin	10 2¾" sticks	12	.3	.1				2.3	1	tr.	100	4	0	tr.	tr.	tr.	0
stick, regular	5 3⅛" sticks	12	.3	.1				2.3	1	tr.	50	4	0	tr.	tr.	tr.	0
Rice, brown	1 lb	1,633	34.0	8.6				351.1	145	7.3	41	971	0	1.52	.24	21.4	0
	1 cup	663	13.8	3.5				142.7	59	3.0	17	395	0	.62	.10	8.7	0
	½ cup cooked	89	1.9	.5				19.1	12	.4	212	53	0	.07	.02	1.1	0
Rice, white, enriched regular	1 lb	1,647	30.4	1.8				364.7	109	13.0	23	417	0	2.00	1.20	16.0	0
	1 cup	670	12.4	.7				148.5	44	5.3	9	170	0	.81	.49	6.5	0
	⅔ cup cooked	112	2.0	.1				24.8	10	.9	383	29	0	.11		1.0	0
parboiled	1 lb	1,674	33.6	1.4				368.8	272	13.0	38	680	0	2.00	1.20	16.0	0
	⅔ cup cooked	93	1.8	.1				20.4	17	.7	313	38	0	.11		1.1	0
instant	1 lb	1,696	34.0	.9				374.2	23	13.0	5	tr.	0	2.10	1.20	16.0	0
	½ cup cooked	90	1.8	tr.				20.0	3	.7	225	—	0	.11		1.1	0
Rice, white, unenriched	1 lb	1,647	30.4	1.8				364.7	109	3.6	23	417	0	.32	.12	7.2	0
	1 cup	670	12.4	.7				148.5	44	1.5	9	170	0	.13	.05	2.9	0
	⅔ cup cooked	112	2.0	.1				24.8	10	.2	383	29	0	.02	.01	.4	0

*Linoleic acid is unsaturated fat.

6. FLOUR, CEREAL GRAINS, AND GRAIN PRODUCTS (cont.)

Food	Measure	Calories	Protein Gm	Total Fat Gm	Saturated Fat Gm	Lino-leic* Acid Gm	Choles-terol Mg	Carbo-hydrate Gm	Calcium Mg	Iron Mg	Sodium Mg	Potassium Mg	A IU	Thiamine Mg	Riboflavin Mg	Niacin Mg	C Mg
Rice polish	1 lb	1,202	54.9	58.1				261.7	313	73.0	tr.	3,239	0	8.35	.82	127.8	0
Rice, granulated	½ cup	300	13.7	14.5				65.4	78	18.2	tr.	832	0	2.09	.20	40.0	0
	3 T (yields ¾ cup cooked)	1,737	27.2	1.4				389.6	41	24.5	—	—	0	1.92	.48	25.4	0
Rice cereals, cold																	
Rice flakes	1 oz	102	1.6	.1				22.9	2	1.4	—	—	0	.11	.03	1.6	0
Rice, puffed	1 lb	1,769	26.8	1.4				397.8	132	7.3	4,477	816	0	1.59	.01	1.5	0
	1 oz (1¼ cups)	111	1.7	.1				24.9	8	.5	280	51	0	.10	.18	20.0	0
Rice, puffed	1 lb	1,810	27.2	1.8				406.0	91	8.2	tr.	454	0	2.00	.01	20.9	0
	1 cup (½ oz)	60	1.0	tr.				13.4	3	.3	—	15	0	.07	—	—	tr.
Rice, puffed, sweetened	1 lb	1,760	19.1	3.2				411.0	209	4.1	3,202	—	0	1.50	—	.8	0
	1 cup (⅔ oz)	66	.7	.1				15.4	8	.2	120	—	0	.06	.05	.6	tr.
Rice, puffed, sweetened, cocoa-flavored	1 lb	1,819	20.4	18.1				393.3	231	15.0	1,624	277	0	1.88	.29	28.6	0
	1 cup (⅔ oz)	68	.8	.7				14.7	9	.6	61	10	0	.07	.23	24.4	0
Rice, shredded	1 lb	1,778	23.6	1.4				402.8	64	8.2	3,837	—	0	1.76	.01	1.1	0
	1 oz	111	1.5	.1				25.2	4	.5	240	—	0	.11	.04	.4	tr.
Rolls																	
Hard roll, enriched	1 med (3")	155	4.9	1.6				29.7	23	1.1	312	48	tr.	.13	—	32.0	0
Hard roll, unenriched	1 med (3")	155	4.9	1.6				29.7	23	.4	312	48	tr.	.03	—	2.0	0
Pan roll, enriched	1 med (3")	85	2.3	1.6				15.0	21	.5	143	27	tr.	.08	.12	1.3	tr.
Pan roll, unenriched	1 med (3")	85	2.3	1.6				15.0	21	.2	143	27	tr.	.02	.03	.2	tr.
Hamburger or frankfurter, enriched	1	119	3.3	2.2				21.2	30	.8	202	38	tr.	.11	.04	.3	tr.
unenriched	1	119	3.3	2.2				21.2	30	.3	202	38	tr.	.02	.06	.4	tr.
Sweet roll	1 3½" roll	134	3.3	3.9				21.9	36	.3	166	53	30	.03	.05	1.1	tr.
Whole-wheat roll	1 med (3")	95	3.7	1.0				19.3	39	.9	208	108	tr.	.13	.06	1.6	tr.
Brown-and-Serve	1 2" roll	85	2.2	1.9				14.3	13	.5	145	26	tr.	.07	.07	.9	tr.

*Linoleic acid is unsaturated fat.

6. FLOUR, CEREAL GRAINS, AND GRAIN PRODUCTS (cont.)

Food	Measure	Calo-ries	Pro-tein Gm	Total Fat Gm	Satu-rated Fat Gm	Lino-* leic Acid Gm	Choles-terol Mg	Car-bohy-drate Gm	Cal-cium Mg	Iron Mg	Sodium Mg	Potas-sium Mg	A IU	Thi-amine Mg	Ribo-flavin Mg	Nia-cin Mg	C Mg
Rye, whole-grain	1 lb	1,515	54.9	7.7				322.9	172	16.8	5	2,118	0	1.94	1.02	7.1	0
Rye flour, light	1 oz (¾ cup)	95	3.4	.5				20.2	11	1.0	tr.	132	0	.12	.06	.4	0
Rye flour, light	1 lb	1,619	42.6	4.5				353.4	100	5.0	5	708	0	.67	.31	2.9	0
Rye flour, medium	1 cup	310	8.2	.9				67.7	19	1.0	5	136	0	.13	.06	.6	0
Rye flour, medium	1 lb	1,588	51.7	7.7				339.3	122	11.8	5	921	0	1.35	.54	11.2	0
Rye flour, dark	1 cup	347	11.3	1.7				74.2	27	2.6	1	201	0	.30	.12	2.4	0
Rye flour, dark	1 lb	1,483	73.9	11.8				308.9	245	20.4	5	3,901	0	2.76	.98	12.2	0
Rye flour, dark	1 cup	405	20.2	3.2				84.3	67	5.6	1	1,065	0	.75	.27	3.3	0
Rye wafers	2	45	1.7	.5				9.9	7	.5	114	78	0	.04	.03	.2	0
Spaghetti, enriched	1 lb	1,674	56.7	5.4				341.1	122	13.0	9	894	0	4.00	1.70	27.0	0
Spaghetti, enriched	1 cup cooked	155	4.8	.6				32.2	11	1.3	1	85	0	.20	.11	1.5	0
Spaghetti, unenriched	1 lb	1,674	56.7	5.4				341.1	122	5.9	9	894	0	.42	.29	7.7	0
Spaghetti, unenriched	1 cup cooked	155	4.8	.6				32.2	11	.6	1	85	0	.01	.01	.4	0
Spaghetti in tomato sauce with cheese, canned	1 lb	345	10.0	2.7				69.9	73	5.0	1,733	549	1,680	.64	.50	8.2	.20
	1 cup	190	5.5	1.4				38.4	40	2.8	953	302	920	.35	.28	4.5	11
Spaghetti and meatballs in tomato sauce, canned	1 lb	467	22.2	18.6				51.7	95	5.9	2,214	445	1,810	.28	.30	4.2	11
	1 cup	257	12.2	10.2				28.4	52	3.2	1,218	245	1,000	.15	.17	2.3	6
Waffles, home recipe, enriched flour	7" waffle	209	7.0	7.4	2	1		28.1	85	1.3	356	109	250	.13	.19	1.0	tr.
Waffles, frozen, enriched flour	3" waffle	60	1.7	1.5				9.9	29	.4	152	37	30	.04	.04	.3	tr.
Waffles, from mix, enriched flour	7" waffle	206	6.6	8.0	3	1		27.2	179	1.0	515	146	170	.10	.17	.7	tr.

*Linoleic acid is unsaturated fat.

6. FLOUR, CEREAL GRAINS, AND GRAIN PRODUCTS (cont.)

Food	Measure	Calories	Protein Gm	Total Fat Gm	Saturated Fat Gm	Lino-leic* Acid Gm	Cholesterol Mg	Carbohydrate Gm	Calcium Mg	Iron Mg	Sodium Mg	Potassium Mg	A IU	Thiamine Mg	Riboflavin Mg	Niacin Mg	C Mg
Wheat flour																	
Whole-wheat	1 lb	1,510	60.3	9.1				322.1	186	15.0	14	1,678	0	2.49	.54	19.7	0
	1 cup	399	15.9	2.4				85.1	49	4.0	4	443	0	.66	.14	5.2	0
	1 T	25	1.0	tr.				5.3	3	.2	tr.	7	0	.04	.01	.3	0
All-purpose, enriched	1 lb	1,651	47.6	4.5				345.2	73	13.0	9	431	0	2.00	1.20	16.0	0
	1 cup unsifted	454	13.1	1.2				95.0	20	3.6	2	119	0	.55	.33	4.4	0
	1 cup sifted	418	12.0	1.1				87.4	18	3.3	2	109	0	.51	.30	4.0	0
	1 T	28	.8	.1				5.9	1	.2	tr.	7	0	.03	.02	.3	0
All-purpose, unenriched	1 lb	1,651	47.6	4.5				345.2	73	3.6	9	431	0	.28	.21	4.1	0
	1 cup unsifted	454	13.1	1.2				95.0	20	1.0	2	119	0	.08	.06	1.1	0
	1 cup sifted	418	12.0	1.1				87.4	18	.9	2	109	0	.07	.05	1.0	0
	1 T	28	.8	.1				5.9	1	.1	tr.	7	0	tr.	tr.	.1	0
Cake or pastry	1 lb	1,651	34.0	3.6				360.2	77	2.3	9	431	0	.14	.14	3.0	0
	1 cup	349	7.2	.8				76.1	16	.5	2	91	0	.03	.03	.6	0
Gluten flour	1 lb	1,715	187.8	8.6				214.1	181	—	9	272	0	—	—	—	0
	1 cup	328	57.9	2.6				66.0	56	—	3	84	0	—	—	—	0
Self-rising, enriched	1 lb	1,597	42.2	4.5				336.6	1,202	13.0	4,894	—	0	2.00	1.20	16.0	0
	1 cup	439	11.6	1.2				92.6	331	3.6	1,346	—	0	.55	.33	4.4	0
Wheat bran	1 lb	966	72.6	20.9				280.8	540	67.6	41	5,085	0	3.25	1.59	95.3	0
	¾ cup	34	2.6	.7				9.9	19	2.4	1	179	0	.11	.06	3.3	0
Wheat germ, raw	1 lb	1,647	120.7	49.4	7	24		211.8	327	42.6	14	3,751	0	9.10	3.09	19.2	0
	1 oz (¼ cup)	103	7.5	3.1	tr.			13.2	20	2.7	1	232	0	.57	.19	1.2	0
Wheat germ, toasted	1 lb	1,774	136.1	52.2	8	25		224.5	213	40.4	1	4,296	500	7.48	1.04	35.4	0
	1 oz (¼ cup)	111	8.5	3.3	tr.	2		14.0	13	2.5	1	268	30	.47	.07	2.2	0
Wheat cereal, hot																	
Rolled wheat	1 lb	1,542	44.9	9.1				354.6	163	14.5	9	1,724	0	1.65	.55	18.6	0
	½ cup (yields 1 cup cooked)	142	4.1	.8				32.6	15	1.3	8	158	0	.15	.05	1.7	0

*Linoleic acid is unsaturated fat.

6. FLOUR, CEREAL GRAINS, AND GRAIN PRODUCTS (cont.)

Food	Measure	Calories	Protein Gm	Total Fat Gm	Saturated Fat Gm	Lino-leic* Acid Gm	Choles-terol Mg	Carbo-hydrate Gm	Calcium Mg	Iron Mg	Sodium Mg	Potas-sium Mg	A IU	Thi-amine Mg	Ribo-flavin Mg	Nia-cin Mg	C Mg
Wheat cereal, hot (cont.)																	
Whole-wheat	1 lb	1,533	61.2	9.1				328.0	204	16.8	9	1,678	0	2.30	.61	21.2	0
	½ cup (yields 1 cup cooked)	141	5.6	.8				30.0	19	1.5	1	154	0	.21	.06	2.0	0
Wheat and malted barley, toasted, quick-cooking	1 lb	1,737	54.4	7.3				356.1	227	11.8	5	—	0	1.54	.29	—	0
	½ cup (yields 1 cup cooked)	160	5.0	.7				32.7	21	1.1	tr.	—	0	1.4	.03	—	0
Wheat cereal, cold																	
Wheat flakes	1 lb	1,606	46.3	7.3				365.1	186	20.0	4,681	—	0	2.92	.62	22.4	0
	1 cup (1 oz)	106	3.1	.6				24.1	12	1.3	309	—	0	.19	.04	1.5	0
Wheat, puffed	1 lb	1,647	68.0	6.8				356.1	127	19.1	18	1,542	0	2.49	1.04	35.4	0
	1 cup (½ oz)	54	2.2	.2				11.8	4	.6	1	51	0	.08	.03	1.2	0
Wheat, puffed, sweetened	1 lb	1,706	27.2	9.5				400.5	118	15.0	730	449	0	2.20	.82	29.3	0
	1 cup (1¼ oz)	120	1.9	.7				28.2	8	1.1	51	32	0	.15	.06	2.1	0
Wheat, shredded	1 lb	1,606	44.9	9.1				362.4	195	15.9	14	1,579	0	1.00	.51	10.0	0
	1 biscuit	88	2.5	.5				19.9	11	.9	1	87	0	.05	.03	1.1	0
Wheat and malted barley flakes	1 lb	1,778	39.9	5.9				382.4	222	11.8	3,538	—	0	2.09	.48	17.7	0
	1 oz (⅔ cup)	111	2.5	.4				23.9	14	.7	221	—	0	.13	.03	1.1	0
Wheat and malted barley granules	1 lb	1,774	45.4	2.7				382.8	240	12.7	3,221	1,043	0	2.09	.32	24.0	0
	1 oz (¼ cup)	111	2.8	.2				23.9	15	.8	201	65	0	.13	.02	1.5	0
Wild rice	1 lb	1,601	64.0	3.2				341.6	86	19.1	32	998	0	2.02	2.87	27.9	0
	4 oz (yields 3 cups cooked)	400	16.0	.8				85.4	21	4.8	8	250	tr.	.50	.72	7.0	0
Zwieback	1 piece	31	.8	.6				5.4	1	tr.	18	11	tr.	tr.	tr.	.1	0

*Linoleic acid is unsaturated fat.

7. LEGUMES AND NUTS

Legumes and nuts are grouped together chiefly because of their similar importance as secondary proteins in the American diet. While meat, fish, poultry, eggs, cheese, and milk are thought of as "protein foods" in this country, throughout South America, Africa, Asia, and the Middle East it is dried beans, nuts, and seeds coupled with grains that provide the daily quota of amino acids.

The term *legumes* encompasses all dried beans, including peas and lentils. With the exception of soybeans, they are considered incomplete proteins and are low in two of the essential amino acids. However, teamed with grains, nuts, or seeds, beans become high-quality proteins with all the essential growth factors. Unlike other beans, soybeans by themselves possess adequate amounts of all the essential amino acids. By adding beans to small quantities of meat, cheese, milk, and other already high-quality protein foods their protein is elevated, making them nutritious budget extenders.

Legumes are also rich in iron, thiamine, niacin, and potassium and are a fair source of calcium and riboflavin. Soybeans are a primary source of calcium in areas where milk is not plentiful. The legume family is an excellent source of some vitamins and minerals which are not included in the table: magnesium, phosphorous, and all the B-complex vitamins with the exception of B_{12}. Unfortunately baking soda, often added to the bean pot to soften the seeds, has a detrimental effect on B-vitamin content.

Legumes are low in fat, but contain more carbohydrate than other traditional protein sources. Although people tend to think of beans as "fattening," on a pound-for-pound basis they are about equal in calories to pork, a choice steak, or loin lamb chops, and contain from $1\frac{1}{4}$ to $1\frac{1}{2}$ times the protein of these meats. Since beans contain no fat or bone waste, one pound goes quite far. (For further comparisons of nutritive value consult the individual tables.) Low sodium levels make beans ideal for low-salt diets.

Although rich in so many food elements beans are not a good source of vitamins A or C. When they are sprouted, however, beans become a low-calorie, low-carbohydrate source of all their original nutrients plus vitamin C. The tiny green leaves on the sprouts indicate stores of vitamin A as well.

Nuts and seeds, such as sesame seeds, pumpkin seeds, and sunflower seeds, are similar in vitamin and mineral content to dried beans; they are well endowed with B vitamins (except riboflavin and B_{12}), iron, magnesium, phosphorous, and vitamin E. Some nuts and seeds, like almonds and sesame seeds, contain considerable amounts of calcium. Of course not all nuts are identical and while some are of excellent protein value (especially when coupled with beans, grains, milk, and milk products), both chestnuts and coconuts have little protein to offer. Carbohydrate content spans a wide range.

Most nuts have a substantial amount of fat, albeit largely the unsaturated kind. This makes them higher in calories per gram of protein than other protein-rich foods in the diet, but gives them "staying power"; a small serving actually slows digestion enough to make nuts valuable as an aid to combating hunger in weight control.

Despite their high nutritive value, nuts and seeds play a minor role in the American diet and because such small quantities are consumed at a time they are not thought of as particularly significant in terms of their ability to promote growth and health. They are most frequently sold roasted (a process more akin to deep-fat frying) and salted, greatly decreasing their health value. In order to promote the role of nuts and seeds in your diet you might try grinding nuts and seeds into meal (or flour) in a blender and using this as a binder or topping on casseroles, ground meat dishes, vegetable or grain combinations, and in baking. Both nuts and seeds can be made into butters, the most popular one being peanut butter. When processed commerically, the addition of hydrogenated fat, salt, and sugar may make nut butters somewhat less desirable, but with the aid of a blender and the addition of small amounts of nut or vegetable oil, any nut or seed can be transformed into a spread in your kitchen.

When eaten as a snack food, nuts and seeds, unlike candies and cookies, offer good nutritional returns for their calorie expenditure.

As a group nuts are low in vitamins A and C.

How to Use the Table

LEGUMES

• Values are given per pound of dried beans and per ½-cup volume of uncooked beans. The approximate volume of cooked beans these measures will make is also given.
• Cooked canned beans can be evaluated from the weight of contents on the label, or from the measured amounts on the table. With the exception of sodium values, canned beans and cooked dried beans are nutritionally alike measure for measure.
• Bean sprouts, soybean derivitives, and several prepared bean products like franks and beans, pork and beans, and chili are also listed on this table. Bean soups, however, are found with other soups in Table 11.

NUTS

• Nuts are analyzed here by the pound, but as they are rarely eaten in such large amounts, smaller units are evaluated as well.
• Nut butters and ground nut meals (flours) are also located on this table.
• The table is unfortunately deficient in the scope of nut products that have been analyzed. If you are using nut butters or ground nut meals that are not listed in these pages you can get a fairly good idea of their nutritional value if you measure and calculate from the amount of nuts or seeds you used in their preparation. Do not fail to take into consideration any deviation in processing from the manner evaluated in the table (such as roasting, salting, dry roasting, or sugar coating), for this will alter the amount of fat, carbohydrate, calories, and sodium.

7. LEGUMES AND NUTS

Food	Measure	Calories	Protein Gm	Total Fat Gm	Saturated Fat Gm	Lino-leic* Acid Gm	Choles-terol Mg	Carbo-hydrate Gm	Calcium Mg	Iron Mg	Sodium Mg	Potassium Mg	A IU	Thiamine Mg	Riboflavin Mg	Niacin Mg	C Mg
Almonds, in shell	1 lb (yields ap. 1⅓ cups shelled)	1,383	43.0	125.4	10	25		45.1	541	10.9	9	1,788	0	.55	2.14	8.1	tr.
Almonds, shelled	1 lb	2,713	84.4	245.9	20	49		88.5	1,061	21.3	18	3,506	0	1.08	4.20	15.9	tr.
	1 cup	848	26.4	76.8	6	15		27.7	332	6.7	6	1,096	0	.34	1.31	5.0	tr.
Almonds, roasted, salted	13-15 nuts	107	3.3	9.7	1	2		3.5	42	.6	1	139	0	.04	.17	.6	tr.
Almond meal, partially defatted	1 lb	2,844	84.4	261.7	21	52		88.5	1,066	21.3	898	3,506	0	.22	4.20	15.9	0
	1 cup	845	25.1	77.8	6	15		26.3	317	6.3	267	1,042	0	.07	1.25	4.7	0
Beans, white, dried	1 lb	1,851	179.2	83.0	7	17		131.1	1,923	38.6	32	6,350	0	1.47	7.61	28.8	tr.
	1 cup	684	66.3	30.7	3	6		48.5	711	14.3	12	2,348	0	.54	2.81	10.6	tr.
	2 T	86	8.3	3.8	tr.	1		6.1	89	1.8	1	293	0	.07	.35	1.3	tr.
	½ cup (yields ap. 1⅓ cups cooked)	1,542	101.2	7.3				278.1	653	35.4	86	5,425	0	2.96	1.02	10.8	—
Beans, white, canned with tomato sauce	1 cup	339	22.3	1.6				61.2	144	7.8	19	1,194	0	.65	.22	2.4	—
Beans, white, canned with pork and tomato sauce	1 lb	544	28.6	2.3				104.3	308	9.1	1,533	1,216	270	.32	.16	2.5	9
	1 cup	305	16.0	1.3				58.5	173	5.1	860	682	150	.18	.09	1.4	5
Beans, red, dried	1 lb	553	27.7	11.8	4	1		86.2	245	8.2	2,100	953	590	.34	.14	2.6	9
	1 cup	310	15.5	6.6	2	1		48.4	137	4.6	1,179	535	330	.19	.08	1.5	5
	½ cup (yields ap. 1⅓ cups cooked)	1,556	102.1	6.8				280.8	499	31.3	45	4,463	90	2.33	.92	10.6	—
Beans, red, canned	1 lb	342	22.5	1.5				61.8	110	6.9	10	982	20	.51	.20	2.3	
	1 cup	408	25.9	1.8				74.4	132	8.2	14	1,198	tr.	.23	.18	2.7	
	½ cup	229	14.5	1.0				41.8	74	4.6	8	672	tr.	.13	.10	1.5	
Beans, pinto, calico and red Mexican, dried	1 lb	1,583	103.9	5.4				288.9	612	29.0	45	4,463	—	3.80	.95	10.0	—
	½ cup (yields ap. 1⅓ cups cooked)	322	21.1	1.1				58.7	124	5.9	9	906	—	.77	.19	2.0	—

*Linoleic acid is unsaturated fat.

7. LEGUMES AND NUTS (cont.)

Food	Measure	Calories	Protein Gm	Total Fat Gm	Saturated Fat Gm	Lino-* leic Acid Gm	Cholesterol Mg	Carbohydrate Gm	Calcium Mg	Iron Mg	Sodium Mg	Potassium Mg	Vitamins A IU	Thiamine Mg	Riboflavin Mg	Niacin Mg	C Mg
Beans, black and brown, dried	1 lb	1,538	101.2	6.8				277.6	612	35.8	113	4,708	140	2.51	.91	9.8	
	½ cup (yields ap. 1 cup cooked)	312	20.6	1.4				56.4	124	7.3	23	956	30	.51	.18	2.0	
Beans, lima, dried	1 lb	1,565	92.5	7.3				290.3	327	35.4	18	6,936	tr.	2.17	.75	8.6	
	½ cup (yields ap. 1½ cups cooked)	342	20.2	1.6				63.5	72	7.7	4	1,518	tr.	.47	.16	1.9	
Beans, mung, dried	1 lb	1,542	109.8	5.9				273.5	535	34.9	27	4,663	360	1.71	.96	11.7	
	½ cup (yields ap. 1¼ cups cooked)	337	24.0	1.3				59.8	117	7.6	6	1,020	80	.37	.21	2.6	
Beans, mung, sprouted	1 lb	159	17.2	.9				29.9	86	5.9	23	1,012	90	.60	.61	3.4	86
	1 cup	35	3.8	.2				6.5	19	1.3	5	221	20	.13	.13	.7	19
Beans and frankfurters, canned	1 lb	653	34.5	32.2				57.2	168	8.6	2,445	1,188	590	.30	.26	5.7	tr.
	1 cup	366	19.4	18.0				32.1	94	4.8	1,372	667	330	.17	.15	3.2	tr.
Brazil nuts, in shell	1 lb (yields ap. 1½ cups shelled)	1,424	31.1	145.6	29	38		23.7	405	7.4	2	1,557	tr.	2.09	.26	3.5	
Brazil nuts, shelled	1 lb	2,967	64.9	303.5	61	79		49.4	844	15.4	5	3,243	tr.	4.35	.54	7.3	
	1 cup	946	20.7	96.8	19	25		15.7	269	4.9	2	1,034	tr.	1.39	.17	2.3	
	4 nuts	98	2.1	10.0	2	3		1.6	13	.5	tr.	107	tr.	.14	.02	.2	
Butternuts, in shell	1 lb	399	15.1					5.3		4.3							
Butternuts, shelled	1 lb	2,853	107.5	277.6				38.1		30.8							
	5 nuts	94	3.5	9.2				1.3		1.0							
Cashew nuts	1 lb	2,545	78.0	207.3	35	15		132.9	172	17.2	68†	2,105	450	1.93	1.12	8.0	
	1 cup	795	24.4	64.8	11	5		41.5	54	5.4	21†	658	140	.60	.35	2.5	
Chestnuts, in shell	1 lb (36 lge nuts)	713	10.7	5.5				154.7	99	6.2	22	1,668		.82	.81	2.2	
Chestnut flour	1 lb	1,642	27.7	16.8				345.6	227	14.5	50	3,842		1.06	1.67	4.3	
	1 oz	103	1.7	1.1				21.6	14	.9	3	240		.07	.10	.3	

*Linoleic acid is unsaturated fat.
†900 milligrams sodium per pound, or 281 milligrams sodium per cup if salted.

7. LEGUMES AND NUTS (cont.)

Food	Measure	Calories	Protein Gm	Total Fat Gm	Saturated Fat Gm	Lino-leic* Acid Gm	Cholesterol Mg	Carbohydrate Gm	Calcium Mg	Iron Mg	Sodium Mg	Potassium Mg	A IU	Thiamine Mg	Riboflavin Mg	Niacin Mg	C Mg
Chickpeas, dried	1 lb	1,633	93.0	21.8	2	8		276.7	680	31.3	118	3,615	230	1.42	.68	9.3	—
	½ cup (yields ap. 1¼ cups cooked)	341	19.4	4.6	tr.	2		57.9	142	6.5	25	756	50	.30	.14	1.9	—
Coconut, in shell	1 lb	816	8.3	83.3	72	tr.		22.2	31	4.0	54	604	0	.13	.05	1.3	7
Coconut meat	1 lb	1,569	15.9	160.1	138	tr.		42.6	59	7.7	104	1,161	0	.24	.10	2.4	14
	2"x2" piece	155	1.6	15.8	14	tr.		4.2	6	.8	10	115	0	.02	.01	.2	4
	1 cup shredded	449	4.5	45.8	39	tr.		12.2	17	2.2	30	332	0	.07	.03	.7	1
Coconut, dried, unsweetened	1 lb	3,003	32.7	294.4	253	tr.		104.3	118	15.0		2,667	0	.27	.20	2.7	0
	1 cup	529	5.8	51.8	45	tr.		18.4	21	2.6		470	0	.05	.04	.5	0
	1 T	33	.4	3.2	3	tr.		1.1	2	.2		29	0	tr.	tr.	tr.	0
Coconut, dried, sweetened	1 lb	2,486	16.3	177.4	153	tr.		241.3	73	9.1		1,601	0	.63	.12	1.6	0
	1 cup	404	2.6	28.8	25	tr.		39.2	12	1.5		260	0	.03	.02	.3	0
	1 T	25	.2	1.8	1	tr.		2.5	1	.1		16	0	tr.	tr.	tr.	0
Cowpeas (blackeye peas), dried	1 lb	1,556	103.4	6.8				279.9	336	26.3	159	4,645	140	4.74	.97	9.8	—
	½ cup	343	22.8	1.5				61.7	74	5.8	35	1,024	30	1.05	.21	2.2	—
	1 cup cooked (yields ap. 1¼ cups cooked)	188	12.6	.7				34.2	42	3.2	20	568	20	.40	.10	.1	—
Filberts (hazelnuts), in shell	1 lb (yields ap. 1¼ cups shelled)	1,323	26.3	130.2	7	21		34.9	436	7.1	4	1,469		.96		2.0	tr.
Filberts (hazelnuts), shelled	1 lb	2,876	57.2	283.0	14	45		75.8	948	15.4	9	3,193		2.08		4.3	tr.
	1 cup	854	17.0	84.1	4	13		22.5	282	4.6	3	949		.62		1.3	tr.
Hickory nuts, in shell	1 lb	1,068	21.0	109.1	9	20		20.3	tr.	3.8							
	8 nuts	67	1.3	6.8	tr.	1		1.3	tr.	.2							
Hickory nuts, shelled	1 lb	3,053	59.9	311.6	25	56		58.1		10.9							
Lentils, dried	1 lb	1,542	112.0	5.0				272.6	358	30.8	136	3,583	270	1.69	.99	9.3	—
	½ cup (yields ap. 1¼ cups cooked)	322	23.4	1.0				57.0	75	6.4	28	749	60	.35	.20	1.9	—
Macadamia nuts, in shell	1 lb	972	11.0	100.7				22.4	67	2.8		371	0	.48	.15	1.8	0

(Minerals group: Calcium, Iron, Sodium, Potassium. Vitamins group: A, Thiamine, Riboflavin, Niacin, C.)

*Linoleic acid is unsaturated fat.

7. LEGUMES AND NUTS (cont.)

Food	Measure	Calories	Protein Gm	Total Fat Gm	Saturated Fat Gm	Linoleic* Acid Gm	Cholesterol Mg	Carbohydrate Gm	Calcium Mg	Iron Mg	Sodium Mg	Potassium Mg	A IU	Thiamine Mg	Riboflavin Mg	Niacin Mg	C Mg
Macadamia nuts, shelled	1 lb	3,134	35.4	324.8				72.1	218	9.1	—	1,198	0	1.54	.48	5.8	0
	7 nuts	196	2.2	20.3				4.5	14	.6	—	75	0	.10	.03	.4	0
Peanuts, raw, in shell	1 lb (yields ap. 2 1/6 cups shelled)	1,868	86.1	157.3	35	46		61.6	228	7.0	17	2,232	—	3.77	.44	56.8	0
Peanuts, raw, shelled	1 lb	2,558	117.9	215.5	47	63		84.4	313	9.5	23	3,057	—	5.16	.60	77.8	0
	1 cup	844	38.9	71.1	16	21		27.9	103	3.1	8	1,009	—	1.70	.20	25.7	0
Peanuts, roasted, in shell	1 lb (yields ap. 2 1/4 cups shelled)	1,769	79.6	148.0	33	43		62.6	219	6.7	15	2,130	—	.97	.41	52.0	0
Peanuts, roasted, shelled	1 lb	2,640	118.8	220.9	49	64		93.4	327	10.0	23	3,180	—	1.45	.61	77.6	0
	1 cup	792	35.6	66.3	15	19		28.0	98	3.0	7	954	—	.44	.18	23.3	0
Peanuts, roasted, salted	1 lb	2,654	117.9	225.9				85.3	336	9.5	1,896	3,057	—	1.45	.60	77.8	0
	1 cup	841	37.3	71.6				27.0	106	3.0	601	969	—	.45	.19	24.7	0
Peanut butter with small amount of added fat and salt	1 lb	2,635	126.1	224.1	42	62		78.0	286	9.1	2,753	3,039	—	.58	.57	71.2	0
	1 T	93	4.4	7.9	1	2		2.7	10	.3	97	107	—	.02	.02	2.5	0
Peanut butter with moderate amount of added fat, sweetener and salt	1 lb	2,672	114.3	229.5	42	62		85.3	268	8.6	2,744	2,844	—	.54	.54	66.6	0
	1 T	94	4.0	8.1				3.0	9	.3	97	100	—	.02	.02	2.3	0
Peanut flour, defatted	1 lb	1,683	217.3	41.7	9	2		142.9	472	15.9	41	5,380	—	3.40	1.01	126.1	0
Peas, whole, dried	1 cup	368	47.5	9.1	2	3		31.3	103	3.5	9	1,177		.74	.22	27.6	0
	1 lb	1,542	109.3	5.9				273.5	290	23.1	159	4,559	540	3.38	1.31	13.7	0
	1/2 cup (yields ap. 1 cup cooked)	308	21.9	1.2				54.7	58	4.6	32	912	110	.68	.26	2.7	0
Peas, split, dried	1 lb	1,579	109.8	4.5				284.4	150	23.1	181	4,060	540	3.38	1.31	13.7	0
	1/2 cup (yields ap. 1 1/4 cups cooked)	370	25.7	1.1				66.7	35	5.4	42	952	130	.79	.30	3.2	0

*Linoleic acid is unsaturated fat.

7. LEGUMES AND NUTS (cont.)

Food	Measure	Calories	Protein Gm	Total Fat Gm	Satu-rated Fat Gm	Lino.* leic Acid Gm	Choles-terol Mg	Carbo-hydrate Gm	Cal-cium Mg	Iron Mg	Sodium Mg	Potas-sium Mg	A IU	Thi-amine Mg	Ribo-flavin Mg	Nia-cin Mg	C Mg
Pecans, in shell	1 lb (yields 2¾ cups shelled)	1,652	22.1	171.2	12	34		35.1	175	5.8	tr.	1,450	310	2.08	.31	2.2	4
Pecans, shelled	1 lb	3,116	41.7	323.0	23	65		66.2	331	10.9	tr.	2,735	590	3.92	.59	4.1	7
	1 cup	741	9.9	76.8	5	15		15.7	79	2.6	tr.	650	140	.93	.14	1.0	2
	12-14 halves	97	1.3	10.1	1	2		2.1	10	.3	tr.	86	20	.12	.02	.1	tr.
Pignolias	1 lb	2,504	141.1	215.0				52.6		23.6				2.83		20.4	
	½ cup	430	24.3	37.0				9.0	54	4.1				.49		3.5	tr.
Piñon	1 lb	2,880	59.0	274.4				93.0	297	16.6			140	5.81	1.04	3.2	tr.
	¾ cup	495	10.1	47.2				16.0	46	2.6			20	1.00	.18	.5	
Pistachio nuts, in shell	1 lb	1,347	43.8	121.8	12	23		43.1	594	33.1		2,204	520	1.52		6.4	0
	½ cup	211	6.8	19.0	2	4		6.7	82	4.6		344	80	.34		.9	0
Pistachio nuts, shelled	1 lb	2,694	87.5	243.6	24	46		86.2	171	37.6		4,409	1,040	3.04	.64	8.1	0
	½ cup	370	12.0	33.5	4	6		11.9	23	5.3		606	143	.42	.09	1.1	0
Pumpkin seeds, in hull	1 lb	1,856	97.4	156.8	28	66		50.4	231	50.8			230	.82	.86	10.8	
	⅔ cup	261	13.7	22.0	4	9		7.1	32	7.1			30	.12	.12	1.5	
Pumpkin seeds, hulled	1 lb	2,508	131.5	211.8	38	89		68.0		47.6			320	1.11	1.08	24.3	
	⅔ cup	353	18.5	29.8	5	13		9.6					40	.16	.07	1.3	
Sesame seeds, whole	1 lb	2,554	84.4	222.7	31	94		98.0	5,262	10.9	272	3,289	140	4.43	.59	24.5	0
	1 oz (3 T)	160	5.3	13.9	6	6		6.1	329		17	206	10	.28		1.5	0
Sesame seeds, hulled	1 lb	2,640	82.6	242.2	34	102		79.8	499	3.0				.80	1.43		0
	1 oz (3 T.)	165	5.2	15.1	2			5.0						.05			
Soybeans, dried	1 lb	1,828	154.7	80.3	12	42		152.0	1,025	38.1	23	7,607	360	4.99	.29	10.1	1
	½ cup (yields ap. 1¼ cups cooked)	371	31.4	16.3	2	8		30.9	208	7.7	5	1,545	70	1.01		2.1	
Soybeans, fermented (miso)	1 lb	776	47.6	20.9	3	11		106.6	308	7.7	13,381	1,515	180	.29	.44	1.3	0
	1 T	24	1.5	.7	tr.	tr.		3.3	10	.2	418	47	10	.01	.01	tr.	0
Soybeans, sprouted	1 lb	209	28.1	6.4				24.0	218	4.5			360	1.03	.88	3.9	58
	1 cup	46	6.1	1.4				5.3	48	1.0			80	.23	.19	.9	13

*Linoleic acid is unsaturated fat.

7. LEGUMES AND NUTS (cont.)

Food	Measure	Calories	Protein Gm	Total Fat Gm	Saturated Fat Gm	Linoleic* Acid Gm	Cholesterol Mg	Carbohydrate Gm	Calcium Mg	Iron Mg	Sodium Mg	Potassium Mg	A IU	Thiamine Mg	Riboflavin Mg	Niacin Mg	C Mg
Soybean curd (tofu)	1 lb	327	35.4	19.1	3	10		10.9	581	8.6	32	191	0	.26	.14	.7	0
	1 cake, 2½"x2½"x1"	82	8.9	4.8				2.7	145	2.2	8	48	0	.07	.04	.2	0
Soybean flour, full-fat	1 lb	1,910	166.5	92.1	14	48		137.9	903	38.1	5	7,530	500	3.85	1.41	9.6	0
	1 oz	119	10.4	5.8	1	3		8.6	56	2.4	tr.	471	30	.24	.09	.6	0
Soybean flour, high-fat	1 lb	1,724	186.9	54.9	8	29		151.0	1,089	40.8	5	8,051	—	4.06	1.61	10.3	0
	1 oz	108	11.7	3.4	tr.	2		9.4	68	2.5	tr.	503	—	.25	.10	.6	0
Soybean flour, low-fat	1 lb	1,615	196.9	30.4	tr.	16		166.0	1,193	41.3	5	8,432	360	3.76	1.63	12.0	0
	1 oz	101	12.3	1.9		1		10.4	75	2.6	tr.	527	20	.23	.10	.7	0
Soybean flour, defatted	1 lb	1,479	213.2	4.1				172.8	1,202	50.3	5	8,256	180	4.97	1.56	11.8	0
	1 oz	92	13.3	.3				10.8	75	3.1	tr.	516	10	.31	.10	.7	0
Soybean milk, powder	1 oz (5 T)	122	11.9	5.8	1	3		7.9	50	1.9	—	—	100	.19	.07	.5	0
Soybean milk, fluid	1 cup	79	8.1	3.6				5.3			—	—	120				
Sunflower seeds, in hull	1 lb	1,372	58.8	115.8	14	73		48.7	294	17.4	73	2,253	10	4.80	.57	13.3	
	½ cup	129	5.5	10.9	1	7		4.6	28	1.6	7	211		.45	.05	1.2	—
Sunflower seeds, hulled	1 lb	2,540	108.9	214.6	26	135		90.3	544	32.2	136	4,173	230	8.90	1.05	24.7	
	½ cup	357	15.3	30.2	4	19		12.7	76	4.5	19	587	30	1.25	.15	3.5	
Sunflower-seed flour, partially defatted	1 lb	1,538	205.0	15.4	2	10		171.0	1,579	59.9	254	4,899	—	16.33	2.11	124.0	—
	1 cup	379	50.5	3.8	tr.	2		42.2	389	14.8	63	1,208	—	4.03	.52	30.6	
Walnuts, black, in shell	1 lb (yields ap. ¾ cup shelled)	627	20.5	59.2		28		14.8	tr.	6.0	3	459	300	.22	.11	.7	
Walnuts, black, shelled	1 lb	2,849	93.0	269.0	16	129		67.1	tr.	27.2	14	2,087	1,360	.99	.49	3.3	
	1 cup	790	25.8	74.6	4	36		18.6	tr.	7.5	4	579	380	.27	.14	.9	
Walnuts, English, in shell	1 lb (yields ap. 2 cups shelled)	1,329	30.2	130.6	9	81		32.2	202	6.3	4	918	60	.67	.26	1.9	4
Walnuts, English, shelled	1 lb	2,953	67.1	290.3	20	180		71.7	449	14.1	9	2,041	140	1.49	.58	4.2	9
	1 cup	646	14.7	63.5	4	39		15.7	98	3.1	2	448	30	.33	.13	.9	2

*Linoleic acid is unsaturated fat.

8. FATS AND OILS

The table for fats and oils provides a listing of those items used in cooking, flavoring, and dressing up other dishes which are often forgotten in the final analysis. Salad dressings are found in this section too, for they are mainly oil-based products.

For the most part there is little protein, vitamin, or mineral value derived from these foods. Their contribution to the diet is mostly in terms of calories and fat. But while equal amounts of butter, oil, and margarine provide about the same number of calories, they are not interchangeable on all counts. Most significantly, their distribution of fatty acids varies widely, with fats of animal origin consisting primarily of saturated fatty acids and those of vegetable origin being higher in unsaturated fats. Coconut and palm oils are exceptions to this rule, both containing considerable amounts of saturated fat.

Butter can contain substantial amounts of vitamin A. The values expressed here cover the overall average of vitamin-A content; butter produced in the winter may be much lower, and butter produced in the summer much higher, than specified here. Margarine is frequently fortified with vitamin A and when labeled as such must contain a minimum of 15,000 IU's per pound.

Unrefined vegetable and nut oils, which are not considered in this table, differ from their refined counterparts in that they are rich in vitamin E.

How to Use the Table

• Values for salad dressing are based on typical bottled formulas. For homemade dressing, compute the food value from your recipe ingredients.
• Since fats are generally added to other foods, this table should be regarded frequently in figuring the total food value of many dishes that have been cooked in fat, spread with fat, or seasoned with fat. If you neglect to add this into the total

value of a food you will be ignoring many calories and fats you have consumed daily.

• To help you figure quickly, the food value of fats and oils is given per tablespoon, but since larger quantities may be used in baking or other food combinations, the food value of butter, oil, margarine, and shortening is given per cup, and, when useful, per pound as well.

8. FATS AND OILS

Food	Measure	Calories	Protein Gm	Total Fat Gm	Satu-rated Fat Gm	Lino-leic* Acid Gm	Choles-terol Mg	Carbo-hydrate Gm	Calcium Mg	Iron Mg	Sodium Mg	Potassium Mg	A IU	Thiamine Mg	Ribo-flavin Mg	Niacin Mg	C Mg
Butter, salted†	1 lb	3,245	2.7	367.0	202	11	1,135	1.8	91	0	4,477	104	15,000	—	—	—	0
	1 cup	1,614	1.4	183.0	101	5	565	.9	46	0	2,226	52	7,460	—	—	—	0
	1 T	100	tr.	11.5	6	tr.	35	tr.	3	0	138	2	470	—	—	—	0
	1 pat	36	tr.	4.0	2	tr.	10	tr.	1	0	50	1	170	—	—	—	0
Lard	1 lb	4,091	0	454.0	172	45	430	0	0	0	0	0	0	0	0	0	0
	1 cup	1,845	0	205.0	78	21	195	0	0	0	0	0	0	0	0	0	0
	1 T	117	0	13.0	5	1	10	0	0	0	0	0	0	0	0	0	0
Margarine, salted, fortified‡ First ingredient on label hydrogenated or hardened fat	1 lb	3,266	2.7	367.0	82	65	0	1.8	91	0	4,477	104	15,000	—	—	—	0
	1 cup	1,627	1.4	183.0	41	32		.9	45	0	2,226	52	7,460	—	—	—	0
	1 T	100	tr.	11.5	3	1		tr.	3	0	138	2	470	—	—	—	0
	1 pat	36	tr.	4.0	1	tr.		tr.	1	0	50	1	170	—	—	—	0
First ingredient on label liquid vegetable oil	1 lb	3,266	2.7	367.0	86	141	0	1.8	91	0	4,477	104	15,000	—	—	—	0
	1 cup	1,627	1.4	183.0	43	70		.9	45	0	2,226	52	7,460	—	—	—	0
	1 T	100	tr.	11.5	3	4		tr.	3	0	138	2	470	—	—	—	0
	1 pat	36	tr.	4.0	1	2		tr.	1	0	50	1	170	—	—	—	0

*Linoleic acid is unsaturated fat.
†Unsalted butter contains less than 45 milligrams sodium and potassium per pound; vitamin-A value is year-round average.
‡Unsalted margarine contains less than 45 milligrams sodium and potassium per pound; vitamin-A value based on minimum federal specifications for fortified margarine.

8. FATS AND OILS (cont.)

Food	Measure	Calo-ries	Pro-tein Gm	Total Fat Gm	Satu-rated Fat Gm	Lino-leic* Acid Gm	Choles-terol Mg	Car-bohy-drate Gm	Cal-cium Mg	Iron Mg	Sodium Mg	Potas-sium Mg	A IU	Thi-amine Mg	Ribo-flavin Mg	Nia-cin Mg	C Mg
Oils																	
Corn	1 cup	1,945	0	220	22	117	0	0	0	0	0	0	—	0	0	0	0
	1 T	124	0	14	1	7		0	0	0	0	0	—	0	0	0	0
Cottonseed	1 cup	1,945	0	220	55	110		0	0	0	0	0	—	0	0	0	0
	1 T	124	0	14	4	7		0	0	0	0	0	—	0	0	0	0
Olive	1 cup	1,945	0	220	24	15		0	0	0	0	0	—	0	0	0	0
	1 T	124	0	14	2	1		0	0	0	0	0	—	0	0	0	0
Peanut	1 cup	1,945	0	220	40	64		0	0	0	0	0	—	0	0	0	0
	1 T	124	0	14	3	4		0	0	0	0	0	—	0	0	0	0
Safflower	1 cup	1,945	0	220	18	158		0	0	0	0	0	—	0	0	0	0
	1 T	124	0	14	1	10		0	0	0	0	0	—	0	0	0	0
Sesame	1 cup	1,945	0	220	31	92		0	0	0	0	0	—	0	0	0	0
	1 T	124	0	14	2	6		0	0	0	0	0	—	0	0	0	0
Soybean	1 cup	1,945	0	220	33	114		0	0	0	0	0	—	0	0	0	0
	1 T	124	0	14	2	7		0	0	0	0	0	—	0	0	0	0
Salad dressings, commercial																	
Bleu cheese, regular	1 T	76	1.0	8	2.0	4		1.0	12	tr.	164	6	30	tr.	.02	tr.	tr.
Bleu cheese, low-calorie	1 T	12	.5	1	.5	tr.		.6	10	tr.	177	5	30	tr.	.01	tr.	tr.
French, regular	1 T	66	tr.	6	1.0	3		3.0	2	.1	219	13	—	—	—	—	—

*Linoleic acid is unsaturated fat.

8. FATS AND OILS (cont.)

Food	Measure	Calories	Protein Gm	Total Fat Gm	Satu-rated Fat Gm	Lino-leic* Acid Gm	Choles-terol Mg	Carbo-hydrate Gm	Calcium Mg	Iron Mg	Sodium Mg	Potassium Mg	Vitamins A IU	Thiamine Mg	Ribo-flavin Mg	Niacin Mg	C Mg
French, low-calorie	1 T	13	tr.	tr.				2.0	2	.1	118	12	tr.				
Italian, regular	1 T	77	tr.	8	1.0	4		1.0	1	tr.	293	2	tr.	tr.	tr.	tr.	
Italian, low-calorie	1 T	7	tr.	1				tr.	tr.	tr.	110	2	tr.	tr.	tr.	tr.	
Mayonnaise	1 T	100	tr.	11	2.0	6		tr.	3	.1	84	5	40	.01	.01	.1	
Russian	1 T	69	tr.	7	1.0	4		1.0	3	.1	122	22	100	.01	.01	.1	1
Salad dressing, mayonnaise-type	1 T	65	tr.	6	1.0	3		2.0	2	tr.	88	1	30	tr.	tr.	tr.	tr.
Thousand Island, regular	1 T	80	tr.	8	1.0	4		2.0	2	.1	112	18	50	tr.	tr.	tr.	tr.
Thousand Island, low-calorie	1 T	29	tr.	2	tr.	1		2.0	2	.1	112	18	50	tr.	tr.	tr.	tr.
Salt pork	1 lb	3,410	17.0	370	141.0	22		0	tr.	2.6	5,278	183	0	.78	.17	3.9	
Suet	1 cup	1,768	tr.	200	46.0	14		0	0	0	0	0		0	0	0	0
Vegetable shortening	1 T	115	0	13	3.0	1		0	0	0	0	0		0	0	0	0

*Linoleic acid is unsaturated fat.

9. SUGARS AND SWEETS

Sugars and sweets add many carbohydrates and calories to the American dietary scheme, but few other nutrients. Small amounts of B vitamins and calcium may be found in some of these items, but for the most part their energy potential is far in excess of their nutritional worth.

Unrefined sweeteners like molasses, honey, and brown sugar (which has molasses added) do show some virtue, especially blackstrap molasses which provides calcium and iron. Unfortunately only the figures for strained honey are available; the unfiltered variety contains considerably more B vitamins.

The candies represented here are equally as empty as the sugar which is their basic ingredient. All items containing chocolate are high in total fat, with little of it in the unsaturated form.

How to Use the Table

• A variety of measures is used to reveal the nutritional make-up of foods in this group. Where weights are given rather than volume or individual units, it is because those items are usually purchased by weight or in a package which includes this information—so be sure to look at the candy wrapper before you throw it away.
• Since candies come in so many varieties you'll have to use your judgment as to which description best fits your selection.

9. SUGARS AND SWEETS

Food	Measure	Calories	Protein Gm	Total Fat Gm	Saturated Fat Gm	Lino-lete* Acid Gm	Choles-terol Mg	Carbo-hydrate Gm	Cal-cium Mg	Iron Mg	Sodium Mg	Potas-sium Mg	A IU	Thi-amine Mg	Ribo-flavin Mg	Nia-cin Mg	C Mg
Cake icing																	
Chocolate	1 cup	1,034	8.8	38.2	22	tr.		185.4	165	3.3	168	536	580	.06	.28	.6	0
Coconut	1 cup	604	3.2	12.8	12	tr.		124.3	10	.8	196	277	0	.02	.07	.3	0
Creamy fudge, from mix with water added	1 cup	831	6.9	15.9	5	3		182.8	96	2.7	568	238	tr.	.05	.20	.7	tr.
White, boiled	1 cup	297	1.3	0				75.5	2	tr.	134	17	0	tr.	.03	tr.	0
Candied cherries	1 oz	96	.1	tr.				24.6									
Candied citron	1 oz	89	.1	.1				22.7	24	.2	82	34					
Candied ginger	1 oz	96	.1	.1				24.7									
Candied orange peel	1 oz	90	.1	.1				22.9									
Candy																	
Butterscotch	1 oz	113	tr.	1.0				26.9	5	.4	19	1	40	0	tr.	tr.	0
Candy corn—see Fondant																	
Caramel, plain or chocolate	1 oz	113	1.1	2.9	1	tr.		21.7	42	.4	64	54	tr.	.01	.05	.1	tr.
Caramel with nuts	1 oz	121	1.3	4.6	2	tr.		20.0	40	.4	58	66	10	.03	.05	.1	tr.
Chocolate-flavored roll	1 oz	112	.8	2.3	2	tr.		23.4	19	.5	56	35	tr.	tr.	.02	.3	tr.
Chocolate, bittersweet	1 oz	135	2.2	11.3	6	tr.		13.3	16	1.4	1	174	10	.01	.05	.2	0
Chocolate, semisweet	1 oz	144	1.2	10.1	6	tr.		16.2	9	.7	1	92	10	.01	.03	.1	0
Chocolate, sweet	1 oz	150	1.3	10.0	6	tr.		16.4	27	.4	9	76	tr.	.01	.04	.1	tr.
Chocolate, milk	1 oz	147	2.2	9.2	6	tr.		16.1	65	.3	27	109	80	.02	.10	.1	tr.
Chocolate, milk with almonds	1 oz	151	2.6	10.1				14.5	65	.5	23	125	60	.02	.12	.2	tr.
Chocolate, milk with peanuts	1 oz	154	4.0	10.8	2	2		12.6	49	.4	19	138	50	.07	.08	1.4	tr.
Chocolate-coated almonds	1 oz	161	3.5	12.4				11.2	58	.8	17	155	tr.	.03	.15	.5	tr.
	1 cup	1,016	22.0	78.1	13	10		70.7	363	5.0	106	975	0	.22	.95	3.1	tr.
Chocolate-coated coconut	1 oz	124	.8	5.0	3	tr.		20.4	14	.3	56	47	tr.	.01	.02	.1	tr.
Chocolate-coated fondant	1 oz	116	.5	3.0	1	tr.		23.0	16	.3	52	26	tr.	.01	.02	.1	tr.
Chocolate-coated fudge, caramel and peanuts	1 oz	123	2.2	5.1	2	1		18.2	51	.4	58	85	tr.	.04	.06	.5	tr.

*Linoleic acid is unsaturated fat.

9. SUGARS AND SWEETS (cont.)

Food	Measure	Calories	Protein Gm	Total Fat Gm	Saturated Fat Gm	Lino-* leic Acid Gm	Cholesterol Mg	Carbohydrate Gm	Calcium Mg	Iron Mg	Sodium Mg	Potassium Mg	A IU	Thiamine Mg	Riboflavin Mg	Niacin Mg	C Mg
Candy (cont.)																	
Chocolate-coated honeycombed hard candy with peanut butter	1 oz	131	1.9	5.5	2	1		20.0	23	.5	46	64	tr.	.02	.03	.8	tr.
Chocolate-coated nougat and caramel	1 oz	118	1.1	3.9	1	tr.		20.6	36	.5	49	60	10	.02	.05	.1	tr.
Chocolate-coated peanuts	1 oz	159	4.7	11.7	3	2		11.1	33	.4	17	143	tr.	.11	.05	2.1	tr.
Chocolate-coated raisins	1 oz	121	1.5	4.9	3	tr.		20.0	43	.7	18	171	40	.02	.06	.1	tr.
Chocolate-coated vanilla creams	1 oz	123	1.1	4.9	2	tr.		19.9	36	.2	52	50	tr.	.01	.02	.1	tr.
Fondant	1 oz	103	tr.	.6				25.4	4	.3	60	1	0	tr.	tr.	tr.	0
Fudge, chocolate	1 oz	113	.8	3.5	1	tr.		21.3	22	.3	54	42	tr.	.01	.03	.1	tr.
Fudge, chocolate with nuts	1 oz	121	1.1	4.9	2	2		19.6	22	.3	49	50	tr.	.01	.02	.1	tr.
Fudge, vanilla	1 oz	113	.9	3.1	2	tr.		21.2	32	.1	59	36	tr.	.01	.04	tr.	tr.
Fudge, vanilla with nuts	1 oz	120	1.2	4.7	1	tr.		19.5	31	.2	53	32	0	.01	.04	tr.	tr.
Gumdrops	1 oz	99	tr.	.2				24.8	2	.1	10	1	0	0	tr.	tr.	0
Hard candy	1 oz	109	0	.3				27.6	6	.5	9	1	0	0	0	0	0
Jellybeans	1 oz	104	tr.	.1				26.4	1	.3	3	tr.	0	0	tr.	tr.	0
Marshmallows	1 oz	90	.6	tr.				22.8	5	.5	11	2	0	0	tr.	tr.	0
Mints—see Fondant																	
Peanut bars	1 oz	146	5.0	9.1	2	3		13.4	13	.5	3	127	0	.12	.02	2.7	0
Peanut brittle	1 oz	119	1.6	3.0	1	1		23.0	10	.7	9	43	0	.05	.01	1.0	0
Sugar-coated almonds	1 oz	129	2.2	5.3	tr.	1		19.9	28	.5	6	72	0	.01	.08	.3	0
Sugar-coated almonds	1 cup	637	10.9	26.0		5		98.0	140	2.6	28	356	0	.07	.38	1.4	0
Sugar-coated chocolate disks	1 oz	132	1.5	5.6	3	tr.		20.6	38	.4	20	71	30	.02	.06	.1	tr.
Chewing gum	1 stick	9						2.8					0	0	0	0	0
Chocolate, baking	1 oz	143	3.0	15.0	8	tr.		8.2	22	1.9	1	235	20	.01	.07	.4	0
Chocolate syrup, thin	2 T	97	.9	.8		tr.		24.9	7	.6	21	112	tr.	.01	.03	.3	0
Chocolate syrup, fudge-type	2 T	131	2.0	5.4	3	tr.		21.4	50	.5	35	113	60	.02	.09	.1	tr.

*Linoleic acid is unsaturated fat.

9. SUGARS AND SWEETS (cont.)

Food	Measure	Calories	Protein Gm	Total Fat Gm	Saturated Fat Gm	Lino-* leic Acid Gm	Choles- terol Mg	Carbo- hydrate Gm	Calcium Mg	Iron Mg	Sodium Mg	Potas- sium Mg	A IU	Thi- amine Mg	Ribo- flavin Mg	Nia- cin Mg	C Mg
Honey, strained	1 T	64	tr.	0				17.2	1	.1	1	11	0	tr.	.01	.1	tr.
	1 cup	983	1.0	tr.				266.0	16	1.6	16	165	tr.	.01	.14	.9	4
Jams or preserves	1 T	54	.1	tr.				12.7	4	.4	3	18	tr.	tr.	tr.	tr.	1
Jelly	1 T	49	tr.	tr.				14.0	4	.3	3	13	tr.	tr.	.01	tr.	1
Marmalade	1 T	51	.1					14.0	7	.1		7				tr.	
Molasses, blackstrap	1 T	43						11.0	137	3.2	19	584		.02	.04	.4	
	1 cup	652						168.0	2,095	49.3	293	8,962		.34	.59	6.1	
Molasses, Barbados	1 T	54						14.0	49					.01	.04		
	1 cup	830						214.7	750					.18	.61		
Popcorn, sugar-coated—see Flour, Cereal Grains, and Grain Products																	
Sugar																	
Brown	1 lb	1,692	0	0				437.3	386	15.4	136	1,560	0	.05	.15	.8	0
	1 T	53	0	0				13.7	12	.5	4	49	0	tr.	tr.	tr.	0
	1 cup	819	0	0				211.7	187	7.5	66	755	0	.02	.07	.4	0
White, granulated	1 lb	1,746	0	0				451.3	0	tr.	5	14	0	0	0	0	0
	1 T	42	0	0				10.9	0	.2	tr.	tr.	0	0	0	0	0
	1 cup	768	0	0				199.0	0	.5	2	6	0	0	0	0	0
White, powdered	1 lb	1,746	0	0				451.3	0	tr.	5	14	0	0	0	0	0
	1 T	23	0	0				6.0	0	.1	tr.	tr.	0	0	0	0	0
	1 cup	461	0	0				119.2	0	.5	1	4	0	0	0	0	0
Maple	piece 1¾" x 1¼" x ½"	118						30.6	49	.5	5	82					
Syrups																	
Cane	1 T	55	0	0				14.2	13	.8	2	89	0	.03	.01	tr.	0
Maple	1 T	53		0				13.6	22			37	0			tr.	0
Sorghum	1 T	54						14.2	36	2.6	14				.02		
Table blend, corn	1 T	61	0	0				15.7	10	.9	1	1	0			tr.	0
Table blend, cane and maple	1 T	53	0	0				13.6	3	tr.	tr.	5	0	0		0	0

*Linoleic acid is unsaturated fat.

10. ALCOHOLIC AND CARBONATED BEVERAGES

There is not much to be said about alcoholic and carbonated beverages, as you will see at a glance from the table which follows. They are simply an embodiment of carbohydrates and calories. The remaining categories of nutrients are largely empty, except for an occasional, barely significant figure here and there. Even the fruit-flavored sodas contain none of the nutritional benefits of fruit, only the simulated flavor.

If you can afford empty calories this is one place to find them.

How to Use the Table

● Food values for this group are expressed in terms of standard-size servings; 1½ fluid ounces (or a jigger) for hard liquor; 3½ fluid ounces (just under ½ cup) for wine; and 8 fluid ounces (one cup) for soft drinks and beer.

10. ALCOHOLIC AND CARBONATED BEVERAGES

Food	Measure	Calories	Protein Gm	Total Fat Gm	Saturated Fat Gm	Lino-leic Acid* Gm	Cholesterol Mg	Carbohydrate Gm	Calcium Mg	Iron Mg	Sodium Mg	Potassium Mg	A IU	Thiamine Mg	Riboflavin Mg	Niacin Mg	C Mg
Beer	8 oz	101	.7	0				9.1	12	tr.	17	60	—	tr.	.07	1.4	—
Gin, rum, vodka, whisky																	
80-proof	1½ oz jigger	97	—	—				tr.	—	—	tr.	—	—	—	—	—	—
86-proof	1½ oz jigger	105	—	—				tr.	—	—	tr.	—	—	—	—	—	—
90-proof	1½ oz jigger	110	—	—				tr.	—	—	tr.	—	—	—	—	—	—
94-proof	1½ oz jigger	116	—	—				tr.	—	—	tr.	—	—	—	—	—	—
100-proof	1½ oz jigger	124	—	—				tr.	—	—	tr.	—	—	—	—	—	—
Club soda	8 oz	0	0	0				0	—	—	—	—	0	0	0	0	0
Cola	8 oz	96	0	0				25	—	—	—	—	0	0	0	0	0
Cream soda	8 oz	106	0	0				27	—	—	—	—	0	0	0	0	0
Fruit-flavored soda and Tom Collins mix	8 oz	114	0	0				30	—	—	—	—	0	0	0	0	0
Ginger ale	8 oz	76	0	0				20	—	—	—	—	0	0	0	0	0
Quinine soda	8 oz	76	0	0				20	—	—	—	—	0	0	0	0	0
Root beer	8 oz	101	0	0				26	—	—	—	—	0	0	0	0	0
Wines, dessert	3½ oz	141	.1	0				8	8	.4	4	77	—	.01	.02	.2	—
Wines, table	3½ oz	87	.1	0				4	9		5	94	—	tr.	.01	.1	—

*Linoleic acid is unsaturated fat.

11. SOUPS

Prepared soups are among the most popular items in the food marketplace so it is important that you understand what you get with your purchase in terms of nutrition. Analysis of common commercial brands provided the sampling in our table. If you wish to know the food value of a soup you create in your own kitchen, add up the nutrients contained in all the ingredients and you will have a pretty good picture of what you have put together. Do not count on receiving the full vitamin-C or thiamine value as they are both easily destroyed by the heat of cooking.

How to Use the Table

● Values are given for one can or package of soup in the dry, frozen, or condensed form and represent an average for several brands. Individual brands may vary somewhat, depending on the amount and quality of the ingredients they use. The manufacturer's nutritional labeling may help clear up any significant differences.
● The nutritional content of 1 cup (8 fluid ounces) of soup prepared with whole milk or water according to package directions is also included.

11. SOUP

Food	Measure	Calories	Protein Gm	Total Fat Gm	Saturated Fat Gm	Linoleic Acid Gm	Cholesterol Mg	Carbohydrate Gm	Calcium Mg	Iron Mg	Sodium Mg	Potassium Mg	A IU	Thiamine Mg	Riboflavin Mg	Niacin Mg	C Mg
Asparagus, cream of																	
condensed																	
prepared with water	1 can, 10½ oz	161	6.0	4.2				25.0	66	1.8	2,441	298	740	.09	.21	1.8	—
prepared with milk	1 cup	64	2.4	1.7				10.0	26	.7	976	119	300	.04	.08	.7	—
Bean with pork, condensed	1 cup	163	7.7	7.0				17.5	206	1.3	1,052	338	510	.08	.34	.8	6
prepared with water	1 can, 11½ oz	437	20.8	15.0				56.4	163	5.9	2,628	1,030	1,700	.35	.19	2.4	2
Beef broth, condensed	1 cup	175	8.3	6.0				22.6	65	2.4	1,051	412	680	.14	.08	1.0	—
prepared with water	1 can, 10½ oz	77	12.5	0				6.6	tr.	1.2	1,941	322	tr.	tr.	.06	3.0	—
Beef noodle, condensed	1 cup	31	5.0	0				2.6	tr.	.5	776	129	tr.	tr.	.02	1.2	—
prepared with water	1 can, 10½ oz	170	9.5	6.6				17.3	18	2.1	2,275	190	150	.12	.15	2.6	3
Beef noodle, dry	1 cup	68	3.8	2.6				6.9	tr.	.8	910	76	60	.05	.06	1.0	1
prepared with water	2 oz pkg	219	7.7	4.2	1		tr.	37.0	27	1.1	1,343	130	70	.30	.16	2.3	2
Bouillon cubes	1 cube	5	.8	.1				.2	9	.4	960	4	20	.10	.05	.8	—
Celery, cream of																	
condensed	1 can, 10½ oz	215	4.2	12.5				22.0	119	1.5	2,370	268	510	.03	.12	1.3	3
prepared with water	1 cup	86	1.7	5.0				8.8	48	.6	948	107	200	.01	.05	.5	1
prepared with milk	1 cup	185	7.0	10.3				16.3	228	.4	1,024	326	410	.05	.31	.6	2
Chicken consommé,																	
condensed	1 can, 10¾ oz	55	8.5	.3				4.6	30	3.0	1,835	—	—	.03	—	—	—
prepared with water	1 cup	22	3.4	.1				1.8	12	1.2	734	—	—	.01	—	—	—
Chicken, cream of,																	
condensed	1 can, 10½ oz	235	7.2	14.3	2	7		20.0	56	1.2	2,409	196	1,040	.03	.13	1.4	3
prepared with water	1 cup	94	2.9	5.7	1	3		8.0	22	.5	964	78	420	.01	.05	.6	1
prepared with milk	1 cup	193	8.2	11.0	4	3		15.5	202	1.1	1,040	297	630	.05	.31	.7	2
Chicken gumbo, condensed	1 can, 10½ oz	137	7.7	3.9				18.2	48	1.5	2,358	265	540	.06	.09	3.2	12
prepared with water	1 cup	55	3.1	1.6				7.3	19	.6	943	106	220	.02	.04	1.3	5

*Linoleic acid is unsaturated fat.

11. SOUP (cont.)

Food	Measure	Calories	Protein Gm	Total Fat Gm	Saturated Fat Gm	Lino-leic* Acid Gm	Choles-terol Mg	Carbo-hydrate Gm	Cal-cium Mg	Iron Mg	Sodium Mg	Potas-sium Mg	A IU	Thi-amine Mg	Ribo-flavin Mg	Nia-cin Mg	C Mg
Chicken noodle, condensed	1 can, 10½ oz	158	8.3	4.8				19.6	21	1.2	2,429	137	90	.03	.06	2.0	tr.
prepared with water	1 cup	63	3.3	1.9				7.8	8	.5	972	55	40	.01	.02	.8	tr.
Chicken noodle, dry	2 oz pkg	217	8.2	5.7				32.9	34	1.4	2,426	83	190	.29	.15	2.4	3
prepared with water	1 cup	54	2.1	1.4				8.2	9	.4	607	21	50	.07	.04	.6	1
Chicken with rice, condensed	1 can, 10½ oz	116	7.7	3.0				14.0	21	.9	2,275	244	390	tr.	.06	1.3	—
prepared with water	1 cup	46	3.1	1.2				5.6	8	.4	910	98	160	tr.	.02	.7	—
Chicken with rice, dry	1½ oz pkg	150	3.8	1.2				26.7	19	.4	1,856	30	tr.	.02	.01	.5	—
prepared with water	1 cup	38	1	.7				6.7	5	.1	464	8	tr.	.01	tr.	.1	—
Chicken with vegetables, condensed	1 can, 10¾ oz	189	10.3	6.1				23.4	46	1.5	2,575	244	5,480	.06	.09	2.8	—
prepared with water	1 cup	76	4.1	2.4				9.4	18	.6	1,030	98	2,190	.02	.04	1.1	—
Clam chowder, Manhattan, condensed	1 can, 10¾ oz	201	5.5	6.4				30.5	89	2.8	2,335	457	2,160	.06	.06	2.8	—
prepared with water	1 cup	80	2.2	2.6				12.2	36	1.1	934	183	860	.02	.02	1.1	—
Clam chowder, New England, frozen, condensed	1 can	455	15.8	2.7				37.0	319	3.4	3,699	787	220	.13	.30	1.7	—
prepared with water	1 cup	152	5.3	.9				12.0	106	1.1	1,233	262	70	.04	.10	.6	—
prepared with milk	1 cup	205	8.1	11.8				16.0	202	1.1	1,274	379	180	.06	.24	.7	—
Minestrone, condensed	1 can, 10½ oz	259	11.9	8.3				34.5	89	1.1	2,420	759	5,660	.18	.15	2.7	—
prepared with water	1 cup	104	4.8	3.3				13.8	36	.8	968	304	2,270	.07	.06	1.1	—
Mushroom, cream of, condensed	1 can, 10½ oz	330	5.6	23.8	3	12		25.0	101	.9	2,367	244	180	.04	.30	1.8	tr.
prepared with water	1 cup	132	2.2	9.5	1	5		10.0	40	.4	947	98	70	.02	.12	.7	tr.
prepared with milk	1 cup	231	7.5	14.8	4	5		17.5	220	1.0	1,023	317	280	.06	.38	.8	1
Onion, condensed	1 can, 10½ oz	161	13.1	6.2				12.8	68	1.2	2,604	256	tr.	tr.	.06	tr.	—
prepared with water	1 cup	64	5.2	2.5				5.1	27	.5	1,042	102	tr.	tr.	tr.	tr.	—
Onion, dry	1½ oz pkg	148	5.9	4.5				22.9	41	.6	2,840	235	30	.05	.03	.3	6
prepared with water	1 cup	37	1.5	1.1				5.7	10	.2	710	59	10	.01	.01	.1	2

*Linoleic acid is unsaturated fat.

11. SOUP (cont.)

Food	Measure	Calories	Protein Gm	Total Fat Gm	Satu-rated Fat Gm	Lino-* leic Acid Gm	Choles-terol Mg	Carbohy-drate Gm	Calcium Mg	Iron Mg	Sodium Mg	Potassium Mg	A IU	Thi-amine Mg	Ribo-flavin Mg	Nia-cin Mg	C Mg
Pea, green, condensed	1 can, 11 oz	331	14.4	5.6				57.4	112	2.2	2,289	499	870	.12	.16	2.8	19
prepared with water	1 cup	132	5.8	2.2				23.0	45	.9	916	200	350	.05	.06	1.1	8
prepared with milk	1 cup	231	11.1	7.5				30.5	225	1.5	992	419	560	.09	.32	1.2	9
Pea, green, dry	3¾ oz pkg	385	23.8	4.4				65.5	64	5.7	2,509	929	130	.46	.49	4.4	1
prepared with water	1 cup	128	7.9	1.5				21.8	21	1.9	836	310	40	.15	.16	1.5	tr.
Pea, green with ham, frozen, condensed	1 can, 15 oz	480	32.3	9.8				68.1	106	6.8	3,189	855	770	.64	.25	4.2	—
prepared with water	1 cup	160	10.8	3.3				22.7	35	2.3	1,063	285	260	.21	.08	1.4	—
prepared with milk	1 cup	213	13.6	6.1				26.7	131	2.3	1,104	402	370	.23	.22	1.5	—
Pea, split, condensed	1 can, 10¾ oz	359	21.4	7.9				51.8	76	3.4	2,338	671	1,100	.60	.36	3.4	3
prepared with water	1 cup	144	8.6	3.2				20.7	30	1.4	935	268	440	.24	.14	1.4	1
prepared with milk	1 cup	243	13.9	8.3				28.2	210	2.0	1,011	487	650	.28	.40	1.5	2
Potato, cream of, frozen, condensed	1 can, 15 oz	370	11.4	18.3				42.6	204	3.0	4,167	787	1,440	.17	.22	1.7	—
prepared with water	1 cup	123	3.8	6.1				14.2	68	1.0	1,389	262	480	.06	.07	.6	—
prepared with milk	1 cup	176	6.6	8.9				18.2	164	1.0	1,430	379	590	.08	.21	.7	—
Shrimp, cream of, frozen, condensed	1 can, 15 oz	565	17.0	42.1				30.7	136	1.7	3,657	617	9,360	.17	.10	6.4	—
prepared with water	1 cup	188	5.7	14.0				10.2	45	.6	1,219	206	3,120	.06	.10	2.1	—
prepared with milk	1 cup	241	8.5	16.8				14.2	141	.6	1,260	323	3,230	.08	.24	2.2	—
Tomato, condensed	1 can, 10½ oz	215	4.8	6.2				37.8	33	1.8	2,358	560	2,410	.15	.09	2.8	30
prepared with water	1 cup	86	1.9	2.5				15.1	13	.7	943	224	960	.06	.04	1.1	12
prepared with milk	1 cup	185	7.2	7.8				22.6	193	1.3	1,019	443	1,170	.10	.30	1.2	13
Tomato vegetable with noodle, dry	2½ oz pkg	247	6.2	5.7				44.5	33	1.4	1,451	123	1,700	.21	.13	1.8	18
prepared with water	1 cup	62	1.6	1.4				11.1	8	.4	363	31	430	.05	.03	.5	5
Turkey noodle, condensed	1 can, 10½ oz	194	10.7	7.2				20.9	35	1.5	2,479	190	480	.12	.12	3.0	tr.
prepared with water	1 cup	78	4.3	2.9				8.4	14	.6	992	76	190	.05	.05	1.2	tr.

*Linoleic acid is unsaturated fat.

11. SOUP (cont.)

Food	Measure	Calories	Protein Gm	Total Fat Gm	Satu-rated Fat Gm	Lino-leic* Acid Gm	Choles-terol Mg	Car-bohy-drate Gm	Cal-cium Mg	Iron Mg	Sodium Mg	Potas-sium Mg	A IU	Thi-amine Mg	Ribo-flavin Mg	Nia-cin Mg	C Mg
Vegetable beef, condensed	1 can, 11 oz	203	13.1	5.6				24.6	31	1.9	2,663	406	6,860	.10	.12	2.5	—
prepared with water	1 cup	81	5.2	2.2				9.8	12	.8	1,065	162	2,740	.04	.05	1.0	—
Vegetable with beef broth, condensed	1 can, 10¾ oz	195	6.7	4.3				33.5	49	2.2	2,103	597	7,620	.09	.06	3.0	—
prepared with water	1 cup	78	2.7	1.7				13.4	20	.9	841	239	3,050	.04	.02	1.2	—
Vegetarian vegetable, condensed	1 can, 10¾ oz	195	5.5	5.2				32.3	49	2.4	2,085	427	7,010	.09	.09	2.2	—
prepared with water	1 cup	78	2.2	2.1				12.9	20	1.0	834	171	2,800	.04	.04	.9	—

*Linoleic acid is unsaturated fat.

12. BABY FOODS

If you prepare food for your infant at home you can compute for yourself just what it is you are serving in terms of nutrition. When the food you serve your child is made in an industrial kitchen it is almost impossible for you to determine what its food value is, unless of course you are given the recipe. Since high-quality infant nutrition is so important, a representative sampling of prepared baby foods has been analyzed.

How to Use the Table

● Prepared foods in jars are expressed in units of 3½ ounces, which is an average jar size (and since weight is given on each jar any variation can be easily adjusted). Cereal is measured by its dry weight and teething biscuits by the individual piece.
● Unfortunately figures are not available for the fatty-acid content of these items. Some clue comes from reading the label; if coconut oil, palm oil, margarine, butter, or shortening are used in the manufacture the food will be higher in saturated fats than if nut and vegetable oils are employed.

12. BABY FOODS

Food	Measure	Calories	Protein Gm	Total Fat Gm	Saturated Fat Gm	Lino-leic Acid Gm	Cholesterol Mg	Carbohydrate Gm	Calcium Mg	Iron Mg	Sodium Mg	Potassium Mg	A IU	Thiamine Mg	Riboflavin Mg	Niacin Mg	C Mg
Cereals, dry form																	
Barley	6 T	97	3.8	.3				20.6	206	14.9	127	116	0	1.04	.34	9.0	0
High-protein	6 T	100	9.9	1.0				13.5	228	17.7	183	302	—	1.03	.32	6.7	0
Mixed	6 T	103	4.2	.8				19.8	230	15.8	132	97	0	.88	.38	6.2	0
Oatmeal	6 T	105	4.6	1.5				18.5	212	13.5	122	105	0	.72	.29	5.6	0
Rice	6 T	104	1.8	.4				22.4	240	14.1	148	58	0	.72	.35	5.5	0
Dinners																	
Beef noodle dinner	3½ oz	48	2.8	1.1				6.8	12	.5	269	159	620	.02	.05	.5	2
Beef with vegetable	3½ oz	87	7.4	3.7				6.0	13	1.2	304	113	1,100	.07	.17	1.6	2
Cereal, egg yolk and bacon	3½ oz	82	2.9	4.9				6.6	29	.8	301	36	520	.05	.06	.4	—
Chicken noodle dinner	3½ oz	49	2.1	1.3				7.2	27	.3	297	42	800	.03	.06	.4	1
Chicken with vegetables	3½ oz	100	7.4	4.6				7.2	22	.9	265	71	1,000	.09	.15	1.6	2
Macaroni, tomatoes, meat, and cereal	3½ oz	67	2.6	2.0				9.6	21	.5	381	77	500	.14	.12	1.0	1
Split peas, vegetables, ham, or bacon	3½ oz	80	4.0	2.1				11.2	29	.7	295	112	600	.08	.05	.5	1
Turkey with vegetables	3½ oz	86	6.7	3.2				7.6	38	.6	348	122	1,000	.13	.13	1.8	2
Veal with vegetables	3½ oz	63	7.1	1.6				5.1	11	.8	323	95	800	.08	.15	2.0	2
Vegetables and bacon, with cereal	3½ oz	68	1.7	2.9				8.7	17	.6	282	130	2,200	.07	.05	.6	1

*Linoleic acid is unsaturated fat.

12. BABY FOODS (cont.)

Food	Measure	Calories	Protein Gm	Total Fat Gm	Satu-rated Fat Gm	Lino-leic* Acid Gm	Choles-terol Mg	Carbo-hydrate Gm	Cal-cium Mg	Iron Mg	Sodium Mg	Potas-sium Mg	A IU	Thi-amine Mg	Ribo-flavin Mg	Nia-cin Mg	C Mg
Dinners (cont.)																	
Vegetables and beef, with cereal	3½ oz	56	2.7	1.6				7.6	17	.8	307	143	2,800	.03	.04	.9	1
Vegetables and chicken, with cereal	3½ oz	52	2.1	1.4				7.7	33	.4	307	55	1,000	.03	.04	.5	tr.
Vegetables and ham, with cereal	3½ oz	64	2.8	2.2				8.3	25	.3	360	90	1,000	.08	.05	.5	3
Vegetables and lamb, with cereal	3½ oz	58	2.2	2.0				7.7	23	.7	269	148	2,200	.03	.05	.7	1
Vegetables and liver, with cereal	3½ oz	47	3.1	.4				7.8	17	2.7	236	162	4,700	.04	.37	1.6	3
Vegetables and liver, with bacon and cereal	3½ oz	57	2.4	1.9				7.5	11	2.6	284	131	4,600	.03	.33	1.3	2
Vegetables and turkey, with cereal	3½ oz	44	2.1	.8				7.2	22	.3	307	46	400	.01	.03	.4	1
Veal with vegetables	3½ oz	63	7.1	1.6				5.1	11	.8	323	95	800	.08	.15	2.0	2
Egg yolks, strained	3½ oz	210	10.0	18.4				.2	81	3.0	273	59	1,900	.12	.22	tr.	tr.
Egg yolks with ham or bacon	3½ oz	208	10.0	18.1				.3	71	2.8	313	82	1,900	.10	.23	.5	—
Fruit and fruit products																	
Apple sauce	3½ oz	72	.2	.2				18.6	4	.4	6	64	40	.01	.02	.1	tr.
Apple sauce with apricots	3½ oz	86	.3	.1				22.6	4	.3	†	105	600	.01	.02	.1	2
Bananas (with added ascorbic acid), strained	3½ oz	80	.4	.2				21.6	13	.2	29	118	70	.02	.02	.2	35

*Linoleic acid is unsaturated fat.
†Varies with sample, from 3 to 45 milligrams sodium per 3½ ounces.

12. BABY FOODS (cont.)

Food	Measure	Calories	Protein Gm	Total Fat Gm	Saturated Fat Gm	Lino-leic Acid Gm	Choles-terol Mg	Carbo-hydrate Gm	Calcium Mg	Iron Mg	Sodium Mg	Potassium Mg	A IU	Thiamine Mg	Ribo-flavin Mg	Niacin Mg	C Mg
Fruits																	
Bananas and pineapple	3½ oz	80	.4	.1				20.7	20	.2	59	72	30	.01	.01	.1	2
Fruit dessert with tapioca	3½ oz	84	.4	.2				21.5	15	.4	53	73	450	.02	.01	.1	4
Peaches	3½ oz	81	.6	.2				20.7	6	.3	t	80	500	.01	.02	.7	3
Pears	3½ oz	66	.3	.2				17.1	7	.2	4	62	30	.02	.02	.2	2
Pears and pineapple	3½ oz	69	.4	.1				17.6	7	.2	t	72	20	.03	.02	.2	2
Plums with tapioca	3½ oz	94	.3	.2				24.3	5	.4	38	44	250	.01	.02	.2	2
Prunes with tapioca	3½ oz	86	.3	.2				22.4	7	.9	33	120	400	.02	.06	.4	4
Meat and poultry																	
Beef, strained	3½ oz	99	14.7	4.0				0	8	2.0	228	183	—	.01	.16	3.5	0
Beef, junior	3½ oz	118	19.3	3.9				0	8	2.5	283	242	—	.02	.20	4.3	0
Beef heart	3½ oz	93	13.5	3.8				.4	5	3.7	208	—	—	.06	.30	3.6	0
Chicken	3½ oz	127	13.7	7.6				0	—	1.9	263	96	—	.02	.16	3.5	0
Lamb, strained	3½ oz	107	14.6	4.9				0	9	2.1	241	181	—	.02	.17	3.3	0
Lamb, junior	3½ oz	121	17.5	5.1				0	13	2.7	294	228	—	.02	.21	4.1	—
Liver, strained	3½ oz	97	14.1	3.4				1.5	6	5.6	253	202	24,000	.05	2.00	7.6	10
Liver and bacon, strained	3½ oz	123	13.7	6.6				1.3	6	4.2	302	192	22,000	.05	1.99	7.8	7
Pork, strained	3½ oz	118	15.4	5.8				0	8	1.5	223	178	—	.19	.20	2.7	—
Pork, junior	3½ oz	134	18.6	6.0				0	8	1.2	237	210	—	.23	.23	2.8	—
Veal, strained	3½ oz	91	15.5	2.7				0	10	1.7	226	214	—	.03	.20	4.3	—
Veal, junior	3½ oz	107	18.8	3.0				0	8	1.6	276	206	—	.03	.22	6.0	—

*Linoleic acid is unsaturated fat.
†Varies with sample, from 4 to 75 milligrams sodium per 3½ ounces.

12. BABY FOODS (cont.)

Food	Measure	Calories	Protein Gm	Total Fat Gm	Saturated Fat Gm	Lino-leic* Acid Gm	Choles-terol Mg	Car-bohy-drate Gm	Cal-cium Mg	Iron Mg	Sodium Mg	Potas-sium Mg	A IU	Thi-amine Mg	Ribo-flavin Mg	Nia-cin Mg	C Mg
Pudding, custard	3½ oz	100	2.3	1.8				18.6	64	.3	150	94	100	.02	.12	.1	1
Pudding, fruit	3½ oz	96	1.2	.9				21.6	27	.3	128	75	100	.03	.05	.1	3
Teething biscuit	1 biscuit	43	1.3	.3				8.8	36	.5	48	28	—	.05	.06	.3	0
Vegetables																	
Beans, green	3½ oz	22	1.4	.1				5.1	33	1.1	213	93	400	.02	.06	.3	3
Beets, strained	3½ oz	37	1.4	.1				8.3	18	.7	212	228	20	.02	.03	.1	3
Carrots	3½ oz	29	.7	.1				6.8	23	.5	169	181	13,000	.02	.03	.4	3
Mixed vegetables	3½ oz	37	1.6	.3				8.5	22	.9	272	170	4,700	.05	.04	.6	1
Peas, strained	3½ oz	54	4.2	.2				9.3	11	1.2	272	100	500	.08	.09	1.2	10
Spinach, creamed	3½ oz	43	2.3	.7				7.5	64	.6	194	142	5,000	.02	.13	.3	6
Squash	3½ oz	25	.7	.1				6.2	24	.4	292	138	2,400	.02	.04	.3	8
Sweet potatoes	3½ oz	67	1.0	.2				15.5	16	.4	187	180	4,800	.04	.03	.4	8
Tomato soup, strained	3½ oz	54	1.9	.1				13.5	24	.4	294	300	1,000	.05	.12	.7	3

*Linoleic acid is unsaturated fat.

13. MISCELLANEOUS

The final table of food content lists all those things that didn't seem to fit in any other food group. This is not to imply that they do not make significant contributions to our diets. Anyone concerned about the sodium content of their diet will find the nutritive value of salt in this category and should add a tablespoon of salt per day to their diet survey if they are heavy salters, and a teaspoon of salt per day if only lightly salted dishes are consumed.

If you have failed to locate an item on the previous tables perhaps you will find it here. But unfortunately not all foods have yet been analyzed by the United States Department of Agriculture. When this is the case, foods that are similar can assist you in making evaluations and knowledgeable choices.

13. MISCELLANEOUS ITEMS

Food	Measure	Calories	Pro-tein Gm	Total Fat Gm	Satu-rated Fat Gm	Lino-leic* Acid Gm	Choles-terol Mg	Car-bohy-drate Gm	Cal-cium Mg	Iron Mg	Sodium Mg	Potas-sium Mg	Vitamins				
													A IU	Thi-amine Mg	Ribo-flavin Mg	Nia-cin Mg	C Mg
Baking powder																	
Phosphate-type	1 T	18	tr.	tr.				4.4	940	—	1,230	25	0	0	0	0	0
Tartrate	1 T	9	tr.	tr.				2.3	0	0	874	455	0	0	0	0	0
S-A-S	1 T	12	tr.	tr.				3.0	757	—	1,198	—	0	0	0	0	0
Barbecue sauce	1 cup	227	3.7	17.2	2.5	10		20.0	52	2.0	2,034	434	900	.02	.03	.8	13
Carob flour	1 lb	816	20.4	6.4				366.1	1,597	—	—	—	—	—	—	—	—
	1 oz	51	.4	.4				22.9	100	—	—	—	—	—	—	—	—
Cocoa powder																	
Breakfast	1 T	15	.8	1.2	1	tr.	tr.	2.4	7	.5	tr.	76	tr.	.01	.02	.1	0
Breakfast, processed with alkali	1 T	15	.8	1.2	tr.	tr.		2.3	8	.5	36	32	tr.	.01	.02	.1	0
Low-fat	1 T	11	1.0	.6				2.7	4	.5	tr.	76	0	.01	tr.		0
Coffee, instant†	1 rounded t	3	tr.	tr.				.7		.1	1	65	0	0	0	.6	0
Gelatin, plain	1 envelope (1 T)	23	6.0	0				0	—	—	—	—	—	—	—	—	—
Gelatin dessert powder	3 oz pkg	316	8.0	0				74.9	—	—	270	—	—	—	—	—	—
Gelatin dessert	½ cup	71	1.8					16.9	—	—	61	—	—	—	—	—	—
Gelatin dessert with fruit added	½ cup	80	1.6	.1				19.6	—	—	41	—	—	—	—	—	—
Mustard, brown	1 T	25	1.6	1.7				1.4	33	.5	352	35					
Mustard, yellow	1 T	20	1.3	1.2				1.7	23	.5	337	35					
Pudding mix																	
Chocolate, regular, starch base	3¼ oz pkg	332	2.8	1.9				84.3	18	1.5	412	88	tr.	.02	.06	.3	0
Chocolate, instant, starch base	3¼ oz pkg	329	2.9	1.5				83.7	226	1.8	372	78	tr.	.01	.05	.3	0
Custard dessert, vegetable-gum base	3¼ oz pkg	354	0	.1				91.1	8	.1	274	23	0	0	0	0	0

*Linoleic acid is unsaturated fat.
†Contains 60 to 80 milligrams caffeine.

13. MISCELLANEOUS ITEMS (cont.)

Food	Measure	Calories	Protein Gm	Total Fat Gm	Saturated Fat Gm	Lino-lele* Acid Gm	Choles-terol Mg	Carbo-hydrate Gm	Calcium Mg	Iron Mg	Sodium Mg	Potassium Mg	A IU	Thiamine Mg	Ribo-flavin Mg	Niacin Mg	C Mg
Pudding, prepared—see Milk and Milk Products																	
Salt	1 T	0	0	0				0	45	tr.	6,962	tr.	0	0	0	0	0
Sherbet	1 cup	258	1.7	2.3				59.3	31	tr.	19	42	120	.02	.06	tr.	4
Soy sauce	1 T	10	.8	.2				1.4	15	.6	5	27	0	0	0	0	0
Tapioca, dry	1 cup	534	.9	.3				131.1	12	.7	1,096	55	0	tr.	.04	.1	0
Tapioca cream pudding	1 cup	221	8.3	8.4				28.2	173	.1	257	223	480	.07	.30	.2	2
Tartar sauce	1 T	74	.2	8.1				.6	3	.1	99	11	30	tr.	tr.	tr.	—
Tea, instant	1 t	1	—	tr.				.4	tr.	tr.	—	23	—	—	tr.	tr.	—
Vegetable main dishes, canned																	
Peanuts and soya	3½ oz	237	11.7	16.9	3	1		13.4	—	—	—	—	—	—	—	—	—
Wheat protein	3½ oz	109	16.3	.8				8.8	—	—	—	—	—	—	—	—	—
Wheat protein, nuts	3½ oz	212	20.3	7.1				17.7	—	—	—	—	—	—	—	—	—
Wheat protein, vegetable oil	3½ oz	189	19.1	10.4				5.2	—	—	—	—	—	—	—	—	—
Wheat and soy protein	3½ oz	104	16.1	1.2				7.6	—	—	—	—	—	—	—	—	—
Wheat and soy protein, vegetable oil	3½ oz	150	16.1	5.6				9.5	—	—	—	—	—	—	—	—	—
Vinegar, cider	1 T	2	tr.	0				.9	1	.1	tr.	15	—	—	—	—	—
Vinegar, distilled	1 T	2	0	—				.7	—	.1	—	2	—	—	—	—	—
Yeast, compressed	1 cake (1 oz)	24	3.4	.1				3.1	4	1.4	5	173	tr.	.20	.47	3.2	tr.
Yeast, dry active	1 T	20	2.6	.1				2.7	3	1.1	4	140	tr.	.16	.38	2.6	tr.
Yeast, brewers'	1 T (¼ oz)	23	3.1	.1				3.0	17	1.4	10	151	tr.	1.25	.34	3.0	tr.
Yeast, torula	1 T	22	3.1	.1				3.0	34	1.5	1	163	tr.	1.12	.40	3.5	tr.

*Linoleic acid is unsaturated fat.

APPENDIX

RECOMMENDED DAILY DIETARY ALLOWANCES
(Revised 1973)

	AGE years	WEIGHT pounds	HEIGHT inches	CALORIES	PROTEIN grams	CALCIUM mg	PHOSPHORUS mg	IODINE mcg*	MAGNESIUM mg	IRON mg	VITAMIN A IU	VITAMIN D IU	VITAMIN E IU	VITAMIN C mg	NIACIN mg	RIBOFLAVIN mg	THIAMINE mg	VITAMIN B6 mg	VITAMIN B12 mcg*	FOLACIN mcg*	ZINC mg
Infants	0-½	14	24	lb x 53	lb x 1.0	360	240	35	60	10	14,400	400	4	35	5	.4	.3	.3	.3	.05	3
	½-1	20	28	lb x 49	lb x .9	540	400	45	70	15	2,000	400	5	35	8	.6	.5	.4	.3	.05	5
Children	1-3	28	34	1,300	23	800	800	60	150	15	2,000	400	7	40	9	.8	.7	.6	1.0	.1	10
	4-6	44	44	1,800	30	800	800	80	200	10	2,500	400	9	40	12	1.1	.9	.9	1.5	.2	10
	7-10	66	54	2,400	36	800	800	110	250	10	3,300	400	10	40	16	1.2	1.2	1.2	2.0	.3	10
Males	11-14	97	63	2,800	44	1,200	1,200	130	350	18	5,000	400	12	45	18	1.5	1.4	1.6	3.0	.4	15
	15-18	134	69	3,000	54	1,200	1,200	150	400	18	5,000	400	15	45	20	1.8	1.5	2.0	3.0	.4	15
	19-22	147	69	3,000	54	800	800	140	350	10	5,000	400	15	45	20	1.8	1.5	2.0	3.0	.4	15
	23-50	154	69	2,700	56	800	800	130	350	10	5,000		15	45	18	1.6	1.4	2.0	3.0	.4	15
	51+	154	69	2,400	56	800	800	110	350	10	5,000		15	45	16	1.5	1.2	2.0	3.0	.4	15
Females	11-14	97	62	2,400	44	1,200	1,200	115	300	18	4,000	400	10	45	16	1.3	1.2	1.6	3.0	.4	15
	15-18	119	65	2,100	48	1,200	1,200	115	300	18	4,000	400	11	45	14	1.4	1.1	2.0	3.0	.4	15
	19-22	128	65	2,100	46	800	800	100	300	18	4,000	400	12	45	14	1.4	1.1	2.0	3.0	.4	15
	23-50	128	65	2,000	46	800	800	100	300	18	4,000		12	45	13	1.2	1.0	2.0	3.0	.4	15
	51+	128	65	1,800	46	800	800	80	300	10	4,000		12	45	12	1.1	1.0	2.0	3.0	.4	15
Pregnant				+300	+30	1,200	1,200	125	450	18+	5,000	400	15	60	+2	+.3	+.3	2.5	4.0	.8	20
Lactating				+500	+20	1,200	1,200	150	450	18	6,000	400	15	80	+4	+.5	+.3	2.5	4.0	.6	25

Published by National Academy of Sciences, National Research Council, Food and Nutrition Board.
*Micrograms.

MINIMUM DAILY REQUIREMENTS
As established by the United States Food and Drug Administration

	VITAMIN A (IU)	VITAMIN D (IU)	VITAMIN C (mg)	THIAMINE (mg)	RIBOFLAVIN (mg)	NIACIN (mg)	CALCIUM (gm)	PHOSPHORUS (gm)	IRON (mg)	IODINE (mg)
Infants	1,500	400	10	.25	.6	*	*	*	*	*
1 to 6 years	3,000	400	20	.50	.9	5.0	750	750	7.5	.1
6 to 12 years	3,000	400	20	.75	.9	7.5	750	750	10.0	.1
12 years or older	4,000	400	30	1.00	1.2	10.0	750	750	10.0	.1
Pregnant or lactating women	4,000	400	30	1.00	1.2	10.0	1,500	1,500	15.0	.1

*No value reported.

Why Eat?
The Elements of Food

HOW FOOD WORKS FOR YOU

Although the human body has a remarkable capacity for self-regeneration and for withstanding abuse, it is nevertheless a composite of irreplaceable systems. Since you are going to be living with these systems for a long time it is wise to have a basic knowledge of how they work.

We all realize that the purpose of food is to nourish the body, but how many people know how this function is carried out? It is this very lack of understanding that has contributed to many of our illnesses and weight problems and allows us to waste money on foods that are appealing to our palate although they may actually undermine good health.

The science of nutrition is concerned with the way in which the body receives and uses food. Although the effect of food has been studied since the beginning of time, it is only recently that actual laboratory research has been able to recognize, isolate, and trace the course of food matter after it has entered the human body. These findings are by no means complete; due to the complexity of the mechanisms in our bodies many of the functions and effects of food are still unknown. But, even with the limited knowledge that we have so far, we can still improve our lives.

All foods can be broken down into seven major components: protein, fats, carbohydrates, vitamins, minerals, enzymes, and water. These elements, referred to as nutrients, are the substances in food which serve the body. They function in three general ways:

1. They provide the body with fuel, which when burned (or oxidized) releases energy for activity.

2. They provide materials for the building and maintenance of body tissues, including the skeletal structure and the soft tissues.

3. They provide materials needed to regulate the body's processess and supply materials the body can use to generate its own regulatory substances.

The full role of each nutrient is not yet determined, but in general terms, protein, fat, and carbohydrate provide the source of food energy; protein and several specific minerals compose body building matter; and vitamins, minerals, and protein are regarded as the body regulators, although current research indicates that fat and carbohydrate are also important for their regulatory effect on the body systems. Water falls into all categories because it enters into almost every bodily function. The remaining group of enzymes, although probably no less vital, leaves a large void in nutritional data. Enzymes have yet to be completely isolated and studied, and so must be recognized as present and essential, but at this time too elusive to be classified in THE TABLES OF FOOD CONTENT.

In the remainder of this chapter you will find some facts you need to know about food that can help you overcome your own misconceptions, the enticing labels, and the advertising promotion when making food choices. Once acquainted with how nutrients are used by your body, you will understand better why they deserve consideration when you select foods for your daily menu.

Calories

A calorie is a unit of measure for the amount of energy available in food. Just as the combustion of gasoline in the engine enables a car to travel a certain distance, the oxidation of food in the body releases a certain amount of measurable energy expressed as calories. A calorie is not a food element. The calories are not really *in* the food or a part *of* the food. They simply represent the amount of heat and energy produced *by* the food.

When food is oxidized (or burned) in the body it generates energy that can be utilized immediately to power the basic body processess or do muscular work; if not needed immediately this energy can be stored for future activities. *All energy (no matter what the source) that is not used when available is stored in the form of fat.* When the body runs out of fresh fuel for its functions it breaks down this stored fat. If fuel is continually supplied in excess of needs this fat remains and increases. Approximately 3,500 stored calories (or extra units of energy) add up to one pound of body fat. It is important to note here that the body does not distinguish between calories from meat and calories from cake—all calories are equal despite the source, and any excess can be turned to fat.

The number of calories provided by a food depends on its nutrient composition. Each gram of carbohydrate in a food can be burned in the body to generate 4 calories; each gram of protein has the potential to generate 4 calories, each gram of fat contains a potential 9 calories. A food can contain one kind of fuel, for example, sugar which is 100 percent carbohydrate; two kinds of fuel, as in beef which is protein and fat; or all three kinds of fuel, as in milk which contains carbohydrates, protein, and fat. Few foods contain only one source of energy, particularly prepared foods composed of several food items in one dish. Therefore, without THE TABLES OF FOOD CONTENT it is impossible to figure how much energy you can expect to obtain (or how much fat you can expect to store) from your food intake.

Although calories are viewed with concern by many people, they provide the energy all of us need to breathe, digest our food, maintain our body heat, and carry out all the other fundamental body functions which comprise our "basal metabolism" or basic life processes. This base energy requirement, coupled with the energy required by muscular activity, determines the amount of calories a person can ingest and burn daily without creating any stored energy, or fat. Energy needs differ for each individual and vary depending on body size, body composition, state of health, mental and physical tension, internal secretions, age, sex, body temperature, and degree of activity. Since age decreases basal metabolism most people require fewer calories as they grow older. To serve as a general guideline, an average of 12 to 15 calories per pound of body weight are needed daily for a moderately active person to exist without weight loss or gain. Naturally the food you ingest, your level of activity, even the efficiency with which food is converted to energy, all fluctuate, but by maintaining a relatively consistent calorie intake body weight can remain stable.

Protein

Protein is the basis of all animal tissues. Each molecule of protein is composed of a series of smaller units known as amino acids, the "building blocks" of protein. In order to create body protein twenty different amino acids must be present, all at the same time. Twelve of these amino acids can be made by the body itself, but eight of them (with a possible ninth in children) must come from external sources. The primary function of proteins in the diet is to supply these essential amino acids.

The amino-acid make-up of foods varies. When all eight of the essential amino acids are present in food in the right proportion for use in our bodies, the food is considered to be a "high-quality" or "complete" protein. Some foods have too little of certain amino acids to make them useful as protein builders in the body. These are termed "low-quality" or "incomplete" proteins. *Foods that contain low-quality protein can be improved by combining them with other incomplete proteins or with small amounts of high-quality protein foods, to create protein of excellent value.* Common examples include cereal with milk, whole-grain bread with peanut butter or cheese, rice and beans.

Body tissue is dynamic, which means it is continually breaking down and being replaced. Since protein is the foundation of all living tissues it must be available at all times. During periods of growth, such as childhood, athletic training, pregnancy, or following a depleting illness, the need for protein increases.

In addition to its role in creating body tissues (which include bones, muscles, hair, and nails), protein is used in the formation of body enzymes, hormones, and antibodies. It is also responsible for the transporting of oxygen and for carrying the genetic code to all body cells.

The exact amount of protein you need to carry out these daily duties has never been determined. Cross-cultural studies indicate that the body can probably adjust within certain levels and reach a state of equilibrium based on customary protein intake. Specific research has concluded that the average adult requires a *minimum* of .5 grams of protein per 2.2 pounds (1 kilogram) of body weight each day. If all this protein is supplied by high-quality protein foods such as meat, fish, poultry, soy, eggs, milk, and cheese, then .3 to .35 grams per kilogram may be sufficient. If lower-quality protein foods—such as beans, whole grains, nuts, and seeds—provide the major source of this nutrient, .65 to .8 grams per kilogram of body weight should be consumed to meet daily needs. In terms of total daily protein, this means an adult on a diet of mixed protein (both high- and low-quality), weighing 110 pounds (50 kilograms), should receive at least 25 grams of protein; at 175 pounds (80 kilograms), 40 grams of protein are necessary. These values, however, are minimal, and, considered in terms of daily calories, about 10 to 15 percent of the total calories in your diet should be provided by protein for optimal efficiency.

Children have a higher protein need, and proper growth depends on at least 2.2 grams of protein per kilogram for an infant, gradually decreasing to 1 gram per kilogram throughout the primary growth years, or until about age fifteen. A five-year-old, weighing 44 pounds (20 kilograms) should be supplied with 36 grams of protein each day.

All protein beyond that needed to support the vital functions is burned for fuel, and if not needed as energy, is stored as fat. Once protein is converted to fat, like all body fat, it cannot be used for anything except energy in the future. But, since protein is composed of carbon, hydrogen, oxygen, and nitrogen, and the creation of energy depends only on carbon, hydrogen, and oxygen, the protein that is used for fuel deposits a nitrogen residue in the bloodstream. This excess nitrogen is transported to the kidneys where it is excreted as waste matter in the urine. High protein consumption therefore means more work for these body organs.

Fat

Fat provides the body with its most concentrated form of fuel. One pound of salad oil (100 percent fat) is about equal in energy value to 2½ pounds of sugar (100 percent carbohydrate).

In addition to its use as energy, the fat you eat retards the digestion of food in the stomach, giving it what is known as "staying power" or "satiety value." By combining fat with other nutrients in the diet, hunger can be allayed longer.

Dietary fat also stimulates the production of fat-digesting enzymes and bile. It aids in the formation of beneficial intestinal bacteria, and it is needed by the brain, nerves, and sex glands. Fat is also a carrier of the vitamins A, D, E, and K, and without it these vitamins cannot be properly absorbed.

Certain kinds of fat in your food contain linoleic, linolenic, and arachidonic acid, three dietary essentials used in the formation of sex hormones and adrenal hormones. Lecithin, also associated with certain fats in food and a product of body synthesis dependent on the presence of linoleic acid, is thought to be useful in the breakdown of undesirable fat deposits in the arteries.

While *body fat*, or adipose tissue, provides a constant source of energy reserves and is needed as padding around internal organs and for the maintenance of body heat, only *dietary fat* can be used for these other purposes.

Each molecule of fat is actually a composite of various fatty substances. The fat found in food is 98 percent to 99 percent triglycerides, with the remainder phospholipids and sterol compounds such as cholesterol. The triglycerides can be further broken down into fatty acids and glyceride. These fatty acids are an important consideration in the selection of fat-containing foods and are found in three forms—saturated, monounsaturated, and polyunsaturated. There is some amount of each type of fatty acid in all fats. Animal fats contain the highest proportion of saturated fats, and vegetable oils contain largely monounsaturated and polyunsaturated fats in varying proportions. In general, the degree of saturation determines the consistency of fat at room temperature. The more saturated fatty acids present in the fat portion of a food, the more solid it is at room temperature.

There appears to be some correlation between the fat in our diet and fat deposits in the arteries, liver, and other body tissues. It is now believed that polyunsaturated fats (which include the essential linoleic acid) help break down body cholesterol and clear the passageways of the bloodstream, while saturated fats actually promote fat deposits. Monounsaturated fats appear to be neutral, neither clogging nor clearing the arterial roadways.

Great concern about the adverse effects fat may have on the body has led to the warning that *no more than* 35 percent of the daily calories should come from the fat in our diet, while actually levels of 25 percent to 30 percent are even more desirable. This is still a good deal higher than the percent of fat in the diet of most non-Western nations, particularly those which exhibit little incidence of heart disease and other fat-related ailments, where as few as 8 percent to 14 percent of the calories are supplied by fat. In addition to the fat ceiling, as much of this fat as possible should be unsaturated. To help you determine the amounts of saturated and unsaturated fats you are getting in your food THE TABLES OF FOOD CONTENT divide the fat portions of food into saturated fatty acid and unsaturated linoleic acid whenever this information is available.

Although dietary fat rapidly adds up to calories, remember that body fat is the end product of unused carbohydrates and proteins as well.

Carbohydrates

Carbohydrates, in the form of sugar and starch, are the primary source of energy in the diet. Cellulose, a more complex form of carbohydrate, remains largely undigested and is an important source of roughage necessary to proper digestion and evacuation. As a fuel source, starch and sugar are interchangeable; in terms of their other functions in the body, however, they are not identical.

Simple pure sugar (white sugar) lacks both building and regulatory materials (vitamins and minerals) and actually increases the appetite for itself, but not the appetite for other foods. Thus sugar consumption, if not carefully controlled, can easily lead to malnutrition.

Sugar tends to irritate the mucous lining when the stomach is empty; therefore, it is preferable to eat it at the end of the meal when other foods are present to protect the stomach walls.

Furthermore, sucrose, the essence of cane sugar, may affect fat deposits in the blood and liver less favorably than glucose and fructose, the basic sugars in honey, fresh fruits, and starch.

Despite these factors and the contention of some scientists that carbohydrates are nonessential to the human diet, most authorities believe that ingesting too little carbohydrate is detrimental to health. Glucose, the end product of carbohydrate metabolism, is the primary source of food for the brain. While some fat and protein can be converted to glucose, carbohydrate itself is needed in the cycle which converts these nutrients to blood sugar. Without sufficient carbohydrates in the diet, fat bodies known as ketones accumulate in the blood. This condition, known as ketosis, may precipitate gout or kidney disorders. Carbohydrates also conserve water and electrolytes to help maintain fluid balance, and they keep body protein from being wasted for energy.

To enjoy all these benefits, one-fifth of your daily calories (or 5 grams of carbohydrate per 100 calories) should be consumed in the form of carbohydrates. If unrefined, foods offering these carbohydrates will provide substantial quantities of vitamins and minerals, and lesser but still valuable amounts of protein.

It should be emphasized here that carbohydrates in themselves have never been proven to be fattening. Long-term studies of various diets aimed at weight loss have shown that, ultimately, a weight loss is a result of *calorie deficit*. It is true, however, that weight loss proceeds more quickly when carbohydrates are restricted, and further investigation indicates that breakdown of body fat is somewhat inhibited by carbohydrate. While this makes low-carbohydrate diets tempting to the dieter, it cannot negate the important role carbohydrate plays in the body.

Minerals

Minerals act in the body both as body materials, found in the hard and soft tissues, and as regulators. It is amazing what the small amounts of minerals we ingest do for us.

Calcium and phosphorous give rigidity to bones and teeth. Phosphorous is found as part of the cell structure. Iron is an important component of hemoglobin in the blood. Chlorine is a component of the gastric juices. Sodium goes into the making of blood and body fluids. Potassium is found in muscles and organs. Magnesium is contained in bones, muscles, and part of the blood. Iodine is found in the thyroid and in the hormone thyroxine. Copper is associated with iron in the tissues.

Minute but essential amounts of minerals are important in the maintenance and growth of body cells. Calcium, sodium, and potassium chloride influence the contractibility of muscles, and their presence in the surrounding fluids controls the rhythm of the heart. Nerve responses are dependent on calcium, potassium, magnesium, and sodium. Calcium influences the clotting of blood and may provide protection against radiation through its ability to reduce strontium 90 levels in the blood.

Potassium and sodium enter into a balance which neutralizes the blood. Phosphorous and iron take part in the oxidation, secretions, development, and reproduction of all cells.

Some of the minerals form part of the chemicals which enter into food metabolism, like iodine and sulphur. Zinc is found in the enzymes of the blood and pancreas; molybdenum in the liver; and magnesium, manganese, cobalt, potassium, iron, and copper in all body enzymes.

Chlorine promotes acidity for digestion of certain foods in the stomach, while other minerals create an alkaline atmosphere for fat digestion in the small intestine.

These same nutrients transport oxygen from the lungs to the tissues, and return carbon dioxide from the tissues to the lungs. They control the movement of all fluids for the assimilation of the products of digestion into the blood and the removal of waste.

Minerals are found in a great variety of foods. They are drawn from the ground by plants and transferred to man in plant foods and in the by-products of animals that feed off plants. The only mineral that can be difficult to obtain even on a plentiful diet is iodine. Iodine is present only in ocean fish, kelp and other seaweed products, and foods grown on iodine-rich soil. To increase the supplies of iodine in the diet, iodized salt is available.

There are many different opinions as to the necessary amount of each mineral. As our use of all food nutrients is interrelated, an increase in one may promote better utilization or an increased need for others. As an example, calcium is best absorbed in an acid medium, so that while the lactic acid in milk aids calcium absorption, oxalic acid in spinach, rhubarb, and chocolate (which all have an alkaline reaction in the stomach) may hinder it. While fat and the presence of vitamin D promote calcium absorption, too much phosphorous can bind it. If dietary supplies are not adequate to meet regulatory needs, calcium will be drawn out of the bones, which is why many old people probably suffer from osteomalacia (softening of the bone marrow). On the positive side, high levels of calcium enhance iron utilization.

Vitamins

While vitamins do not enter directly into body reactions, they are catalysts (or accelerators) that must be present for nutrients to be effectively converted to energy or used in the building and maintenance of cells and tissues. Like the regulatory minerals, vitamins are needed in relatively minute quantities. However, no one food can supply them all, and with few exceptions they cannot be synthesized in the body.

The level of vitamins actually required to prevent overt signs of deficiency has been established in certain instances by animal experimentation and deficiencies induced on a highly controlled diet. While the base need for many vitamins has thus been demonstrated, it is more difficult to set optimum levels due to personal differences in health, ability to absorb and utilize various vitamins, and the presence of other dietary factors which often dictate vitamin requirements. For many vitamins which are known to be essential, neither minimum nor recommended levels have yet been set.

There are, however, several factors that should be considered when evaluating your vitamin intake. Substantial loss of food or body fluids through diarrhea and vomiting can be responsible for vitamin deficiencies. Vitamins, sensitive to heat and oxygen, are often destroyed during food preparation. The B vitamins and vitamin C are soluble in water and may seep out of a food and into the surrounding liquid during cooking. Vitamins A, D, E, and K, which are commonly associated with lipids in food, are fat soluble and can only be absorbed in a fat medium. On the other hand, frequent use of mineral oil (not an uncommon habit), which acts as a lubricant and is not digested, will carry fat-soluble vitamins in suspension out of the body. While excess water-soluble vitamins are excreted in the urine and therefore must be replenished daily, fat-soluble vitamins can be stored for short periods in body fat so that their daily consumption may be less crucial.

VITAMIN A

Two forms of this vitamin exist in foods—pure vitamin A found in foods of animal origin, and provitamin A or carotene which is found in plants. Carotene is converted to vitamin A in the human body and THE TABLES OF FOOD CONTENT take this conversion factor into consideration in listing the amount of this vitamin available from food.

Vitamin A affects the development of the cells on the outer layer of skin and the cells that are used for body secretions. Without enough vitamin A these secretions cannot take place, bacteria growth increases, and the body loses one of its methods of self-protection. For this reason vitamin A is considered important in resisting infection. Vitamin A is also responsible for the production of visual purple for sight, particularly night vision; is influential in the laying of bone and tooth enamel; is needed for production of red and white blood corpuscles; helps stimulate the appetite; and eases digestion.

To prevent overt signs of deficiency a minimum of 2,500 IU's must be available to the body daily. This is considerably below the amounts needed for good health. In addition, fat must be present for vitamin A to be absorbed, and both vitamin E and the B vitamin choline can enhance its utilization. Low-protein diets markedly reduce vitamin-A absorption into the intestines, where carotene is converted to a usable form of the vitamin.

Individual need for vitamin A depends on body weight and also varies with the amount of use your eyes receive and the intensity of light under which you work. Although excess vitamin A can be stored for future use, massive doses (above 50,000 IU's daily) can be toxic.

VITAMIN D

Vitamin D promotes calcium absorption and phosphorous retention, and thereby acts in the body for good bone development. It is particularly important during periods of rapid growth, but is vital for adults as well, since a lack of vitamin D can result in softening of the bone structure in later life.

Vitamin D can be synthesized in the body by the interaction of ultraviolet sun rays and the oils on your skin. Unfortunately clothing, fog, dust, clouds, pollution, and other obstructing factors can cut down on this process. Because of this internal vitamin D production, it is difficult to ascertain what the demand for this vitamin actually is. Since very few foods contain vitamin D, the only way to meet this need, other than exposure to sunlight, is by drinking fortified milk or supplementing the diet with fish-liver oils. In the latter case it should be noted that daily doses over a period of time of 4,000 units in infants and 10,000 to 20,000 units in adults have caused adverse effects.

VITAMIN E

Actually a group of vitamins known collectively as tocopherols, vitamin E, acclaimed by many for its rejuvenating properties, works to protect unsaturated fatty acids, vitamin A, and sex hormones from destruction by oxygen. Hence, it is known as an antioxidant. In addition to this known usage, vitamin E is probably involved in the healing of scar tissue and in the soothing of burns and itching. In animal studies it has been connected with fertility and with muscular and heart functions, although these studies are not yet considered conclusive in terms of human nutrition. One of the most widely occurring symptoms of vitamin-E deficiency in animals is muscular dystrophy.

Although there is no disputing the fact that vitamin E is essential to good health, research has never been able to determine how much of it we need. But as the whole grains, nuts, seeds, and unrefined oils once widespread in the American diet are replaced by foods dependent on chemically extracted oils, refined flours and cereals, and roasted nuts, this vitamin is slowly being processed out of our diets.

Like the other fat-soluble vitamins, vitamin E cannot be absorbed without the simultaneous inclusion of fat in the diet.

VITAMIN K

Vitamin K is needed to make prothrombin, an essential factor in blood clotting. Because this vitamin is synthesized in the body, the amount of K which must be supplied by food has never been determined.

VITAMIN B COMPLEX

The vitamin B complex consists of eleven different vitamins, each related in function, yet unique. They often occur together in foods and a deficiency in one is usually accompanied by a deficiency in all, although one in particular may predominate in the condition. There is still much to be learned about this group of vitamins, but they are regarded as the anti-stress vitamins and are considered insurance against such diseases as diabetes, high blood pressure, cancer, toxemia of pregnancy, heart and kidney ailments. Consumption of one or more of the B vitamins increases the need for the others; favorable dietary conditions can promote production of some B vitamins in the intestine. Also, B vitamins are chiefly involved with carbohydrate metabolism, so that sugar increases the need for these vitamins while at the same time is probably decreasing your appetite for foods which offer them.

The three B vitamins which have been most regularly isolated in foods, and which are computed in THE TABLES OF FOOD CONTENT, are thiamine, niacin, and riboflavin. They all participate in the conversion of food to energy which makes them important in combating fatigue, depression, and mental cloudiness.

Thiamine is additionally related to motility in the gastrointestinal tract, proper heart functioning, and nervous responses. Since it is an intermediary in the conversion of glucose to energy, the need for thiamine is related to the daily expenditure of calories. The minimum level for adults is set at .27 to .33 milligrams per 1,000 calories used in daily activities. However, it is not advisable to allow thiamine intake to fall below 1 milligram daily.

Riboflavin requirement is determined by calorie intake. For adults .25 to .27 milligrams per 1,000 calories is viewed as a base level, but upward of 1 milligram daily is preferable to meet normal needs. The recommended daily allowance provides .6 milligrams per 1,000 calories. From two to five times this amount can be absorbed before the tissues are fully saturated.

Niacin is related to body weight as well as to the amount of the amino acid tryptophan in the diet and total calorie intake. A minimum of 4.4 milligrams per 1,000 calories is needed to maintain body levels of niacin and prevent deficiency symptoms. However, 8.8 milligrams should be considered a base level even if your energy intake is below 2,000 calories.

Vitamin B_6 (pyridoxine) is associated with fat and amino acid metabolism. It is somehow involved with brain functioning since its lack can cause migraines and convulsions. B_6 deficiency also reduces antibody formation. No formal recommendations have ever been made for vitamin-B_6 allotment since a diet sufficient in the other B vitamins is believed to provide adequate B_6 as well, but it is known that an increase in dietary protein brings an increased need for B_6.

Pantothenic acid is also involved in fat and carbohydrate metabolism and enters into the formation of hemoglobin. Since it helps to produce cortisone it is considered important in the synthesis of adrenal hormones and in fighting arthritis. How much we need is undetermined, however, it is widely furnished in the plant and animal kingdoms.

Vitamin B_{12} stimulates the regeneration of blood and is instrumental in preventing pernicious anemia. It is almost uniquely supplied in foods of animal origin, with brewers' yeast, kelp, and wheat germ being the exceptions.

The function of *Para-Amino Benzoic Acid*, or PABA, has not yet been pinpointed. It is thought to influence the growth of the intestinal bacteria responsible for the production of folic acid. Folic acid in turn enhances the assimilation of pantothenic acid. PABA is easily provided in a diet including liver, milk, beef, pork, whole wheat, wheat germ, and molasses, but if you are taking any sulfa drugs, which are similar to PABA in chemical composition, it is quite possible to incur a deficiency, for the drugs compete with, and often displace this B vitamin in the body.

Nothing grows without *Folacin* (also known as folic acid), for it triggers cell division. Once again, its availability is determined by adequate levels of other B vitamins in the diet.

Biotin, another intermediary of glucose metabolism, is synthesized by bacteria in the body. This synthesis is believed to cover all needs, although a diet containing many raw egg whites, which prohibit biotin absorption, can bring about a deficiency.

Choline, along with *Inositol* and B_6, enhances fat metabolism and prevents fat accumulation in the liver. Both choline and inositol are partially synthesized in the body so that additional needs have never been determined.

In general your need for B vitamins hinges on your size, the amount of energy in your food supply, activity, daily stress, and the other foods in your diet. Some of these factors can actually inhibit proper absorption and to compensate it is best to keep your intake of the entire complex high and let your body determine how much it can use. Since the B vitamins are all water soluble, any excess is excreted in the urine so that there is no danger of toxicity. Deficiency can be induced, however, by large supplementation of one without a corresponding balance of the others. If one is continually fatigued it is a good idea to add more B-vitamin-rich foods to the menu.

VITAMIN C

Finally we come to vitamin C, considered by many a defense against the common cold. While the debate over its actual ability to prevent colds continues, it is an established fact that vitamin C aids in the formation of antibodies necessary to fight infection. It is also needed for the formation of collagen, the cement between body cells, and it speeds healing of wounds and bones. Vitamin C is believed to enhance iron use and absorption and is thereby effective in maintaining normal blood and hemoglobin levels.

Smoke, smog, DDT, viral infections, and drugs all destroy this highly unstable vitamin, so that your exposure to these variables helps determine your need. It is not stored in the body, but it can be absorbed into the tissues like a sponge; huge doses can be accepted readily, yet once body tissues are saturated all excess will be expelled.

Nutrition and Your Diet

With the exception perhaps of vitamin D, food is your best source of all these nutrients. Under some circumstances additional supplementation is warranted, and if kept under control is rarely detrimental—except to the budget.

Let THE TABLES OF FOOD CONTENT be your guide to the amount of each nutrient you are receiving from your diet, and if you feel you would like to increase your levels of any food element consult the tables for convenient food sources of this extra nutriment.

Your present level of food nutrients can also help you decide how much of a supplement you might want to add from nonfood sources. Learning to evaluate your diet can help you with these decisions.

A Summary of Nutrients

———◆———

Following are the foods which provide the primary source of these nutrients in your diet:

Protein

>Meats
>Fish
>Poultry
>Eggs
>Milk and cheese
>Dried beans (legumes)
>Nuts and nut butters
>Wheat germ
>Brewers' yeast

Fat

>Saturated—
>>Butter
>>Cream, whole milk, and related products
>>Chocolate
>>Meat
>>Coconut and palm oils
>>Margarine
>>Animal fats in general
>>Pastry
>Unsaturated—
>>Vegetable and most nut oils
>>Salad dressing
>>Mayonnaise
>>Margarine
>>Nuts and nut butters

Cholesterol—
>	Meats, especially glandular meats
>	Butter
>	Cheese
>	Egg yolks
>	Shellfish

Carbohydrate
>	Flour and grain products, including cereals, pasta, and baked foods
>	Sugar, honey, molasses, corn syrup, maple syrup
>	Candy, jam and jellies
>	Fruits, particularly those canned in syrup
>	Vegetables, particularly potatoes, peas, corn, winter squash

Calcium
>	Milk and milk products, including ice cream and cheese
>	Dark green leafy vegetables
>	Canned sardines and canned salmon
>	Almonds
>	Sesame seeds
>	Soy beans, soy flour, and soy products
>	Blackstrap molasses
>	Oats
>	Egg yolks

Iron
>	Lean meats
>	Glandular meats
>	Chicken, especially dark meat
>	Shellfish
>	Dried beans (legumes)
>	Dried fruits, especially raisins, prunes, and apricots
>	Blackstrap molasses
>	Egg yolks
>	Whole-grain and enriched flour and grain products

Sodium
>	Prepared foods
>	Canned vegetables
>	Meats

Pickles
Salted butter and margarine
Salt-water fish
Table salt
Milk
Cheese
Eggs
Baking soda and baking powder
Fresh carrots, beets, spinach, and celery

Potassium

Bananas
Oranges
Avocados
Vegetables, particularly potatoes, winter squash, to-
matoes, and leafy greens
Nuts, particularly peanuts and peanut butter
Dried beans (legumes)
Soy flour
Brewers' yeast
Molasses
Meats
Dried fruit
Cocoa powder

Magnesium

Bananas
Whole-grain products
Dried beans (legumes)
Milk
Dark green leafy vegetables
Nuts

Phosphorous

Whole-grain products
Bran
Cheese
Milk
Dried beans (legumes)
Eggs
Meats
Peanuts and peanut butter

Iodine

        Iodized and sea salt
        Kelp and other seaweed
        Seafood (salt-water varieties)

Zinc

        Beef
        Eggs
        Liver
        Herring
        Oysters
        Barley
        Brown rice
        Oatmeal
        Sunflower seeds
        Kelp and other seaweed
        Pure maple syrup
        Carrots
        Peas

Vitamin A

        Deep yellow and orange fruits and vegetables, especially carrots, sweet potatoes, apricots, winter squash, pumpkin, and cantaloupe
        Yellow corn and whole, unbolted yellow cornmeal
        Whole milk, cream, butter, and whole-milk cheese
        Liver
        Fortified margarine
        Dark green vegetables, especially broccoli, escarole, spinach, and parsley
        Tomatoes and tomato products

Thiamine

        Pork
        Heart, kidneys, and liver
        Dried beans (legumes)
        Whole-grain and enriched flour and grain products
        Wheat germ
        Brewers' yeast
        Nuts, especially peanuts and peanut butter

Riboflavin

      Meats, especially liver, kidneys, and heart
      Milk and cheese
      Dark leafy greens
      Brewers' yeast
      Enriched flour and grain products

Niacin

      Lean meats, particularly liver
      Poultry
      Fish
      Dried beans (legumes)
      Whole-grain and enriched flour and grain products
      Wheat germ
      Brewers' yeast
      Nuts, especially peanuts and peanut butter

Vitamin B_6

      Bananas
      Whole-grain products
      Chicken
      Dried beans (legumes)
      Egg yolks
      Dark green leafy vegetables
      Fish and shellfish
      Meats
      Nuts
      Potatoes
      Prunes and raisins
      Brewers' yeast
      Wheat germ

Folacin

      Liver
      Dark green vegetables
      Dried beans (legumes)
      Nuts

Pantothenic Acid

      Organ meats
      Eggs
      Bran

Peanuts
Oats
Whole wheat
Wheat germ
Pork
Beef

Vitamin B₁₂

Meats, particularly glandular meats
Milk and cheese
Fish
Eggs and egg yolks
Wheat germ
Brewers' yeast
Kelp and other seaweed

Vitamin C

Fruits and vegetables, particularly citrus fruits, green
and red pepper, tomatoes, potatoes cooked in their
jackets, cantaloupe, strawberries, raw cabbage, brussel
sprouts, broccoli

Vitamin D

Fortified milk
Egg yolks
Fish-liver oils
Sunshine

Vitamin E

Vegetable oils
Wheat germ and wheat-germ oil
Whole-grain products
Peanuts
Dark leafy greens

Index

Adrenalin, 66
Ailments: cleansing fast as relief for, 36-37; protection of body from harmful bacteria, intoxicants, and pollutants, 45 *see also* Physical ailments, control or causes of
Air Force diet, 19, 22
Alcoholic and carbonated beverages, 274-75 (*table*)
Allergies, 111-13
Almonds, 257
American Heart Association, 95
American meals, typical, 46-47, 70-92
Amino acids, 54, 72, 77, 237, 256
Anemia, 76, 305
Antibiotics, harmful, 52, 56, 67
Artificial sweeteners, 17, 27
Atherosclerosis, 94, 101
Atkins diet, 19, 20, 24-26, 29

Baby foods, 281, 282-85 (*tables*)
Baby's formula, 87-89
Bacteria, beneficial, 66
Bacterial infections, 48
Baked goods, 97, 198, 236
Baking soda, 222, 256
Balanced diet and the RDA, 70-75
Balanced meals, daily, 46-51
Banana and skimmed milk diet, 32
Banting diet, 19
Barley, 236
Basal metabolic rate, 39

"Basic four" food groups, 72, 74, 75
Beans, 108, 109, 111, 256, 257
Biotin, 198, 307
Bircher-Benner, Dr. M.O., 65, 67, 68
Bircher-Benner diet, 65-69
Birth defects, factors increasing risk of, 80
Blood cells, 66
Blood cholesterol, 26, 94-97 *see also* Cholesterol
Bloodstream, 114
Blood sugar: low, 26, 45, 101, 106, 108, 114, 115 *see also* Hypoglycemia; maintaining, increasing, and controlling, 101, 107-10
Blood triglycerides, 26, 95, 298
Body fat and fat tissue, 19-20, 26
Boston Police diet, 25
Brain cells, fetal, 77
Brain energy, 114
Breads: whole-grain, 54, 100; white, 236 *see also* Baked goods
Brewers' yeast, 36, 47, 54
Butter, 67, 89, 98, 257, 265

Cakes and pastries, 237-38
Calcium, 18, 27, 36, 47, 54-56, 60, 63, 67, 99, 198, 200, 236, 256-57, 270; supplementation, 48
Calorie: expenditure and needs, 9-10, 18, 26, 39, 40, 73, 294-96;

intake, 40, 59, 73, 97, 102, 294-96; reduction and level, 10-12, 18, 20, 59, 97

Calories and caloric values, 4, 7-8, 10-11

Calories-Don't-Count diet, 19

Calories, "empty," 40

Cancer, and artificial sweeteners, 27

Candies, 270

Canned: fish, 186; and frozen vegetables, 222; fruits and fruit juices, 208, 209; or frozen food, 44, 98, 222

Carbohydrates, 25-26, 28-29, 40, 47, 50, 72, 73, 101-4, 108-10, 220, 237, 257, 299-300; "empty," 97-98, 100

Carbonated and alcoholic beverages, 274-75 (table)

Carotene, 303

Cells, human body, structure and nourishment of, 45, 72

Cereal and flour enrichment, 43, 98, 100, 236

Cereal grains, grain products, and flour, 236-38, 239-55 (tables)

Cereals, 66, 89, 90, 98

Cheeses, 54, 58, 79, 89, 90, 97, 111, 201

Chemical: fertilizers, 44, 46; food additives, 43, 45

Chemicalized food items, dangers of, 17, 56

Chemicals, air- and food-borne, 48

Children, feeding young, 86-88; foods liked by, 89-92

Chocolate, 270

Cholesterol, 26, 56, 59, 64, 94-99, 201, 298

Choline, 307

Cocoa, 111

Coffee, 106, 108, 111

Constipation, 27

Cooking, for retaining of nutrients, 44

Cortisone, 306

Cottage cheese diet, 32, 33

Counting calories, 10-11, 18, 29, 30

Cow's milk, compared to mother's, 86, 87

Crash diets, 6, 31-34

Cyclamates, 27

Daily diet allowances, 46, 70-75, 102, 108, 291 (table)

Dairy foods, 53, 54, 55, 58, 67, 99, 108

Dairy and milk products, 200-206 (tables)

Davis, Adelle, 44, 48

Dehydration, 63

Depression and mental confusion, 117

Diabetes, 101-105

Diet allowances, daily, 46, 70-75, 102, 108, 291-93 (tables)

Diet, balanced, and the RDA and USDA, 70-75

Diet, designing your own, 143-44 (table), 145-48

"Diet foods," 17

Diet for weight gain, 38-42

Diet for weight loss, see Weight (loss) control

Diet, homemade (sample), 148-51 (tables), 152-53

Diet, learning to evaluate your, 121-42; record of food intake, 122-26 (table), 127-28 (table), 129-30 (table); nutrient intake, 135-38 (table), 139; three-day sample daily record, 139-42

Diet, nutrition and, 308-14

Diet survey food charts, 126, 128, 130, 138, 144, 149, 151, 158, 324

Diet, well-rounded, 71-75

Diet for a Small Planet (Lappé), 52

Dr. Atkins' Diet Revolution, 19, 25

Dr. Stillman's diets: liquid semifast, 35, 36; Quick-Inches-Off, 31; Quick-Weight-Loss, 19, 20-23, 24

Drinking Man's diet, 19, 22

Drugs, unwise use of, 48, 80

Dry-milk powder, 47, 200, 201

Du Pont diet, 19

Eating American-style, 70-92

Eating, the "whys" of, 3

Egg and grapefruit diet, 32, 33

Eggs, 53, 54, 58-59, 61, 79, 98, 111; nutritive value of, 198-99 (*table*)

Elements of food, 293-305

Energy: food sources of, 71-72; input and outflow, affecting weight reduction, 7-8, 20, 26; requirements, applying to weight gain, 39

Enzymes, 66, 207, 208

Fasting, as relief for ailments and disorders, 36-37

Fat: animal, 47, 101-2; body, and fat tissue, 19-20, 26; good and harmful effects of, 40; in the diet, 17, 24, 46, 72, 73, 96-97, 101, 102, 270, 298-99; symptoms caused by dietary fat, 26

Fat-mobilizing hormone, 20, 22

Fat-soluble vitamins, 47

Fats and oils, 265-66, 267-69 (*tables*)

Fats: hydrogenated, 47, 257; saturated, 50, 56, 59, 64, 96, 97, 99, 198, 201, 237, 265, 281; unsaturated, 40, 42, 47, 50, 97, 257

Fatty acids: 20, 26, 109, 265, 298; and skin health, 25; essential, 80; unsaturated, 67

Feeding young children, 86-88; foods liked by kids, 89-92

Fiber content, *see* Roughage

Fish, 61, 67, 79, 108, 111, 164, 165, 186; tables of food content (nutritive value), 187-97; canned fish, 186

Flour, cereal grains, and grain products, 236-38, 239-55 (*tables*)

Flour and cereal enrichment, 43, 98, 100, 236

Flour, whole-wheat, 100

Fluorine, 165

Folacin, 220, 307

Folic acid, 307

Food and Nutrition Board of the National Research Council, 70, 71

Food: canned or frozen, 44, 98, 186, 208, 209, 222; content, *see* Nutritive value of foods; elements of, 293-305; for health, 93-117; groups, "basic four," 72, 74, 75; habits leading to overweight, 4; intake, your own record of, 122-30 (*tables*), 134-38 (*table*), 139; three-day sample record, 139-42; metabolism, rates of, 116; miscellaneous, 286-88 (*tables*); sensitivity, 111-13; supplementation vs. natural foods, 43-46; whole quality, foods chosen for their, 46-51

Foods: liked by kids, 89-92; preferable or rejectable by you, 145 (*table*), 144-46

Formula for baby, 87, 88, 89

Frozen or canned foods, 44, 98, 186, 208, 209, 222

Fruit: 74, 108, 109; and fruit products, 207-9, 210-19 (*ta-*

bles); canned fruit and fruit juices, 208-9

Gain weight, how to, 38-42
Game, 61, 111
Glucose, 26, 101, 106, 114
Glycogen, 101
Gout, 110-11
Grains and grain products, 61, 62, 63, 67, 98, 108, 109, 111, 236-55 (tables)
Greens, 98

Health: food for, 93-117; diet (hypothetical), 133-34; hazards involved in being overweight or in dietary plans, 3, 10, 17
Heart ailments, control of, 94-100
Hemoglobin production, 76
High blood pressure, 94-96
High-protein diet, 20, 21, 24, 26, 28
Honey, 270
Hormone: balance, 113; fat-mobilizing, 20, 22; production, 24, 76, 306
Hormones, harmful, 56
Hydrogenated fats, 47, 257
Hypertension, 94, 95, 96
Hypoglycemia, 106-10

Infants, solid food for, 87-89
Infections, bacterial, 48
Inositol, 307
Insulin: production, 22, 27, 106-7, 108, 114; shock, 101; treatments, 105
Iodine, 51, 76, 79, 99, 165, 220
Iron, 36, 47, 54, 60, 63, 67, 76, 77, 111, 198, 207, 220, 256, 257, 270

Jolliffe, Dr. Norman, 13
Juices, fruit, canned, 208-9

Kelp, 55, 220
Ketone bodies, 20, 25, 109
Ketosis, 26

Lactose, 87
Lappé, Frances, 52
Lecithin, 96
Legumes: and leafy vegetables, 54, 58, 61, 63, 74, 98; and nuts, 256-64 (tables)
Linolenic acid, 47, 105
Liquid diets, 35-37
Lose weight, see Weight (loss) control
Low-calorie dieting, 6-12, 26, 27, 132-33
Low-carbohydrate dieting, 19-30
Low-salt dieting, 40, 45, 50, 79, 88, 95, 98, 99, 256

Macrobiotics diet, 61-65
Macrobiotics: An Invitation to Health and Happiness (Ohsawa), 62
Magnesium, 27, 47, 51, 55, 63, 67, 96, 98, 108, 109, 111, 114, 220, 237, 256, 257
Margarine, 265
Mayo Clinic diet, 19, 21-22
Meals: American-style, 46-47, 70-92; for control of hypoglycemia, 107-8; skipping or spacing of, 6, 109, 115-17; well-balanced daily, 46-51
Measurement of foods during diet survey, 134-35
Measures, standard table of, 163
Meat, 97, 98, 108; for babies, 89
Meat, poultry, and fish, as primary sources of protein and other nutrients, 164; meat and poultry, food content of (nutritive value), 167-85 (tables); fish, content of (nutritive value), 187-97 (tables)
Meatless menu, 53-56, 67

Meats, organ and muscle, 79, 97, 111, 164

Menstruation, 113

Mental health, how food affects, 113-17

Menu planning, 146-47

Metabolic disturbances, foods free from, 44

Metabolic rate, basal, 39

Metabolism, 19-20, 25, 26, 38, 39, 49, 66, 72, 97, 98, 101, 104, 108, 114, 116, 307; rates of food metabolism, 116

Metrecal plan, 35

Milk and dairy products, 200-206 (tables)

Milk and milk products: 54, 55, 67, 108, 111; dry-milk powder, 47, 200, 201; fermented, 67; nonfat, 58; raw, 58; skim or nonfat dry, 15, 17, 18, 89, 201

Milk, mother's, compared to cow's, 86, 87

Mind, feeding your, 115

Minerals, 30, 36, 39, 40, 42, 43, 44, 47, 48, 50, 51, 52, 55, 63, 66, 72, 108, 114, 116, 208, 301-2

Minimum Daily Requirements, 292 (table)

"Miracle eggnog diet," 32

Miscellaneous foods, 286, 287-88 (tables)

Molasses, 270

Multiple vitamins, 25

Muscle and organ meats, 79, 97, 111, 164

National Heart and Lung Institute, 95

National Research Council, 39-40, 84

Natural foods: balanced diet, 46-51; basic, 44-51; vs. food supplementation, 43-46

Natural, whole, and organic food diets, 43-69

Niacin, 55, 102, 109, 111, 256, 306

Nidetch, Jean, 13

Nitrogen metabolism, 66

Nursing mother, diet for, 83 (table)-85

Nutrient intake, 126 (table), 128 (table), 135-38 (table), 139

Nutrient intake tables, individual (in numerical order): meat, poultry, and fish, 326; eggs, 327; milk and dairy products, 328; fruit and fruit products, 329; vegetables and vegetable products, 330; flour, cereal grains, and grain products, 331; legumes and nuts, 332; fats and oils, 333; sugars and sweets, 334; alcoholic and carbonated beverages, 335; soups, 336; baby foods, 337; miscellaneous, 338

Nutrients: essential, 43-46; summary of, 309-14

Nutrition and Your Mind (Watson), 115, 116

Nutrition: and your diet, 308-10; in pregnancy, 76-78 (table), 79-81

Nutritional deficiencies, as cause of many diseases, 45

Nutritive value of foods, tables, (in numerical order): meat and poultry, 167-85; fish, 187-97; eggs, 198-99; milk and dairy products, 202-6; fruit and fruit products, 207-19; vegetables and vegetable products, 220-35; flour, cereal grains, and grain products, 236-55; nuts and legumes, 256-64; fats and oils, 265-69; sugars and sweets, 270-73; alcoholic and carbonated beverages, 274-75;

soups, 276-80; baby foods, 281-85; miscellaneous, 286-88

Nuts and legumes, 256-64 (*tables*)

Nuts and seeds, 53, 54, 58, 59, 61, 63, 67, 98, 111, 256, 257

Obesity Clinic, at N.Y.C. Dept. of Health, 13

Ohsawa, George, 61, 62

Oils, 67, 80, 89, 97, 257

Oils and fats, 265-69 (*tables*)

On-Off diet, 32

One-sided diets, *see* Crash diets

Organ and muscle meats, 79, 97, 111, 164

Organic, natural, and whole food diets, 43-69

Organically grown foods, 44

Oxalic acid, 220

Pancreas, 107, 114

Pantothenic acid, 26, 198, 306

Para-Amino Benzoic Acid, 307

Pasta, 100, 237

Pastries and cakes, 237-38

Peanut butter, 257

Pesticides, 44, 52, 67

Phosphorus, 47, 55, 109, 237, 256, 257

Physical ailments, control of, or causes of, related to dieting, 10, 26, 27, 36-37
    see also Allergies; Diabetes; Gout; Heart ailments; Hypoglycemia

Placenta, 77

Plants, as sources of protein, vitamins, and minerals, 52, 54

Polyunsaturates, 105
    see also Unsaturated and polyunsaturated fats

Potassium, 18, 27, 55, 62, 67, 96, 100, 108, 109, 111, 220, 237, 256

Poultry, 79, 108, 165-66; 167-85, 187-97 (*tables*)

Pregnancy, nutrition in, 76-78 (*table*), 79-81

Prepared foods, 97, 98, 198

Processed, synthetic, and chemicalized foodstuffs, 45, 49, 55

Protection from harmful bacteria, viruses, intoxicants, and pollutants, 45

Protein, 20, 21, 24, 26, 28, 36, 39, 40, 43, 46, 47, 51-55, 60, 63, 66, 67, 72, 73, 77, 79, 101, 111, 198, 200, 257, 296-97; primary sources of, 164, 167-85 (*tables*), 187-97 (*tables*)

Protein diet, high, 20, 21, 24, 26, 28

Psychonutritional therapy, 115-17

Pumpkin seeds, 257

Purines, 110

Quick-Inches-Off diet, 31

Quick-Weight-Loss diet, 19, 20-24

Raw foods, 43, 65-69

Recipe breakdown (baked macaroni and cheese), 136-38 (*table*)

Recipe evaluation, 138 (*table*)

Recommended Daily Allowances (RDA), and basic natural foods plan, 46; balanced diet and, 70-75; diabetes and, 102; hypoglycemia and, 108; 291 (*table*)

Record and measurement of foods eaten by you, during diet survey, 134-35

Refining of food, 43-44

Reject list of foods, 144, 145

Residual fatty acids, *see* Fatty acids

Riboflavin, 55, 99, 102, 111, 198, 220, 236, 256, 306

Rice: brown, 54, 62; white, 98

Rice diet, 32, 236

Rockefeller diet, 35

Rodale, J. J., 44, 48

Roughage, 27, 61, 72, 74, 80

Saccharin, 27

Salad dressing, 265

Salt, as injurious to the body, 40, 45, 50, 79, 88, 95, 98, 99, 256 see also Low-salt dieting

Saturated fats, 50, 56, 59, 64, 96, 97, 99, 198, 201, 237, 265, 281

Schizophrenia, 113

Seasonings, 58, 66

Seaweed, 220

Seeds and nuts, 53, 54, 58, 59, 61, 63, 67, 98, 111, 256, 257

Sensitivity to food, 111-13

Sesame seeds and products, 54, 63, 257

Skim milk, or nonfat dry milk 15, 17, 18, 89, 201

Skin health, and fatty acids, 25

Smoking, 48, 94

"Snack dieting," 9, 18, 50, 108, 257

Sodium, 18, 62, 67, 95, 96, 98, 100, 220, 256

Solid food for infants, 87-89

Soups, 89, 276-80 (tables)

Soy beans and products, 47, 54, 256

Specific dynamic action, 20

Starches, 104, 106

Stillman, Dr. Irwin M., 35; diets of: Quick-Inches-Off, 31; Quick-Weight-Loss, 19, 20, 23-24; Two-week liquid semifast, 35, 36

Stress, 5-6, 10, 48, 94, 113

Sugar, as injurious to the body, 40, 45, 50, 59, 65-66, 106, 108

Sugar: brown, 270; concentrated, 64; natural, 59

Sugars and sweets, 270-73 (tables)

Sulfa drugs, 307

Sunflower and sesame seeds, 54, 63, 257

Supplementation, food, vs. natural foods, 43-46

"Sweet-tooth diet," 32

Sweets, 50, 104, 107

Sweets and sugars, 270-73 (tables)

Synthetic, processed, and chemicalized foodstuffs, 45, 99

Table of standard measures, 163

Tables of food content, see Nutritive value of foods tables

Tea, 111

Teething foods, 90

Thiamine, 26, 36, 55, 77, 102, 109, 111, 221, 256, 306

Three-day: sample menu, 153-58 (table); sample record (diet survey), 130 (table), 139-42

Thyroid: gland, 76; supplement, 25

Torula yeast, 54

Trace minerals, 47, 67, 109

Triglycerides, 26, 95, 298

Two-week liquid semifast, 35, 36

Underweight, how to remedy, 38-42

United States Dept. of Agriculture, 70, 72, 161, 286

Unsaturated and polyunsaturated fats, 40, 42, 47, 50, 96, 97, 105, 237, 257

Unsaturated fatty acids, 67

Uric acid, 26, 110, 111

Urine, 20, 25

Vegetables: and legumes, 54, 58, 61, 63, 74, 90, 108, 109, 111; and vegetable products, 220-35 (*tables*); canned and frozen, 222

Vegetarian diet, 133

Vegetarianism, 51-56, 61

Vitamin: supplementation, 48, 50-52, 55, 66, 72, 116; toxicity, 49

Vitamins, 300-306; Vitamin A, 18, 27, 29, 40, 42, 47, 48, 49, 55, 67, 74, 77, 90, 99, 103, 198, 207, 220, 265, 303, 304; Vitamin B and B complex, 26, 29, 36, 40, 42, 47, 51, 54, 55, 60, 63, 67, 80, 98, 100, 106, 108, 109, 114, 165, 198, 200, 220, 236, 237, 256, 257, 270, 305-7; Vitamin B_6, 96, 100, 198, 207, 306, 307; Vitamin B_{12}, 55, 111, 165, 198, 200, 256, 306-7; Vitamin C, 27, 29, 36, 47, 55, 67, 74, 77, 90, 103, 109, 200, 207, 208, 220, 257, 308; Vitamin D, 17, 47, 49, 67, 90, 198, 304, 308; Vitamin E, 47, 48, 49, 55, 79, 97, 100, 106, 109, 114, 236, 237, 257, 265, 304-5; Vitamin K, 47, 67, 305

Vitamins: fat-soluble, 47; multiple, 25; need for, 302-308

Watson, Dr. George, 115, 116

Weight gain, how to achieve, 38-42

Weight (loss) control, 3-6, 50; and low-calorie dieting, 6-12; and Weight Watchers diet, 12-18; and low-carbohydrate dieting, 19-30; crash diets, 31-34; liquid diets, 35-37; and yoga diet, 59; and Bircher-Benner diet, 68

Weight Watchers diet, menus, and recipes, 12-18

Weights, table of desirable, 5

Wheat germ, 36, 47, 54, 55, 90, 98

Whole, natural, and organic food diets, 43-69

Wine and eggs diet, 32

Yeast, nutritional, 36, 47, 54, 55

Yin-Yang foods, 62-64

Yoga foods, 57-60

Yogurt, 46, 54, 58, 59, 80, 89, 201

Zero-carbohydrate diet, 20, 26

Diet Survey Forms

———◆———

DIET SURVEY CHART

Food	Measure	Calories	Protein Gm	Total Fat Gm	Saturated Fat Gm	Linoleic Acid Gm	Cholesterol Mg	Carbohydrate Gm	Calcium Mg	Iron Mg	Sodium Mg	Potassium Mg	A IU	Thiamine Mg	Riboflavin Mg	Niacin Mg	C Mg

(Column groups: **Minerals** covers Calcium, Iron, Sodium, Potassium; **Vitamins** covers A, Thiamine, Riboflavin, Niacin, C)

Food categories:

1 Meat, Poultry, Fish
2 Eggs
3 Milk and Dairy Products
4 Fruit and Fruit Products
5 Vegetables and Vegetable Products
6 Flour, Cereal Grains, and Grain Products
7 Legumes and Nuts
8 Fats and Oils
9 Sugars and Sweets
10 Alcoholic and Carbonated Beverages
11 Soup
12 Baby Foods
13 Miscellaneous

Total
Average Daily
Nutrient Intake

DIET SURVEY CHART

Food	Measure	Calories	Protein Gm	Total Fat Gm	Saturated Fat Gm	Linoleic Acid Gm	Cholesterol Mg	Carbohydrate Gm	Calcium Mg	Iron Mg	Sodium Mg	Potassium Mg	A IU	Thiamine Mg	Riboflavin Mg	Niacin Mg	C Mg
							Minerals					Vitamins				

Food	Measure	Calories	Protein Gm	Total Fat Gm	Saturated Fat Gm	Linoleic Acid Gm	Cholesterol Mg	Carbohydrate Gm	Calcium Mg	Iron Mg	Sodium Mg	Potassium Mg	A IU	Thiamine Mg	Riboflavin Mg	Niacin Mg	C Mg
1 Meat, Poultry, Fish																	
2 Eggs																	
3 Milk and Dairy Products																	
4 Fruit and Fruit Products																	
5 Vegetables and Vegetable Products																	
6 Flour, Cereal Grains, and Grain Products																	
7 Legumes and Nuts																	
8 Fats and Oils																	
9 Sugars and Sweets																	
10 Alcoholic and Carbonated Beverages																	
11 Soup																	
12 Baby Foods																	
13 Miscellaneous																	
Total Average Daily Nutrient Intake																	

INDIVIDUAL NUTRIENT INTAKE CHART: GROUP 1. MEAT, POULTRY, AND FISH

Food	Measure	Calo-ries	Pro-tein Gm	Total Fat Gm	Satu-rated Fat Gm	Lino-leic Acid Gm	Choles-terol Mg	Car-bohy-drate Gm	Cal-cium Mg	Iron Mg	Sodium Mg	Potas-sium Mg	A IU	Thi-amine Mg	Ribo-flavin Mg	Nia-cin Mg	C Mg
Total																	

326

INDIVIDUAL NUTRIENT INTAKE CHART: GROUP 2. EGGS

Food	Measure	Calories	Protein Gm	Total Fat Gm	Saturated Fat Gm	Linoleic Acid Gm	Cholesterol Mg	Carbohydrate Gm	Calcium Mg	Iron Mg	Sodium Mg	Potassium Mg	A IU	Thiamine Mg	Riboflavin Mg	Niacin Mg	C Mg

Total

INDIVIDUAL NUTRIENT INTAKE CHART: GROUP 3. MILK AND DAIRY PRODUCTS

Food	Measure	Calo-ries	Pro-tein Gm	Total Fat Gm	Satu-rated Fat Gm	Lino-leic Acid Gm	Choles-terol Mg	Car-bohy-drate Gm	Cal-cium Mg	Iron Mg	Sodium Mg	Potas-sium Mg	A IU	Thi-amine Mg	Ribo-flavin Mg	Nia-cin Mg	C Mg
Total																	

INDIVIDUAL NUTRIENT INTAKE CHART: GROUP 4. FRUIT AND FRUIT PRODUCTS

Food	Measure	Calo-ries	Pro-tein Gm	Total Fat Gm	Satu-rated Fat Gm	Lino-leic Acid Gm	Choles-terol Mg	Car-bohy-drate Gm	Cal-cium Mg	Iron Mg	Sodium Mg	Potas-sium Mg	A IU	Thi-amine Mg	Ribo-flavin Mg	Nia-cin Mg	C Mg

Minerals | Vitamins

Total

INDIVIDUAL NUTRIENT INTAKE CHART: GROUP 5. VEGETABLES AND VEGETABLE PRODUCTS

Food	Measure	Calories	Protein Gm	Total Fat Gm	Saturated Fat Gm	Linoleic Acid Gm	Cholesterol Mg	Carbohydrate Gm	Calcium Mg	Iron Mg	Sodium Mg	Potassium Mg	A IU	Thiamine Mg	Riboflavin Mg	Niacin Mg	C Mg
Total																	

INDIVIDUAL NUTRIENT INTAKE CHART: GROUP 6. FLOUR, CEREAL GRAINS, AND GRAIN PRODUCTS

Food	Measure	Calo-ries	Pro-tein Gm	Total Fat Gm	Satu-rated Fat Gm	Lino-leic Acid Gm	Choles-terol Mg	Car-bohy-drate Gm	Cal-cium Mg	Iron Mg	Sodium Mg	Potas-sium Mg	A IU	Thi-amine Mg	Ribo-flavin Mg	Nia-cin Mg	C Mg
Total																	

INDIVIDUAL NUTRIENT INTAKE CHART: GROUP 7. LEGUMES AND NUTS

Food	Measure	Calories	Protein Gm	Total Fat Gm	Saturated Fat Gm	Linoleic Acid Gm	Cholesterol Mg	Carbohydrate Gm	Calcium Mg	Iron Mg	Sodium Mg	Potassium Mg	A IU	Thiamine Mg	Riboflavin Mg	Niacin Mg	C Mg
Total																	

INDIVIDUAL NUTRIENT INTAKE CHART: GROUP 8. FATS AND OILS

Food	Measure	Calo-ries	Pro-tein Gm	Total Fat Gm	Satu-rated Fat Gm	Lino-leic Acid Gm	Choles-terol Mg	Car-bohy-drate Gm	Cal-cium Mg	Iron Mg	Sodium Mg	Potas-sium Mg	A IU	Thi-amine Mg	Ribo-flavin Mg	Nia-cin Mg	C Mg

Total

INDIVIDUAL NUTRIENT INTAKE CHART: GROUP 9. SUGARS AND SWEETS

Food	Measure	Calo-ries	Pro-tein Gm	Total Fat Gm	Satu-rated Fat Gm	Lino-leic Acid Gm	Choles-terol Mg	Car-bohy-drate Gm	Cal-cium Mg	Iron Mg	Sodium Mg	Potas-sium Mg	A IU	Thi-amine Mg	Ribo-flavin Mg	Nia-cin Mg	C Mg

Total

334

INDIVIDUAL NUTRIENT INTAKE CHART: GROUP 10. ALCOHOLIC AND CARBONATED BEVERAGES

Food	Measure	Calories	Protein Gm	Total Fat Gm	Saturated Fat Gm	Linoleic Acid Gm	Cholesterol Mg	Carbohydrate Gm	Minerals Calcium Mg	Iron Mg	Sodium Mg	Potassium Mg	Vitamins A IU	Thiamine Mg	Riboflavin Mg	Niacin Mg	C Mg

Total

INDIVIDUAL NUTRIENT INTAKE CHART: GROUP 11. SOUP

Food	Measure	Calo-ries	Pro-tein Gm	Total Fat Gm	Satu-rated Fat Gm	Lino-leic Acid Gm	Choles-terol Mg	Car-bohy-drate Gm	Cal-cium Mg	Iron Mg	Sodium Mg	Potas-sium Mg	A IU	Thi-amine Mg	Ribo-flavin Mg	Nia-cin Mg	C Mg
Total																	

INDIVIDUAL NUTRIENT INTAKE CHART: GROUP 12. BABY FOODS

Food	Measure	Calo-ries	Pro-tein Gm	Total Fat Gm	Satu-rated Fat Gm	Lino-leic Acid Gm	Choles-terol Mg	Car-bohy-drate Gm	Cal-cium Mg	Iron Mg	Sodium Mg	Potas-sium Mg	A IU	Thi-amine Mg	Ribo-flavin Mg	Nia-cin Mg	C Mg
Total																	

INDIVIDUAL NUTRIENT INTAKE CHART: GROUP 13. MISCELLANEOUS

Food	Measure	Calo- ries	Pro- tein Gm	Total Fat Gm	Satu- rated Fat Gm	Lino- leic Acid Gm	Choles- terol Mg	Car- bohy- drate Gm	Cal- cium Mg	Iron Mg	Sodium Mg	Potas- sium Mg	A IU	Thi- amine Mg	Ribo- flavin Mg	Nia- cin Mg	C Mg
Total																	

338

About the Authors

Nikki and David Goldbeck live in Woodstock, New York, where they collaborate on books and articles concerning food and nutrition. When not at home, they are on the road lecturing and teaching. *The Dieter's Companion* is the third book they have written together; their two previous published books are *The Supermarket Handbook* and *The Good Breakfast Book*.

Nikki Goldbeck, who holds a degree in nutrition from Cornell University's School of Human Ecology, is the author of *Cooking What Comes Naturally*. David Goldbeck is a lawyer and teacher.

More of the Best on Nutrition and Diet from SIGNET

☐ **LET'S EAT RIGHT TO KEEP FIT by Adelle Davis.** Sensible, practical advice from America's foremost nutrition authority as to what vitamins, minerals and food balances you require, and the warning signs of diet deficiencies. (#E7245—$2.25)

☐ **LET'S COOK IT RIGHT by Adelle Davis.** Revised and updated, the celebrated cookbook dedicated to good health, good sense and good eating. Contains 400 easy-to-follow, basic recipes, a table of equivalents and an index. (#E7246—$2.25)

☐ **THE STORY OF WEIGHT WATCHERS by Jean Nidetch as told to Joan Rattner Heilman.** Here is the full, unexpurgated Weight Watchers program and story described by Jean Nidetch herself. If you are overweight and diet defeats you, this can be the most important book you will ever read. (#W6665—$1.50)

☐ **SECRETS FOR STAYING SLIM by Lelord Kordel.** Diet Naturally! A famous nutritionist, and author of EAT AND GROW YOUNGER, offers an organically correct guide to quick weight loss that keeps you trim and healthy. (#W7164—$1.50)

☐ **CALORIES AND CARBOHYDRATES by Barbara Kraus.** This dictionary contains over 8,000 brand names and basic foods with their caloric and carbohydrate counts. Recommended by doctors, nutritionists, and family food planners as an indispensable aid to those who must be concerned with what they eat, this book will become an important diet reference source. (#J6670—$1.95)

THE NEW AMERICAN LIBRARY, INC.,
P.O. Box 999, Bergenfield, New Jersey 07621

Please send me the SIGNET BOOKS I have checked above. I am enclosing $_____(check or money order—no currency or C.O.D.'s). Please include the list price plus 35¢ a copy to cover handling and mailing costs. (Prices and numbers are subject to change without notice.)

Name_____

Address_____

City_____State_____Zip Code_____
Allow at least 4 weeks for delivery